# Editorial Board

Contributor

**J. Douglas Cameron, MD, MBA**

*Professor, Department of Ophthalmology and Visual Neurosciences, Director of Research, The University of Minnesota, Minneapolis, MN*

# Table of Contents

# Journals Represented

Journals represented in this YEAR BOOK are listed below.

Acta Ophthalmologica
AJNR American Journal of Neuroradiology
American Journal of Ophthalmology
Annals of Neurology
British Journal of Ophthalmology
Clinical Ophthalmology
Cornea
European Journal of Paediatric Neurology
Eye
Eye (London)
Human Pathology
Investigative Ophthalmology & Visual Science
Japanese Journal of Ophthalmology
Journal of Athletic Training
Journal of Cataract and Refractive Surgery
Journal of Clinical Endocrinology and Metabolism
Journal of Clinical Oncology
Journal of Neurology, Neurosurgery, and Psychiatry
Journal of Pediatric Ophthalmology and Strabismus
Journal of Refractive Surgery
Journal of the American Association for Pediatric Ophthalmology and Strabismus
Journal of the American Medical Association Ophthalmology
Laryngoscope
Nature Communications
Neurology
New England Journal of Medicine
Ophthalmic Plastic and Reconstructive Surgery
Ophthalmic Surgery, Lasers & Imaging Retina
Ophthalmology
Retina

## STANDARD ABBREVIATIONS

The following terms are abbreviated in this edition: acquired immunodeficiency syndrome (AIDS), cardiopulmonary resuscitation (CPR), central nervous system (CNS), cerebrospinal fluid (CSF), computed tomography (CT), deoxyribonucleic acid (DNA), diopter (D), electrocardiography (ECG), health maintenance organization (HMO), human immunodeficiency virus (HIV), intensive care unit (ICU), intramuscular (IM), intravenous (IV), magnetic resonance (MR) imaging (MRI), ribonucleic acid (RNA), ultrasound (US), and ultraviolet (UV).

## NOTE

The YEAR BOOK OF OPHTHALMOLOGY® is a literature survey service providing abstracts of articles published in the professional literature. Every effort is made to assure the accuracy of the information presented in these pages. Neither the editors nor the publisher of the YEAR BOOK OF OPHTHALMOLOGY® can be responsible for errors in the original materials. The editors' comments are their own opinions. Mention of specific products within this publication does not constitute endorsement.

To facilitate the use of the YEAR BOOK OF OPHTHALMOLOGY® as a reference tool, all illustrations and tables included in this publication are now identified as they appear in the original article. This change is meant to help the reader recognize that any illustration or table appearing in the YEAR BOOK OF OPHTHALMOLOGY® may be only one of many in the original article. For this reason, figure and table numbers will often appear to be out of sequence within the YEAR BOOK OF OPHTHALMOLOGY®.

# 1 Cataract Surgery

---

## Multifocal intraocular lenses: Relative indications and contraindications for implantation

Braga-Mele R, for the ASCRS Cataract Clinical Committee (Univ of Toronto, Ontario, Canada)

*J Cataract Refract Surg* 40:313-322, 2014

---

This article presents an extensive overview of best clinical practice pertaining to selection and use of multifocal intraocular lenses (IOLs) currently available in the United States. Relevant preoperative diagnostic evaluations, patient selection criteria, counseling, and managing expectations are reviewed, as well as how to approach patients with underlying ocular intricacies or challenges and best practices for intraoperative challenges during planned implantation of a multifocal IOL. Managing the unhappy multifocal IOL patient if implantation has been performed is also addressed (Fig 1).

▶ This is a detailed review of the many factors affecting postoperative success of diffractive multifocal intraocular lens (MFIOL) implantation. It summarizes key

**Positive Characteristics**

- Keenly interested in spectacle independence for most distance and near tasks
- Easy-going personality with a positive demeanor
- Would accept a small compromise in distance acuity
- Willing to understand that it is not a procedure with a guaranteed outcome
- Generally more interested in working with you in something of a partnership
- Near tasks include mostly reading
- Moderate to high hyperopia without heavy dependence on computer work or moderate to high myopia, although the latter will tend to be relatively less satisfied

**Negative Characteristics**

- Does not mind wearing glasses
- The hypercritical patient with unrealistic expectations will never be satisfied
- If the sharpest clearest vision is their main concern, then it is back to monofocals
- Avoid those with a heavy dependence on intermediate vision, night vision, or specific job requirements; eg, commercial pilots, public service vehicle, taxi, or truck drivers
- Avoid low myopes in general as they are used to excellent uncorrected reading vision that will be difficult to match or surpass

FIGURE 1.—Positive and negative characteristics to aid in the selection of suitable multifocal IOL candidates. (Reprinted from Journal of Cataract & Refractive Surgery. Braga-Mele R, for the ASCRS Cataract Clinical Committee. Multifocal intraocular lenses: Relative indications and contraindications for implantation. *J Cataract Refract Surg.* 40:313-322, with permission from ASCRS and ESCRS.)

"pearls" from multiple sources and experienced clinicians. These guidelines are not found in this level of detail anywhere else in the peer-reviewed literature. Strict adherence to preoperative selection criteria as detailed here should help improve satisfaction of patients receiving these implants and reduce the rate of IOL exchange due to dissatisfaction with visual performance. Guidelines for personality and other nonclinical factors predictive of success or failure with MFIOLs are outlined in Fig 1. This is a must-read article for any cataract surgeon who is currently or plans to begin implanting MFIOLs.

**M. F. Pyfer, MD**

**Effect of high pressurization versus normal pressurization on changes in intraocular pressure immediately after clear corneal cataract surgery**

Hayashi K, Yoshida M, Manabe S-I, et al (Hayashi Eye Hosp, Fukuoka, Japan)
*J Cataract Refract Surg* 40:87-94, 2014

*Purpose.*—To compare changes in intraocular pressure (IOP) immediately after clear corneal incision (CCI) cataract surgery between eyes in which IOP was adjusted to a high or normal range at the conclusion of surgery.

*Setting.*—Hayashi Eye Hospital, Fukuoka, Japan.

*Design.*—Comparative case series.

*Methods.*—Either eye of patients scheduled for phacoemulsification was randomized to 1 of 2 groups as follows: eyes that were to be adjusted to (1) high IOP (22 to 40 mm Hg) or (2) normal IOP (10 to 21 mm Hg). The IOP was measured using a rebound tonometer preoperatively; at the conclusion of surgery; and 15, 30, 60, 120, and 180 minutes and 24 hours postoperatively. The Seidel test and anterior segment optical coherence tomography (AS-OCT) were performed.

*Results.*—The mean IOP at the conclusion of surgery was 31.3 mm Hg in the high IOP group and 17.1 mm Hg in the normal IOP group. The IOP decreased to approximately 15 mm Hg by 15 minutes and did not change until 60 minutes in either group. The mean IOP did not differ significantly between groups throughout the observation period ($P \geq .0634$). Hypotony of 5 mm Hg or less was not detected in any eye. The Seidel test was negative and based on AS-OCT, the wound was closed at 60 minutes in all eyes.

*Conclusions.*—After adjusting IOP to a high or normal range, the IOP normalized within 15 minutes postoperatively and was stable for 24 hours. The wound was closed within 60 minutes postoperatively.

▶ This straightforward and well-designed study provides strong evidence that moderate overinflation of the anterior chamber at the conclusion of sutureless clear corneal incision phacoemulsification cataract surgery is not detrimental. This simple maneuver may help seal the incision and prevent influx of ocular surface contaminants in the first few minutes after surgery. One concern with temporary overpressurization is that the incision could subsequently leak after several minutes when the intraocular pressure (IOP) drops to a normal level. It is prudent to verify a watertight incision at normal IOP first, then hyperinflate through the side port and recheck the incision before ending the case.

An interesting extension of this study using rabbit eyes would be to apply India ink externally at the conclusion of surgery, then examine for influx of ink particles in both cases, normal pressure and high pressure, after 30 to 60 minutes. A similar study has been done using human cadaver eyes,[1] but physiologic sealing of the incision may be limited because of endothelial dysfunction after death.

**M. F. Pyfer, MD**

*Reference*

1. Taban M, Sarayba MA, Ignacio TS, Behrens A, McDonnell PJ. Ingress of India ink into the anterior chamber through sutureless clear corneal cataract wounds. *Arch Ophthalmol.* 2005;123:643-648.

## Outcomes of Femtosecond Laser Cataract Surgery With a Diffractive Multifocal Intraocular Lens

Lawless M, Bali SJ, Hodge C, et al (Vision Eye Inst, Chatswood, Australia)
*J Refract Surg* 28:859-864, 2012

*Purpose.*—To report the visual and refractive outcomes in an initial series of eyes undergoing femtosecond laser cataract surgery with implantation of a diffractive multifocal intraocular lens (IOL).

*Methods.*—The first 61 consecutive eyes undergoing femtosecond laser cataract surgery and ReSTOR (Alcon Laboratories Inc) +3.00-diopter (D) add IOL implantation between May and July 2011 were enrolled in the study (LCS group). The control group consisted of a retrospective consecutive cohort of 29 eyes that underwent manual phacoemulsification cataract surgery and ReSTOR +3.00-D add IOL implantation (MCS group) between December 2010 and April 2011. Visual and refractive parameters were collected pre- and postoperatively at 1 and 3 months.

*Results.*—Mean postoperative spherical equivalent refraction was $-0.01 \pm 0.35$ D and $-0.06 \pm 0.30$ D in the LCS and MCS groups, respectively ($P = .492$). Mean absolute refractive prediction error (PE) was $0.26 \pm 0.25$ D for the LCS group and $0.23 \pm 0.16$ D for the MCS group ($P = .489$). Mean arithmetic refractive PE was $0.06 \pm 0.44$ D and $-0.02 \pm 0.30$ D for the LCS and MCS groups, respectively ($P = .388$). No significant difference was noted in mean postoperative uncorrected distance visual acuity or uncorrected near visual acuity between groups. No eyes in either group had surgical complications or loss of corrected distance visual acuity in the follow-up period.

*Conclusions.*—Mean spherical equivalent refraction and visual acuity of our initial group of patients undergoing laser cataract surgery are comparable to the manual phacoemulsification cohort for the AcrySof ReSTOR +3.00-D add IOL.

▶ The significant result here is that an initial unselected consecutive cohort of patients treated with femtosecond laser-assisted cataract surgery and multifocal interocular lens implant achieved an equivalent refractive result to manual surgery. The manual technique had been highly refined, with a reproducible 5-mm capsulorhexis and custom A constant. The femto group was the first treated at this center and did not include refinement of technique or customization of prediction formulas. This suggests that further improvements in outcome may be expected from femto-assisted surgery with more experience. The best study for comparing femto to manual surgery, a randomized intraindividual trial, has yet to be published. Until then, there is no unequivocal and unbiased evidence that femto-assisted surgery achieves superior results to traditional manual phacoemulsification cataract surgery.

**M. F. Pyfer, MD**

---

### Time and cost of teaching cataract surgery

Taravella MJ, Davidson R, Erlanger M, et al (Univ of Colorado, Aurora)
*J Cataract Refract Surg* 40:212-216, 2014

---

*Purpose.*—To compare the differences in the time of completion of cataract surgery for residents and attending surgeons and to assign a dollar cost.

*Setting.*—University of Colorado teaching hospital, Aurora, Colorado, USA.

*Design.*—Comparative case series.

*Methods.*—Cataract cases were divided into 3 levels of difficulty for comparison. Main outcome measures were total case time (incision to patch) and degree of difficulty.

*Results.*—Nine residents and 6 attending surgeons participated in the study. Case times were collected for 324 resident cases and 319 attending surgeon cases. The mean attending surgeon case time was 25.75 minutes ± 12.32 (SD) and the mean resident case time, 46.35 ± 16.75 minutes. There was no significant difference in the degree of difficulty between resident cases and attending surgeon cases. Approximately 600 total cases were performed by 4 residents during 3 years of residency training. Taking into account the mean time of case completion for attending surgeons versus residents, the total difference in time if attending surgeons had performed 600 cataracts would be 12 360 minutes. Using a dollar cost of approximately $11.24 per minute at the institution, the cost difference was calculated to be $138 926.40.

*Conclusion.*—There was a significant time and dollar cost incurred in teaching cataract surgery.

▶ Teaching institutions in medicine are critical to ensuring a future supply of qualified physicians and surgeons. Ophthalmic specialists are no exception. It is well established that there is a cost penalty for resident-performed procedures compared with experienced attending physicians because of longer procedure times, greater use of resources and materials, and more frequent complications. This cost can be quantified in a careful study such as this one. In this article, attending surgeon case times are somewhat longer than expected compared with reports from the most efficient cataract surgeons, but they are fairly typical relative to nationwide average data. A similar study[1] published in 2012 found significantly longer resident case times only for the first half of the academic year. This article also reports a reduction in resident cataract surgery case times with greater experience, but even those with more than 100 cases still took significantly longer than the average attending surgeon. Accurate information regarding the added expense of resident education is necessary for allocating government and private funding for medical training.

**M. F. Pyfer, MD**

*Reference*

1. Hosler MR, Scott IU, Kunselman AR, Wolford KR, Oltra EZ, Murray WB. Impact of resident participation in cataract surgery on operative time and cost. *Ophthalmology.* 2012;119:95-98.

**Achieving Target Refraction after Cataract Surgery**

Simon SS, Chee YE, Haddadin RI, et al (Massachusetts Eye and Ear Infirmary, Boston)

*Ophthalmology* 121:440-444, 2014

*Purpose.*—To evaluate the difference between target and actual refraction after phacoemulsification and intraocular lens implantation at an academic teaching institution's Comprehensive Ophthalmology Service.

*Design.*—Retrospective study.

*Participants.*—We examined 1275 eye surgeries for this study.

*Methods.*—All consecutive cataract surgeries were included if they were performed by an attending or resident surgeon from January through December 2010. Postoperative refractions were compared with preoperative target refractions. Patients were excluded if they did not have a preoperative target refraction documented or if they did not have a recorded postoperative manifest refraction within 90 days.

*Main Outcome Measures.*—The main outcome measure was percentage of cases achieving a postoperative spherical equivalent ± 1.0 diopter (D) of target spherical equivalent.

*Results.*—We performed 1368 cataract surgeries from January through December of 2010. Of these, 1275 (93%) had sufficient information for analysis. Of the included cases, 94% (1196 of 1275) achieved ±1.0 D of target refraction by 90 days after cataract surgery.

*Conclusions.*—This paper establishes a new benchmark for a teaching hospital, where 94% of patients achieved within 1.0 D of target refraction after cataract surgery. The refractive outcomes after cataract surgery at this academic teaching institution were higher than average international benchmarks.

▶ This article establishes a new benchmark in refractive accuracy for a teaching hospital after cataract surgery. This was achieved by careful preoperative biometry using optical coherence interferometry for axial length whenever possible and optimizing intraocular lens power calculations. It is a retrospective study and eliminates patients who were not refracted at 3 months or who had no target refraction identified in the chart. This may introduce bias in the results. However, it is significant that the analysis included both resident and attending surgeons' cases. Other studies have examined mainly a single attending surgeon, and most achieved less than 94% within 1 diopter of target.

Although this type of refractive accuracy is laudable, more work needs to be done to achieve LASIK-like refractive predictability in cataract surgery. New instrumentation, such as intraoperative aberrometry, may help to reach this goal in the future.

**M. F. Pyfer, MD**

---

**Glued Trans-scleral Intraocular Lens Exchange for Anterior Chamber Lenses in Complicated Eyes: Analysis of Indications and Results**

Kumar DA, Agarwal A, Jacob S, et al (Dr Agarwal's Eye Hosp and Eye Res Centre, Chennai, Tamil Nadu)

*Am J Ophthalmol* 156:1125-1133.e2, 2013

---

*Purpose.*—To determine the clinical outcomes after glued trans-scleral posterior chamber intraocular lens (IOL) exchange for anterior chamber (AC) IOL.

*Design.*—Retrospective case series.

*Methods.*—Eyes with AC IOL explantation with glued IOL implantation in a single setting at the Dr Agarwal Eye Hospital and Eye Research Centre, Chennai, India, from 2008 through 2012 were included. Data were collected from the patient records.

*Main Outcome Measures.*—Corrected distance visual acuity (CDVA) in logarithm of the minimal angle of resolution units, intraocular pressure, AC reaction, AC depth, central corneal thickness, central macular thickness, endothelial cell density, and endothelial cell loss (percentage) were determined before and after IOL exchange.

*Results.*—Thirty-eight eyes with mean follow-up of 24.1 ± 15.4 months (range, 8 to 60 months) were analyzed. The indications were corneal decompensation (39.4%), malpositioned AC IOL (28.9%), uveitis (15.7%), glaucoma (13.1%), and broken haptic (2.6%). There was significant improvement in the postoperative CDVA ($P = .000$) and central corneal thickness ($P = .000$) after AC IOL removal. CDVA better than 20/60 was obtained in 65.7% eyes. Thirty-four (86.8%) eyes showed an increase in the CDVA after IOL exchange. The mean endothelial cell loss was 3.4 ± 2.4% (range, 0.13% to 10.5%). There was significant correlation between the CDVA and the central corneal thickness ($P = .000$). There was significant change in the AC depth ($P = .000$), the intraocular pressure ($P = .005$), and the AC inflammation ($P = .000$) after IOL exchange. The preoperative macular edema in 3 eyes resolved after surgery (mean central macular thickness, 205.6 ± 7.2 μm).

*Conclusions.*—Glued trans-scleral fixated posterior chamber IOL exchange for AC IOL can be an excellent alternative in eyes with ocular complications related to AC IOL.

▶ Sutureless intrascleral haptic fixation aided by fibrin glue is an increasingly popular technique for posterior chamber fixation of intraocular lenses (IOL) in the absence of capsular support. This study shows that the technique has good long-term outcomes with a low incidence of complications. The surgical maneuvers can be challenging but well within the skill set of the anterior segment surgeon. I have found that this technique is also effective for refixation of a subluxed 3-piece IOL without removal from the eye through a small incision, as long as adequate vitrectomy is performed around the IOL. It is often quicker than suture refixation because there is no need for complex needle docking and ab externo guidance procedures. Instead, the haptics can be grasped under direct visualization through a small sclerotomy under a flap using micro-forceps and externalized temporarily before inserting in the intrascleral tunnel. Very long-term follow-up for intrascleral fixation has not yet been documented, but this study extends out to 5 years with no cases of loss of fixation. Scleral-sutured IOLs may be complicated by late suture breakage or erosion.

**M. F. Pyfer, MD**

**Pain and cooperation in patients having dominant-side or nondominant-side phacoemulsification**

Aslankurt M, Aslan L, Başkan AM, et al (Sutcu Imam Univ, Kahramanmaraş, Turkey; Uğur Eye Hosp, Kahramanmaraş, Turkey)

*J Cataract Refract Surg* 40:199-202, 2014

*Purpose.*—To evaluate the relationship between laterality and perceived pain and cooperation during phacoemulsification under combined topical and intracameral anesthesia.

*Setting.*—University ophthalmology clinic and eye hospital, Kahramanmaraş, Turkey.

*Design.*—Cohort study.

*Methods.*—Seventy-eight patients with senile cataracts who had ocular surgery were included prospectively. The dominant side was determined with the Edinburg Handedness Inventory. Phacoemulsification and intraocular lens implantation were performed. The surgeon graded the patient's cooperation from 0 (best) to 3 (worst). The duration of surgery was recorded. Another researcher rated perceived pain from 0 (no pain) to 10 (unbearable pain) using a visual analogue scale (VAS). Pain scores and the degree of cooperation for dominant-side and nondominant-side surgery were the primary outcomes.

*Results.*—Forty-six patients had surgery in the dominant eye and 32 in the nondominant eye. The 2 groups were similar in age, sex, and severity and type of cataract. The mean VAS score was significantly higher in patients having dominant-side surgery than in those having nondominant-side surgery ($P < .01$). Similarly, the mean cooperation score was significantly poorer in the patients having dominant-side surgery ($P < .05$). Visual analogue scores were correlated with patient cooperation ($r = 0.890$, $P < .0001$).

*Conclusion.*—Pain scores were higher in dominant-side surgery for cataract under topical and intracameral anesthesia, which should be kept in mind when selecting anesthesia and in studies in which pain is scored.

▶ Patients frequently report greater sensation or discomfort during the second eye surgery, regardless of dominant side status. This study contradicts that conventional wisdom. In this study, no oral or intravenous (IV) sedation was used, whereas most surgeons using topical and intracameral anesthetics also employ supplemental IV sedation. This is usually administered by an anesthetist who also monitors the patient's cardiorespiratory status and comfort level during the procedure and adjusts medication accordingly. Sedation is likely to alter the patient's sensory perception during the procedure and memory afterward. However, in studies that grade level of sensation or discomfort during surgery, it is prudent to control for both dominant side and first- or second-eye surgery. When sedation is not used, surgeons should expect greater patient discomfort and movement when operating on the dominant side. Because patient movement during surgery can increase the likelihood of intraoperative complications, it would be interesting to study the correlation between surgical complications and dominant side.

**M. F. Pyfer, MD**

---

**Visual Impairment Corrected Via Cataract Surgery and 5-Year Survival in a Prospective Cohort**

Fong CS-U, Mitchell P, Rochtchina E, et al (Univ of Sydney, New South Wales, Australia)

*Am J Ophthalmol* 157:163-170.e1, 2014

---

*Purpose.*—To compare mortality risk between cataract surgical patients with corrected and persistent visual impairment.

*Design.*—Cohort study.

*Methods.*—A total of 1864 consecutive patients, aged ≥64 years, undergoing phacoemulsification surgery at Westmead Hospital were followed annually for 5 years postoperatively. Visual impairment status in the surgical eye was categorized as none (presenting visual acuity [VA], ≥20/40), mild (VA <20/40-20/60), or moderate-severe (VA <20/60). All-cause mortality was obtained from the Australian National Death Index.

*Results.*—Of 901 patients with moderate-severe visual impairment before surgery, 60.4% (n = 544), 15.5% (n = 140), and 24.1% (n = 217) had no, mild, or moderate-severe visual impairment in the surgical eye, respectively, 1 month postoperatively. Age-standardized 5-year mortality rates were nonsignificantly lower in patients with either mild (24.7%, 95% confidence interval [CI] 16.5%-32.9%) or no visual impairment (24.1%, 95% CI 19.9%-28.4%) post surgery compared to that in patients whose moderate-severe visual impairment persisted (30.6%, 95% CI 23.3%-37.9%). After adjusting for age, sex, smoking, body mass index, and individual comorbid conditions, such as hypertension, diabetes, angina, myocardial infarction, stroke, transient ischemic attack, and kidney disease, patients with no visual impairment 1 month postoperatively had a lower mortality risk (HR 0.73, 95% CI 0.52-1.01) compared to those with persistent moderate-severe visual impairment after surgery. This finding was significant (HR 0.71, 95% CI 0.51-0.99) after additional adjustment for number of medications taken (continuous variable) and number (≥3 vs <3) of comorbid conditions.

*Conclusion.*—Correcting moderate-severe visual impairment in older patients with phacoemulsification surgery was associated with a lower mortality risk, compared to surgical patients whose visual impairment persisted postoperatively.

▶ Vision impairment has been reasonably well established as an independent risk factor for death from all causes.[1] When correcting for major health issues such as cardiovascular disease and diabetes, which are associated with visual impairment, the association persists but is somewhat weaker. Presumably, an important predictor of mortality is the risk of accidental injury, which is increased by poor vision in at least 1 eye.[2] This study found a slight reduction in mortality 5 years after cataract surgery, compared with patients whose vision did not improve after surgery. The difference became significant only when adjusting for comorbid health conditions such as cardiovascular disease and number of medications taken. The study did not attempt to measure quality of life. Although the converse was not specifically tested, we can reasonably conclude that cataract surgery in patients whose vision did not improve, due to other ocular diseases such as macular degeneration or diabetic retinopathy, did not achieve a benefit in survival over the 5-year study period. Because risk of death from injury is relatively low in the developed world, it may take longer than 5 years follow-up to elicit a more significant survival benefit. I hope the authors will conduct a follow-up study at 10 years in this population.

**M. F. Pyfer, MD**

*References*

1. McCarty CA, Nanjan MB, Taylor HR. Vision impairment predicts 5 year mortality. *Br J Ophthalmol.* 2001;85:322-326.
2. McCarty CA, Fu CL, Taylor HR. Predictors of falls in the Melbourne visual impairment project. *Aust N Z J Public Health.* 2002;26:116-119.

**Influence of axial length and corneal power on the astigmatic power of toric intraocular lenses**

Savini G, Hoffer KJ, Carbonelli M, et al (G.B. Bietti Foundation IRCCS, Rome, Italy; Studio Oculistico d'Azeglio, Bologna, Italy; Univ of California, Los Angeles)

*J Cataract Refract Surg* 39:1900-1903, 2013

*Purpose.*—To assess the influence of the anterior chamber depth (ACD), predicted by corneal power (keratometry [K]), and axial length (AL) on the astigmatic power of toric intraocular lenses (IOLs).

*Setting.*—Private practice, Bologna, Italy.

*Design.*—Noninterventional theoretical study.

*Methods.*—Meridional analysis (based on the Hoffer Q formula) was applied to an eye model with K ranging from 38.0 to 48.0 diopters and AL ranging from 20 to 30 mm. For each diopter (D) of K and each millimeter of AL, the ratio between the toricity at the IOL plane and the toricity at the corneal plane was computed. Several simulations with the Acrysof toric IOL were performed.

*Results.*—The ratio between toricity at the IOL plane and toricity at the corneal plane depended on the predicted ACD. The highest value (1.86) was found with the steepest K (48.0 D) and longest AL (30.0 mm) and the lowest value (1.29), with the flattest K (38.0 D) and shortest AL (20.0 mm). When applied to the toric IOL, the results suggest that a low ratio (≤1.41) led to overcorrection of astigmatism relative to the value reported by the manufacturer's online calculator. In contrast, a high ratio (>1.60) led to undercorrection of the astigmatism.

*Conclusion.*—The ACD influenced the ratio between the cylinder power in the IOL plane and the cylinder power in the corneal plane and should be accounted for when selecting a toric IOL in an eye whose K and AL are far from the average values (Fig 1).

▶ Conversion of the astigmatism power in a toric intraocular lens (IOL) from the IOL plane to the corneal plane depends on the IOL position. It has been well established that effective IOL position will vary with the biometry of the eye. Adjusting for this variation should help improve the accuracy of astigmatism correction when using a toric implant. This adjustment is especially important in eyes that deviate significantly from the population median in axial length or corneal curvature. The online toric IOL pleural from AMO and Staar already make this adjustment. Until the other toric lens selection programs do so, it is prudent

Corneal power (D)

| | | | | | | | | | | | |
|---|---|---|---|---|---|---|---|---|---|---|---|
| 48 | 1.47 | 1.50 | 1.53 | 1.57 | 1.61 | 1.66 | 1.70 | 1.75 | 1.79 | 1.83 | 1.86 |
| 47 | 1.44 | 1.47 | 1.50 | 1.54 | 1.58 | 1.63 | 1.67 | 1.71 | 1.75 | 1.79 | 1.82 |
| 46 | 1.42 | 1.45 | 1.48 | 1.52 | 1.56 | 1.60 | 1.64 | 1.68 | 1.72 | 1.75 | 1.78 |
| 45 | 1.40 | 1.43 | 1.46 | 1.49 | 1.53 | 1.57 | 1.61 | 1.65 | 1.69 | 1.72 | 1.74 |
| 44 | 1.38 | 1.41 | 1.44 | 1.47 | 1.51 | 1.54 | 1.58 | 1.62 | 1.65 | 1.68 | 1.70 |
| 43 | 1.37 | 1.39 | 1.42 | 1.45 | 1.48 | 1.52 | 1.55 | 1.59 | 1.62 | 1.65 | 1.67 |
| 42 | 1.35 | 1.37 | 1.40 | 1.43 | 1.46 | 1.50 | 1.53 | 1.56 | 1.60 | 1.62 | 1.64 |
| 41 | 1.33 | 1.36 | 1.38 | 1.41 | 1.44 | 1.47 | 1.51 | 1.54 | 1.57 | 1.60 | 1.61 |
| 40 | 1.32 | 1.34 | 1.36 | 1.39 | 1.42 | 1.45 | 1.48 | 1.52 | 1.54 | 1.57 | 1.59 |
| 39 | 1.31 | 1.33 | 1.35 | 1.38 | 1.40 | 1.43 | 1.46 | 1.49 | 1.52 | 1.54 | 1.56 |
| 38 | 1.29 | 1.31 | 1.33 | 1.36 | 1.39 | 1.41 | 1.44 | 1.47 | 1.50 | 1.52 | 1.54 |
| | 20 | 21 | 22 | 23 | 24 | 25 | 26 | 27 | 28 | 29 | 30 |

Axial length (mm)

FIGURE 1.—Ratio of toricity at the IOL plane to toricity at the corneal plane as a function of axial length (AL) and corneal power (K). Values in *gray* cells on the right show combinations of AL and K leading to a ratio >1.46 (the mean value used by the manufacturer). Values in *white* on the left show combinations of AL and K leading to a ratio of <1.46. (Reprinted from Journal of Cataract & Refractive Surgery. Savini G, Hoffer KJ, Carbonelli M, et al. Influence of axial length and corneal power on the astigmatic power of toric intraocular lenses. *J Cataract Refract Surg*. 2013;39:1900-1903, Copyright 2013, with permission from ASCRS and ESCRS.)

for the surgeon to make the correction manually by applying the conversion factor to the lens toricity derived in this article (see Table in the original article).

**M. F. Pyfer, MD**

---

**Correcting astigmatism with toric intraocular lenses: Effect of posterior corneal astigmatism**

Koch DD, Jenkins RB, Weikert MP, et al (Baylor College of Medicine, Houston, TX)

*J Cataract Refract Surg* 39:1803-1809, 2013

---

*Purpose.*—To evaluate the impact of posterior corneal astigmatism on outcomes with toric intraocular lenses (IOLs).

*Setting.*—Cullen Eye Institute, Baylor College of Medicine, Houston, Texas, USA.

*Design.*—Case series.

*Methods.*—Corneal astigmatism was measured using 5 devices before and 3 weeks after cataract surgery. Toric IOL alignment was recorded at surgery and at the slitlamp 3 weeks postoperatively. The actual corneal astigmatism was calculated based on refractive astigmatism 3 weeks postoperatively and the effective toric power calculated with the Holladay 2

TABLE 3.—Baylor Toric IOL Nomogram (target range up to 0.40 D WTR). Values in the table are the Vector Sum of the Anterior Corneal and Surgically Induced Astigmatism. Examples: (1) If the Cornea has 3.70 D WTR and Surgically Induced Astigmatism is 0.20 D WTR, use the Value of 3.9 D to select IOL toricity. (2) If the Cornea has 1.90 D ATR and Surgically Induced Astigmatism is 0.20 D WTR, Use the Value of 1.70 D to Select IOL Toricity

| Effective IOL Cylinder Power at Corneal Plane (D) | WTR (D) | ATR (D) |
|---|---|---|
| 0.00 | ≤1.69 (PCRI if >1.00) | <0.39 |
| 1.00 | 1.70–2.19 | 0.40*–0.79 |
| 1.50 | 2.20–2.69 | 0.80–1.29 |
| 2.00 | 2.70–3.19 | 1.30–1.79 |
| 2.50 | 3.20–3.79 | 1.80–2.29 |
| 3.00 | 3.80–4.39 | 2.30–2.79 |
| 3.50 | 4.40–4.99 | 2.80–3.29 |
| 4.00 | 5.00– | 3.30–3.79 |

ATR = against the rule; IOL = intraocular lens; PCRI = peripheral corneal relaxing incision; WTR = with the rule.
*Especially if spectacles have more ATR.

formula. The prediction error was calculated as the difference between the astigmatism measured by each device and the actual corneal astigmatism. Vector analysis was used in all calculations.

*Results.*—With the IOLMaster, Lenstar, Atlas, manual keratometer, and Galilei (combined Placido-dual Scheimpflug analyzer), the mean prediction errors (D) were, respectively, 0.59 @ 89.7, 0.48 @ 91.2, 0.51 @ 78.7, 0.62 @ 97.2, and 0.57 @ 93.9 for with-the-rule (WTR) astigmatism (60 to 120 degrees), and 0.17 @ 86.2, 0.23 @ 77.7, 0.23 @ 91.4, 0.41 @ 58.4, and 0.12 @ 7.3 for against-the-rule (ATR) astigmatism (0 to 30 degrees and 150 to 180 degrees). In the WTR eyes, there were significant WTR prediction errors (0.5 to 0.6 diopters [D]) by all devices. In ATR eyes, WTR prediction errors were 0.2 to 0.3 D by all devices except the Placido-dual Scheimpflug analyzer (all $P < .05$ with Bonferroni correction).

*Conclusions.*—Corneal astigmatism was overestimated in WTR by all devices and underestimated in ATR by all except the Placido-dual Scheimpflug analyzer. A new toric IOL nomogram is proposed (Table 3).

▶ This landmark work may explain some unpredicted results when toric lenses are implanted and offers the potential for fine-tuning these results. The best technique of course would be to actually measure the total corneal astigmatism including posterior surface before surgery, but this is not practical with current instrumentation. Intraoperative wavefront aberrometry comes the closest to this goal but may be confounded by changes induced by surgery that resolve after healing. The most promising technique for detailed corneal mapping including the effect of the posterior corneal surface is high-resolution anterior segment ocular coherence tomography, but this feature is not available commercially at present. Until then, I advise cataract surgeons treating astigmatism by implanting toric lenses to follow the nomogram outlined in this article (see Table 3). In simple terms, we should undercorrect with-the-rule astigmatism by about 1.0 diopter and overcorrect against-the-rule astigmatism by about 0.5 diopter, when measurements are based on conventional keratometers that measure anterior corneal curvature only.

**M. F. Pyfer, MD**

**Macular Edema Following Cataract Surgery in Eyes with Previous 23-Gauge Vitrectomy and Peeling of the Internal Limiting Membrane**

Mylonas G, on Behalf of the Macula Study Group Vienna (Med Univ of Vienna, Austria)

*Am J Ophthalmol* 155:253-259.e2, 2013

*Purpose.*—To investigate intraretinal changes after successful cataract surgery in patients with previous pars plana vitrectomy (PPV) and indocyanine green-assisted peeling of epiretinal membrane and internal limiting membrane (ILM).

*Design.*—Prospective nonrandomized controlled clinical study.

*Methods.*—Twenty eyes of 20 patients with cataract with previous 23-gauge PPV and ILM peeling (PPV group) and 15 consecutive eyes with senile cataract with a healthy macula (control group) were included. Best-corrected visual acuity (BCVA), spectral-domain optical coherence tomography (OCT), infrared fundus imaging, and biomicroscopy were performed at baseline and at week 1, month 1, and month 3 after cataract surgery. OCT raster scans were further analyzed regarding the central millimeter thickness (CMMT), area of retinal thickening size on the topographic map, and changes in retinal structural morphology.

*Results.*—The baseline mean visual acuity in the PPV group was 0.3 ± 0.18 Snellen lines, which improved significantly to 0.85 ± 0.18 ($P < .05$) 3 months after cataract surgery. CMMT was 393 (±44) μm at baseline and increased to 408 (±47) μm at month 3 ($P < .05$). One patient was not seen at the final visit, so data of 19 patients was used. In the PPV group, 8 of 19 patients (42%) developed an increase in CMMT more than 35 μm 1 month after cataract surgery; 5 of these 8 patients (26%) developed macular edema with cyst formation. Three months after surgery, the area of retinal thickening was significantly larger in most patients compared with baseline values. No cystoid macular edema was observed in the control group.

*Conclusions.*—This study provides evidence that patients with previous PPV and membrane and ILM peeling often develop macular edema after successful cataract surgery (Fig 2).

▶ This is a small prospective study that provides useful clinical information. Patients undergoing cataract surgery after pars plans vitrectomy with membrane peeling (PPV/MP) are at much greater than average for postoperative cystoid macular edema (CME). In this study, the rate of clinically significant CME for post-PPV/MP patients was 26%, much higher than the 2% to 5% expected

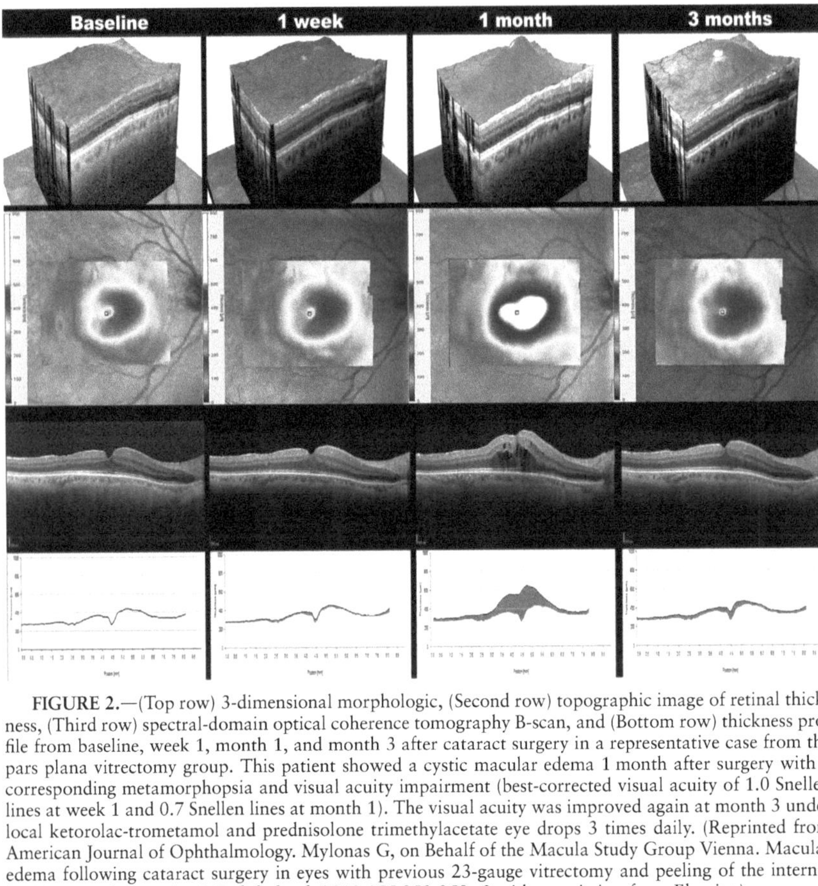


FIGURE 2.—(Top row) 3-dimensional morphologic, (Second row) topographic image of retinal thickness, (Third row) spectral-domain optical coherence tomography B-scan, and (Bottom row) thickness profile from baseline, week 1, month 1, and month 3 after cataract surgery in a representative case from the pars plana vitrectomy group. This patient showed a cystic macular edema 1 month after surgery with a corresponding metamorphopsia and visual acuity impairment (best-corrected visual acuity of 1.0 Snellen lines at week 1 and 0.7 Snellen lines at month 1). The visual acuity was improved again at month 3 under local ketorolac-trometamol and prednisolone trimethylacetate eye drops 3 times daily. (Reprinted from American Journal of Ophthalmology. Mylonas G, on Behalf of the Macula Study Group Vienna. Macular edema following cataract surgery in eyes with previous 23-gauge vitrectomy and peeling of the internal limiting membrane. *Am J Ophthalmol.* 2013;155:253-259.e2,with permission from Elsevier.)

for routine phacoemulsification cataract surgery. These patients need close postoperative monitoring and effective prophylaxis against CME to prevent reduced visual acuity, which can be permanent. Prophylactic measures should include longer duration of topical steroid and nonsteroidal medications for all patients, and perhaps earlier intervention with intravitreal steroid or anti-vascular endothelial growth factor agents in those who exhibit macular thickening on ocular coherence tomography (OCT) between 1 and 3 months after cataract extraction that does not resolve with topical medications. Fig 2 shows typical OCT findings in a post-PPV/MP patient who developed CME within 3 months after uncomplicated cataract surgery.

**M. F. Pyfer, MD**

**Surgical Outcomes and Safety of Femtosecond Laser Cataract Surgery: A Prospective Study of 1500 Consecutive Cases**

Roberts TV, Lawless M, Bali SJ, et al (Vision Eye Inst, Chatswood, Australia)

*Ophthalmology* 120:227-233, 2013

*Objective.*—To report the surgical outcomes and safety of femtosecond (FS) laser cataract surgery (LCS) with greater surgeon experience, modified techniques, and improved technology.

*Design.*—Prospective, interventional case series.

*Participants.*—Fifteen hundred consecutive eyes undergoing FS laser cataract and refractive lens exchange surgery in a single group private practice.

*Intervention.*—Femtosecond LCS.

*Methods.*—All eyes undergoing LCS between April 2011 and March 2012 were included in the study. Cases underwent anterior capsulotomy, lens fragmentation, and corneal incisions with the Alcon/LenSx FS laser (Alcon/LenSx, Aliso Viejo, CA). The procedure was completed by phacoemulsification and insertion of an intraocular lens. The cases were divided into 2 groups: Group 1, initial experience consisting of the first 200 cases; and group 2, the subsequent 1300 cases performed by the same surgeons.

*Main Outcome Measures.*—Intraoperative complication rates and comparison between groups.

*Results.*—Both groups were comparable for baseline demographic parameters. Anterior capsule tears occurred in 4% and 0.31% of eyes, posterior capsule tears in 3.5% and 0.31% of eyes, and posterior lens dislocation in 2% and 0% of eyes in groups 1 group 2, respectively ($P < 0.001$ for all comparisons). Number of docking attempts per case (1.5 vs 1.05), incidence of post-laser pupillary constriction (9.5% vs 1.23%), and anterior capsular tags (10.5% vs 1.61%) were significantly lower in group 2 ($P < 0.001$ for all comparisons).

*Conclusions.*—In the authors' experience, the surgical outcomes and safety of LCS improved significantly with greater surgeon experience, development of modified techniques, and improved technology (Table 3).

▶ This is an impressively large series of femtosecond laser-assisted cataract surgery (FS-LCS) cases. The authors demonstrate a significant learning curve, but with low incidence of intraoperative complications after the initial 200 cases. As laser-assisted cataract surgery gains acceptance and becomes more widely adopted, a key first step is to demonstrate at least parity with the current manual procedure regarding outcomes and potential complications. Here, the first 200 cases had a higher complication rate than manual cataract surgery, but group 2 (the next 1300 cases) had an equal or lower complication rate compared with manual (see Table 3). The authors assert that with experience, most FS-LCS complications become predictable and therefore largely preventable. Further improvements in laser hardware and software design will help to decrease the rate of early complications. Also, this study considered only 1 model of FS laser. Others may have a longer or shorter learning curve. Only further research will determine if

TABLE 3.—Comparison of Intraoperative Complications between Groups

| Complications | Group 1 (n = 200), n (%) | Group 2 (n = 1300), n (%) | *P* Value |
|---|---|---|---|
| Suction breaks | 5 (2.5) | 8 (0.61) | 0.023 |
| Manual corneal incisions | 26 (13) | 25 (1.92) | <0.001 |
| Pupillary constriction | 19 (9.5) | 16 (1.23) | <0.001 |
| Anterior capsule tags | 21 (10.5) | 21 (1.62) | <0.001 |
| Anterior radial tears | 8 (4) | 4 (0.31) | <0.001 |
| Posterior capsule tears | 7 (3.5) | 4 (0.31) | <0.001 |
| Posterior lens dislocation | 4 (2) | 0 (0) | <0.001 |

femtosecond laser assistance improves the outcome of cataract surgery beyond manual techniques sufficiently to justify the increased cost.

**M. F. Pyfer, MD**

**Capsular bag opacification with a new accommodating intraocular lens**

Floyd AM, Werner L, Liu E, et al (Univ of Utah, Salt Lake City)

*J Cataract Refract Surg* 39:1415-1420, 2013

*Purpose.*—To evaluate the biocompatibility and capsular bag opacification of an accommodating intraocular lens (IOL) containing large haptic elements that separate the anterior and posterior capsules.

*Setting.*—John A. Moran Eye Center, University of Utah, Salt Lake City, Utah, USA.

*Design.*—Experimental study.

*Methods.*—Bilateral phacoemulsification with IOL implantation was performed in 6 New Zealand rabbits. Each animal received a study (accommodating) IOL and a control (1-piece hydrophobic acrylic) IOL. Eyes were examined at the slitlamp from 1 day through 6 weeks postoperatively. The globes were then enucleated and evaluated grossly. Capsular bag opacification was scored from the posterior aspect (Miyake-Apple view). The eyes were then processed for complete histopathologic evaluation.

*Results.*—At 6 weeks, the mean posterior capsule opacification (PCO) clinical score was 0.5 ± 0.3 (SD) in the study group and 3.0 ± 0.9 in the control group ($P$ =.001, 2-tail paired $t$ test). Anterior capsule opacification was practically absent in the study group and mild in the control group. Miyake-Apple posterior view showed a mean central PCO score of 0 ± 0 in the study group and 3.0 ± 1.1 in the control group ($P$ =.001), peripheral PCO score of 0.7 ± 0.4 and 3.5 ± 0.8 ($P$ =.0006), respectively, and Soemmerring ring score of 2.3 ± 0.8 and 7.0 ± 2.8 ($P$ =.01), respectively. Histopathology showed no signs of toxicity in any eye.

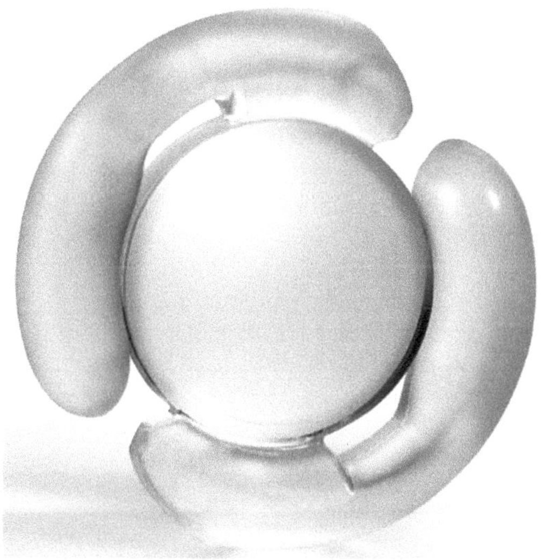

FIGURE 1.—Overall design of the study IOL (image provided by Powervision, Inc.). (Reprinted from Floyd AM, Werner L, Liu E, et al. Capsular bag opacification with a new accommodating intraocular lens. *J Cataract Refract Surg*. 2013;39:1415-1420, with permission from ASCRS and ESCRS.)

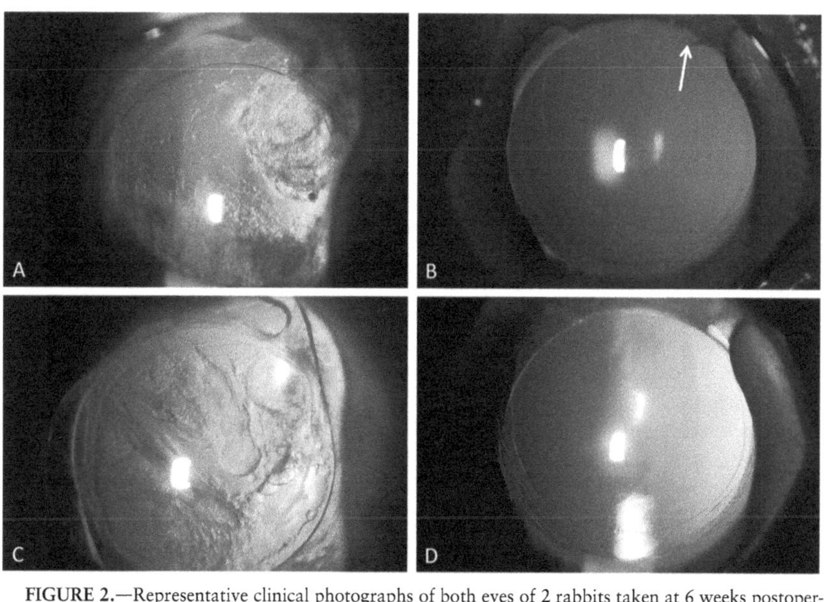


FIGURE 2.—Representative clinical photographs of both eyes of 2 rabbits taken at 6 weeks postoperatively. *A* and *B*: Rabbit 3. *C* and *D*: Rabbit 6. Eyes with the study IOL (*B* and *D*) had clear anterior and posterior capsules. The arrow shows a mild amount of proliferative material protruding anteriorly through the gap between both haptics. Eyes with the control IOL (*A* and *C*) developed diffuse PCO starting at the optic–haptic junctions. (Reprinted from Journal of Cataract & Refractive Surgery. Floyd AM, Werner L, Liu E, et al. Capsular bag opacification with a new accommodating intraocular lens. *J Cataract Refract Surg*. 2013;39:1415-1420, Copyright 2013, with permission from ASCRS and ESCRS.)

*Conclusions.*—The study IOL maintained an expanded capsular bag secondary to the large size of the haptic elements, which appears to prevent capsular bag opacification (Figs 1 and 2).

▶ Posterior capsular opacification (PCO), fibrosis, and cellular proliferation remain the most common postoperative complications of cataract extraction with intraocular lens (IOL) implantation. Effective treatment with yttrium aluminium garnet laser capsulotomy is available, but prevention of this complication is preferable if possible, especially with accommodating lenses that depend on maintenance of capsule elasticity for optimum performance. This experimental study found almost complete absence of PCO in rabbit eyes using a novel accommodating IOL design (Fig 1). This is especially remarkable, as rabbits typically show early and severe PCO with conventional IOLs (Fig 2). Keeping the capsular bag open with access to aqueous flow long term appears to prevent PCO in this study and others recently.[1] This is a key discovery that should ultimately lead to improved IOL designs if human trials are successful.

**M. F. Pyfer, MD**

*Reference*

1. Leishman L, Werner L, Bodnar Z, et al. Prevention of capsular bag opacification with a modified hydrophilic acrylic disk-shaped intraocular lens. *J Cataract Refract Surg*. 2012;38:1664-1670.

## Effects of Multivitamin Supplement on Cataract and Age-Related Macular Degeneration in a Randomized Trial of Male Physicians

Christen WG, Glynn RJ, Manson JE, et al (Brigham and Women's Hosp and Harvard Med School, Boston, MA)
*Ophthalmology* 121:525-534, 2014

*Purpose.*—To test whether long-term multivitamin supplementation affects the incidence of cataract or age-related macular degeneration (AMD) in a large cohort of men.

*Design.*—Randomized, double-blind, placebo-controlled trial.

*Participants.*—A total of 14 641 US male physicians aged ≥50 years.

*Intervention.*—Daily multivitamin or placebo.

*Main Outcome Measures.*—Incident cataract and visually significant AMD responsible for a reduction in best-corrected visual acuity to 20/30 or worse based on self-reports confirmed by medical record review.

*Results.*—During an average of 11.2 years of treatment and follow-up, a total of 1817 cases of cataract and 281 cases of visually significant AMD were confirmed. There were 872 cataracts in the multivitamin group and 945 cataracts in the placebo group (hazard ratio [HR], 0.91; 95% confidence interval [CI], 0.83–0.99; $P = 0.04$). For visually significant AMD, there were 152 cases in the multivitamin group and 129 cases in the placebo group (HR, 1.19; 95% CI, 0.94–1.50; $P = 0.15$).

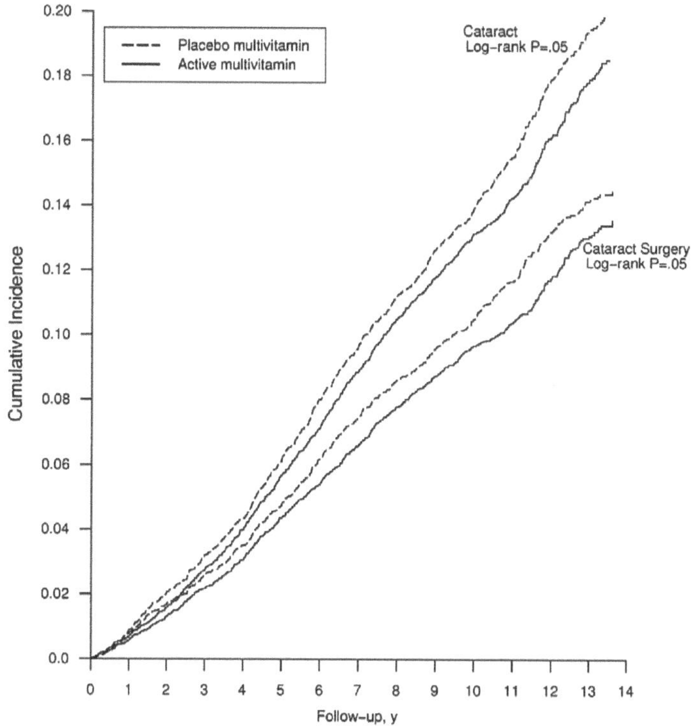


No. at Risk of Cataract

| | | | | | | | | | | | | | | |
|---|---|---|---|---|---|---|---|---|---|---|---|---|---|---|
| Placebo | 5761 | 5687 | 5594 | 5483 | 5373 | 5212 | 5050 | 4897 | 4734 | 4588 | 4451 | 2758 | 1843 | 1615 |
| Active | 5736 | 5668 | 5582 | 5483 | 5376 | 5224 | 5100 | 4939 | 4805 | 4671 | 4536 | 2835 | 1905 | 1656 |

No. at Risk of Cataract Surgery

| | | | | | | | | | | | | | | |
|---|---|---|---|---|---|---|---|---|---|---|---|---|---|---|
| Placebo | 5761 | 5691 | 5614 | 5516 | 5420 | 5290 | 5150 | 5017 | 4874 | 4749 | 4628 | 2901 | 1977 | 1746 |
| Active | 5736 | 5675 | 5598 | 5515 | 5429 | 5297 | 5195 | 5064 | 4951 | 4833 | 4712 | 2985 | 2023 | 1765 |

FIGURE 2.—Cumulative incidence rates of cataract in the multivitamin and placebo groups in the Physicians' Health Study II. Y = year. (Reprinted from Christen WG, Glynn RJ, Manson JE, et al. Effects of multivitamin supplement on cataract and age-related macular degeneration in a randomized trial of male physicians. *Ophthalmology.* 2014;121:525-534, Copyright 2014, with permission from the American Academy of Ophthalmology.)

*Conclusions.*—These randomized trial data from a large cohort of middle-aged and older US male physicians indicate that long-term daily multivitamin use modestly and significantly decreased the risk of cataract but had no significant effect on visually significant AMD (Fig 2).

▶ The Physicians Health Study is a very large, long-term, randomized, double-blind trial comparing multivitamin supplements with placebo in male physicians over 50 years old. This article reports a 9% reduction in the incidence of visually significant cataract (20/30 or worse) or cataract surgery over 11 years (Fig 2). Findings were confirmed by examining the medical records for patients who reported having a cataract diagnosed. Nuclear cataract was the type that showed a small but statistically significant decreased occurrence in the patients who took vitamin supplements. A potential error source in the study is that the formulation of the multivitamin supplement was changed to add lutein midway through the term, and for the first half of the study, the multivitamin patients also took extra vitamin C and vitamin E. Strengths of the study are the large number of subjects (almost 15 000), long duration of follow-up, and the double-blind, placebo-controlled design. This is the first study of its kind to show a modest reduction in cataract risk with daily over-the-counter multivitamin supplementation. Interestingly, the incidence of age-related macular degeneration was also examined here, and no benefit to vitamins was found for this condition in the study population.

**M. F. Pyfer, MD**

---

**Posterior capsule opacification and neodymium:YAG rates with 2 single-piece hydrophobic acrylic intraocular lenses: Three-year results**

Leydolt C, Kriechbaum K, Schriefl S, et al (Med Univ Vienna, Austria)

*J Cataract Refract Surg* 39:1886-1892, 2013

---

*Purpose.*—To compare the incidence and intensity of posterior capsule opacification (PCO) between 2 similar 1-piece foldable hydrophobic acrylic intraocular lenses (IOLs) over 3 years.

*Setting.*—Department of Ophthalmology, Medical University Vienna, Vienna, Austria.

*Design.*—Randomized prospective patient- and examiner-masked clinical trial with intraindividual comparison.

*Methods.*—Patients with bilateral age-related cataract had cataract surgery and implantation of a Tecnis ZCB00 continuous-optic-edge IOL in 1 eye and an Acrysof SA60AT interrupted-optic-edge IOL in the other eye. Postoperative examinations were performed at 6 months and 3 years. Digital retroillumination images were taken of each eye. The amount of PCO (score 0 to 10) was assessed subjectively at the slitlamp and objectively using automated image-analysis software.

*Results.*—The study comprised 54 patients (108 eyes). The mean objective PCO score was 1.3 ± 1.7 (SD) for the continuous-optic-edge IOLs and 0.9 ± 1.3 for the interrupted-optic-edge IOLs ($P = .10$). Three years postoperatively, a neodymium:YAG (Nd:YAG) capsulotomy was performed in 26.1% of eyes with the continuous-optic-edge IOL and 21.7% with the interrupted-optic-edge IOL ($P = .56$). There was no significant difference in corrected distance visual acuity, capsulorhexis–IOL overlap, capsule folds, or anterior capsule opacification 3 years after surgery.

*Conclusions.*—Both IOLs had comparable PCO and Nd:YAG rates 3 years postoperatively. The optimized barrier function of the continuous-optic-edge IOL and the material properties of the interrupted-optic-edge

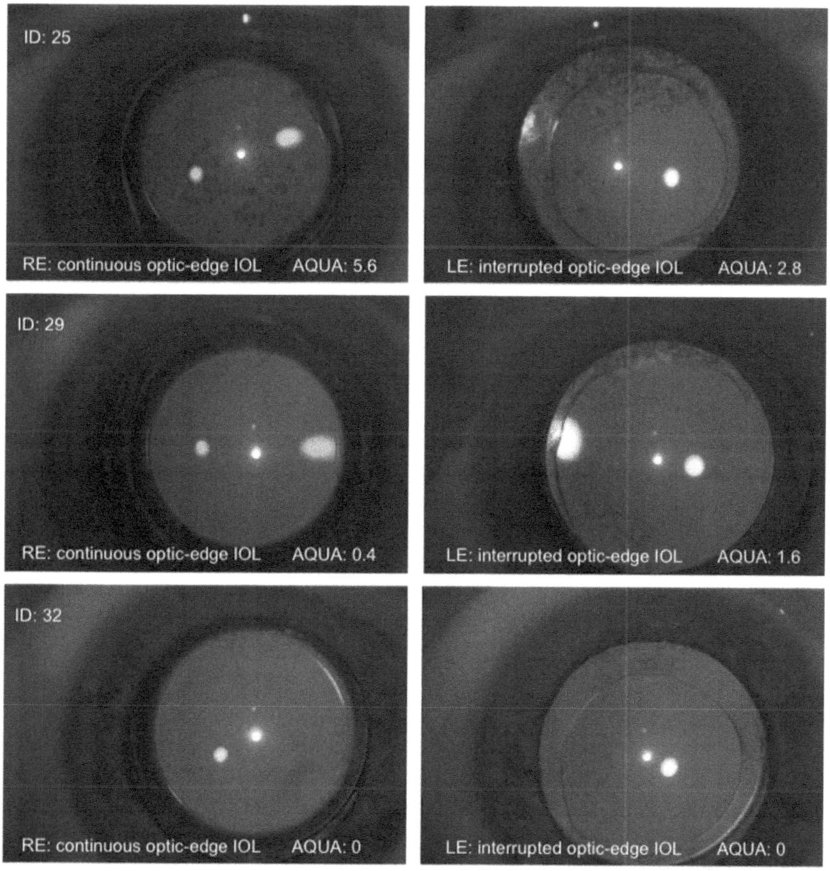


**FIGURE 3.**—Retroillumination images of 3 representative patients (IOL = intraocular lens; LE = left eye; RE = right eye). (Reprinted from Journal of Cataract & Refractive Surgery. Leydolt C, Kriechbaum K, Schriefl S, et al. Posterior capsule opacification and neodymium:YAG rates with 2 single-piece hydrophobic acrylic intraocular lenses: three-year results. *J Cataract Refract Surg*. 2013;39:1886-1892, Copyright 2013, with permission from ASCRS and ESCRS.)

IOL seemingly outbalanced the effect on lens epithelial cell migration and proliferation beneath the optic (Fig 3).

▶ One-piece hydrophobic acrylic intraocular lenses (IOLs) are very popular because of ease of insertion through a small incision, good centration, and predictably stable optical performance in the eye. Posterior capsule opacification (PCO) remains the most common postoperative complication of cataract surgery. Square posterior optic edge design is found to decrease PCO rate by mechanical inhibition of lens epithelial cell (LEC) migration from the peripheral capsular bag. This study compared the PCO rate of the 2 most popular one-piece acrylic IOL designs, finding them equivalent. Significant strengths of this study are randomization, double-blinding, and intraindividual comparison (Fig 3).

Both IOLs studied have a square posterior optic edge, but the SA60AT has a discontinuity in the edge where the haptic meets the optic, and the ZCB00 does not. The authors theorize that the increased inhibitory effect of the continuous edge of the ZCB00 may be offset by a variation in material that makes the SA60AT better for inhibiting LEC migration, but this assertion is unproven. The haptic design, angulation, or another physical property of the ZCB00 may allow the posterior edge to lose contact with the capsule, permitting LEC access behind the optic. More work is necessary, including imaging and postmortem examination of these IOLs in the capsular bag to prove these theories.

**M. F. Pyfer, MD**

---

**Phacoemulsification versus Trabeculectomy in Medically Uncontrolled Chronic Angle-Closure Glaucoma without Cataract**

Tham CCY, Kwong YYY, Baig N, et al (The Chinese Univ of Hong Kong, Hong Kong SAR, People's Republic of China)

*Ophthalmology* 120:62-67, 2013

---

*Objective.*—To compare phacoemulsification versus trabeculectomy with adjunctive mitomycin C in medically uncontrolled chronic angle-closure glaucoma (CACG) without cataract.

*Design.*—Prospective, randomized clinical trial.

*Participants.*—Fifty medically uncontrolled CACG eyes without cataract of 50 patients.

*Intervention.*—Patients were randomized into undergoing either phacoemulsification or trabeculectomy with adjunctive mitomycin C. After surgery, patients were followed up every 3 months for 2 years.

*Main Outcome Measures.*—Intraocular pressure (IOP) and requirement for glaucoma drugs.

*Results.*—Twenty-six CACG eyes were randomized to receive phacoemulsification, and 24 eyes underwent trabeculectomy with mitomycin C. Phacoemulsification and trabeculectomy resulted in significant and comparable IOP reduction at 24 months after surgery (reduction of 8.4 mm Hg or 34% for phacoemulsification vs. 8.9 mm Hg or 36% for trabeculectomy; $P = 0.76$). Over first 24 months, trabeculectomy-treated eyes required on average 1.1 fewer drugs than phacoemulsification-treated eyes ($P < 0.001$). However, trabeculectomy was associated with significantly more surgical complications than phacoemulsification (46% vs. 4%; $P = 0.001$). Eight (33%) of 24 trabeculectomy eyes demonstrated cataract during follow-up.

*Conclusions.*—Both phacoemulsification and trabeculectomy are effective in reducing IOP in medically uncontrolled CACG eyes without cataract. Trabeculectomy is more effective than phacoemulsification in reducing dependence on glaucoma drugs, but is associated with more complications (Fig 1).

▶ This prospective, randomized study has the potential to change the management of medically uncontrolled chronic angle closure glaucoma.

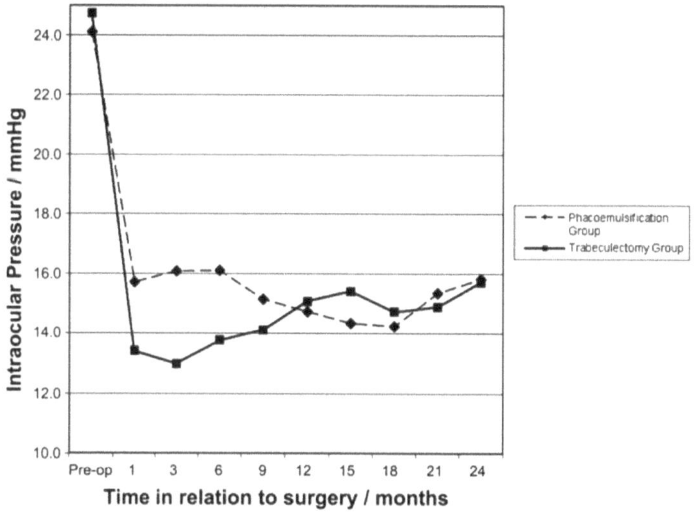


FIGURE 1.—Graph showing intraocular pressure (IOP) profiles of the phacoemulsification group and the trabeculectomy group. Pre-op = before surgery. (Reprinted from Tham CCY, Kwong YYY, Baig N, et al. Phacoemulsification versus trabeculectomy in medically uncontrolled chronic angle-closure glaucoma without cataract. *Ophthalmology.* 2013;120:62-67, Copyright 2013, with permission from the American Academy of Ophthalmology.)

Phacoemulsification lens extraction resulted in equivalent intraocular pressure control compared with trabeculectomy with mitomycin C for 2 years after surgery (Fig 1). The phaco eyes required, on average, 1 additional glaucoma medication to achieve that control. Significant advantages to lens extraction are a much lower complication rate (10 times lower in this study) and avoidance of a second surgery in one-third of trabeculectomy patients who went on to require cataract extraction within 2 years. The trabeculectomy eyes also had a greater incidence of loss of best-corrected vision (25% vs 15%) compared with lens extraction. Prior studies[1] have found that lens extraction is an effective treatment for acute angle closure glaucoma, and now we have additional evidence of the success of lens extraction alone for poorly controlled chronic angle closure.

**M. F. Pyfer, MD**

## *Reference*

1. Husain R, Gazzard G, Aung T, et al. Initial management of acute primary angle closure: a randomized trial comparing phacoemulsification with laser peripheral iridotomy. *Ophthalmology.* 2012;119:2274-2281.

## Anterior chamber flare after femtosecond laser–assisted cataract surgery

Abell RG, Allen PL, Vote BJ (Launceston Eye Inst, Tasmania, Australia)

*J Cataract Refract Surg* 39:1321-1326, 2013

*Purpose.*—To determine whether postoperative ocular inflammation is less after femtosecond laser-assisted cataract surgery than after conventional phacoemulsification (manual) cataract surgery.

*Setting.*—Private clinic, Launceston, Tasmania, Australia.

*Design.*—Prospective consecutive investigator-masked nonrandomized parallel cohort study.

*Methods.*—Consecutive cataract patients who had femtosecond laser-assisted cataract surgery or manual cataract surgery by the same surgeon at a single center were assessed. The primary endpoint was postoperative aqueous flare measured by laser flare photometry at 1 day and 4 weeks. Secondary endpoints included retinal thickness measured by optical coherence tomography and slitlamp examination findings at 4 weeks.

*Results.*—The per-protocol population comprised 176 patients (100 in laser group; 76 in manual group). Postoperative aqueous flare was significantly greater in the manual cataract surgery group at 1 day ($P = .0089$) and at 4 weeks ($P = .003$). There was a significant correlation between effective phacoemulsification time and 1-day postoperative aqueous flare ($r = 0.35$, $P < .0001$). The increase in outer zone thickness measured by optical coherence tomography was less in the laser group ($P = .007$).

*Conclusion.*—Anterior segment inflammation was less after femtosecond laser-assisted cataract surgery than after manual cataract surgery, and this appeared to be due to a reduction in phacoemulsification energy (Fig 1).

▶ This well-constructed study compares a series of about 100 patients treated using manual phacoemulsification cataract extraction with a consecutive series by the same surgeon pretreated with femtosecond laser capsulotomy and lens fragmentation before manual phaco surgery. Although not a primary study end point, effective phaco time (EPT) and total irrigating fluid use during surgery was recorded and found to be lower in the femto laser group. The authors initially theorized that fragmentation of the lens using the femto laser, along with the delay time of about 30 minutes between laser pretreatment and lens removal surgery, may result in increased inflammation postoperatively, especially at day 1. The opposite was found; there was less flare (see Fig 1) and macular thickening in the femto group. No significant difference was found between groups in slit-lamp grading of cell and flare or corneal edema. The study employed good control between groups, the same postoperative medications were used, and flare meter readings were taken under the same conditions. Also, patients with conditions known to predispose them to increased inflammation were excluded from analysis in both groups. However, it was not a randomized study. Patients who declined surgery with the femto laser underwent traditional manual phaco surgery. A much stronger study would be to randomly select 1 eye of each patient for laser-assisted surgery, then perform a within-patient comparison of measurements.

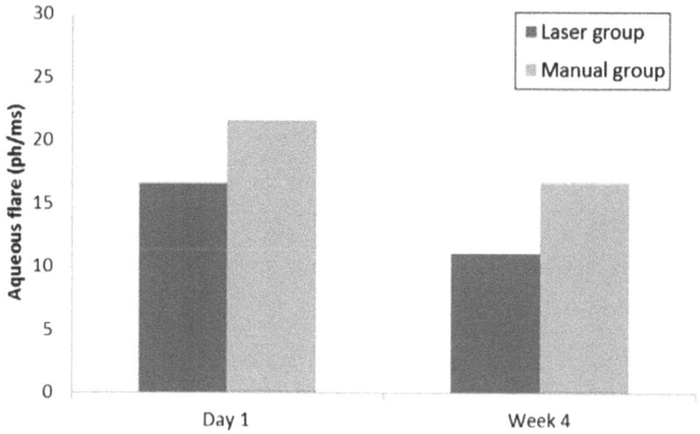


FIGURE 1.—Mean aqueous flare in the laser group and manual group 1 day and 4 weeks after cataract surgery (ph/ms = photons per millisecond). (Reprinted from Journal of Cataract & Refractive Surgery. Abell RG, Allen PL, Vote BJ. Anterior chamber flare after femtosecond laser-assisted cataract surgery. *J Cataract Refract Surg.* 2013;39:1321-1326, Copyright 2013, with permission from ASCRS and ESCRS.)

Until such a study is conducted, findings of superiority for femto-assisted cataract surgery will be subject to claims of unintentional bias because the laser owner has a large financial investment at stake.

**M. F. Pyfer, MD**

---

**Effect of Femtosecond Laser Fragmentation on Effective Phacoemulsification Time in Cataract Surgery**

Conrad-Hengerer I, Hengerer FH, Schultz T, et al (Ruhr Univ Eye Hosp, Bochum, Germany)

*J Refract Surg* 28:879-883, 2012

---

*Purpose.*—To compare the effect of femtosecond laser—assisted cataract surgery on effective phacoemulsification time (EPT) with standard cataract surgery.

*Methods.*—This prospective clinical trial evaluated the feasibility of using a femtosecond laser system (Catalys Precision Laser System, OptiMedica) to perform capsulotomy and lens fragmentation in the treatment of patients with senile cataract. Patients were evaluated preoperatively with the Lens Opacities Classification System III (LOCS III). Fifty-two patients underwent standard cataract surgery and 57 patients underwent femtosecond laser-assisted cataract surgery in December 2011. Both groups underwent phacoemulsification using pulsed ultrasound energy and EPT was evaluated.

*Results.*—Preoperative LOCS III grades were 3.4 ± 0.9 in the femtosecond laser-assisted cataract surgery group and 3.1 ± 0.9 in the standard

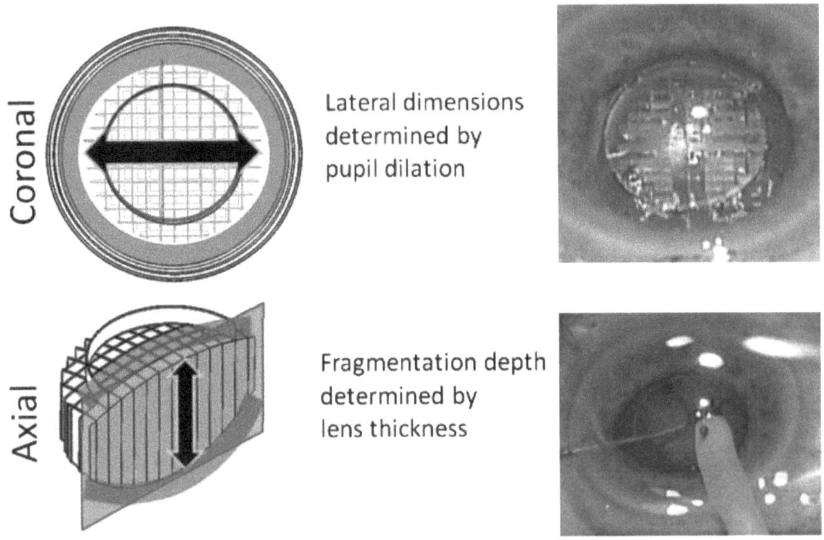


FIGURE 1.—Fragmentation volume customized to patient anatomy. (Courtesy of OptiMedica.) (Reprinted from Conrad-Hengerer I, Hengerer FH, Schultz T, et al. Effect of femtosecond laser fragmentation on effective phacoemulsification time in cataract surgery. *J Refract Surg*. 2012;28:879-883, with permission from SLACK Incorporated.)

group. In the femtosecond laser-assisted cataract surgery group, mean laser treatment time was 54.9 seconds and EPT was 0.16 ± 0.21 seconds compared to 4.07 ± 3.14 seconds in the standard group.

*Conclusions.*—The use of the femtosecond laser-assisted system in cataract surgery led to a lower EPT compared to the standard procedure (Fig 1).

▶ This is the first study to report a significant reduction in ultrasound energy required for cataract removal in patients undergoing femtosecond laser-assisted cataract surgery using the Catalys Precision Laser System (AMO/OptiMedica). This laser allows fragmentation of the entire crystalline lens into small vertical cuboidal cylinders (see Fig 1). The trial was prospective but nonrandomized, although the preoperative nuclear density in both femto and manual groups was similar. Lower ultrasound energy dissipated into the eye during surgery is known to result in less endothelial cell loss after phacoemulsification cataract surgery. Limitations of this study are that endothelial cell count was not measured or reported and that total irrigation fluid used, which has also been correlated with endothelial cell loss, was not reported. Further experience with this laser, along with optimization of phaco machine fluidics and tip geometry, should allow removal of most cataracts up to LOCS III density with essentially zero ultrasound power.

**M. F. Pyfer, MD**

**Anterior Capsulotomy Integrity after Femtosecond Laser-Assisted Cataract Surgery**

Abell RG, Davies PEJ, Phelan D, et al (Tasmanian Eye Inst, Launceston, Tasmania, Australia; Newcastle Eye Hosp Res Foundation, New South Wales, Australia; Univ of Newcastle, Callaghan, New South Wales, Australia; et al)
*Ophthalmology* 121:17-24, 2014

*Objective.*—To compare the incidence of anterior capsular tears after femtosecond laser-assisted cataract surgery (FLACS) versus phacoemulsification cataract surgery (PCS) and to assess the ultrastructural features of anterior capsulotomy specimens (FLACS and PCS) using electron microscopy.

*Design.*—Prospective, multicenter, comparative cohort case series.

*Participants.*—Consecutive patients undergoing FLACS or PCS.

*Methods.*—A prospective cohort study of all patients (n = 1626) undergoing FLACS or PCS by 2 surgeons from centers A and B was undertaken to compare the incidence of anterior capsule tears. Anterior lens capsules were collected by 4 surgeons from centers A, B, C, and D using 3 different commercially available femtosecond platforms, each with latest version upgrades. Lens capsule tissue was prepared for scanning electron microscopy (SEM) using a total of 10 samples for patients undergoing PCS, and 40 samples for patients undergoing FLACS.

*Main Outcome Measures.*—Incidence of anterior capsule tear and comparative ultrastructural features of capsular samples from both PCS and FLACS cases.

*Results.*—There was a significantly increased rate of anterior capsule tears in the FLACS group (15/804 [1.87%]) when compared with the PCS group (1/822 [0.12%]; $P = 0.0002$, Fisher exact test). In 7 cases, the anterior capsule tear extended to the posterior capsule. Because all cases had occurred in complete capsulotomy, the integrity of the anterior capsule was questioned in the FLACS group. Subsequent SEM sampling showed irregularity at the capsule margin, as well as multiple apparently misplaced laser pits in normal parts of the tissue. Aberrant pits were approximately 2 to 4 μm apart and occurred at a range of 10 to 100 μm radially from the capsule edge.

*Conclusions.*—Laser anterior capsulotomy integrity seems to be compromised by postage-stamp perforations and additional aberrant pulses, possibly because of fixational eye movements. This can lead to an increased rate of anterior capsule tears, and extra care should be taken during surgery after femtosecond laser pretreatment has been performed. A learning curve may account for some of the increased complication rate with FLACS. However, the SEM features raise safety concerns for capsular integrity after FLACS and warrant further investigation (Fig 4).

▶ This is a well-conducted study of the microscopic configuration of the anterior capsulotomy created by several models of femtosecond lasers. Clinical concern that the anterior capsule edge is more prone to radial tears than manual continuous

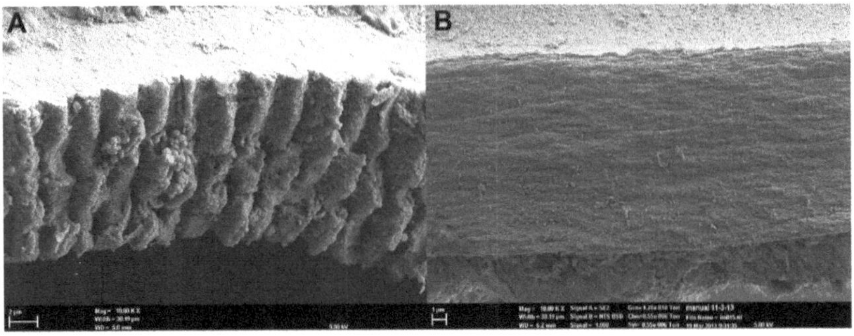

**FIGURE 4.**—**A**, Edge treated with the Catalys femtosecond laser (OptiMedica, Sunnyvale, CA) is serrated, resembling a micro–can-opener structure from the laser photodisruption, each estimated here to be just less than 2 μm across (original magnification, ×10 000). **B**, Manually torn capsule (original magnification, ×10 000). (Reprinted from Abell RG, Davies PEJ, Phelan D, et al. Anterior capsulotomy integrity after femtosecond laser-assisted cataract surgery. *Ophthalmology.* 2014;121:17-24, Copyright 2014, with permission from the American Academy of Ophthalmology.)

capsulorhexis is legitimate. More experience and monitoring are necessary to determine if this is clinically significant or will require adjustment in laser spot density or energy to decrease risk for radial tears. Early reports of intraoperative complications in femto laser-assisted cataract cases have shown a slight increase in the incidence of anterior capsule tears, at least in the first 200 cases.[1] This study provides evidence that postage-stamp-like microscopic perforations in the capsule are created by the femtosecond laser, compared with the relatively smooth edge of a manual capsulorhexis (see Fig 4). Whether this configuration results in relative capsule edge weakness or increased tendency to tear outward with stress has yet to be determined. My personal experience indicates that as long as the laser capsulotomy is complete, there is no associated capsule edge weakness. The surgeon should pay careful attention to complete cortical and lens epithelial cell removal in femto-assisted cases to prevent early anterior capsule fibrosis.

**M. F. Pyfer, MD**

*Reference*

1. Roberts TV, Lawless M, Bali SJ, Hodge C, Sutton G. Surgical outcomes and safety of femtosecond laser cataract surgery: a prospective study of 1500 consecutive cases. *Ophthalmology.* 2013;120:227-233.

# 2 Refractive Surgery

**Sources of Medical Error in Refractive Surgery**

Moshirfar M, Simpson RG, Dave SB (Univ of Utah, Salt Lake City; Univ of Arizona College of Medicine, Phoenix; Northwest Eye Health, Portland, OR; et al)

*J Refract Surg* 29:303-310, 2013

*Purpose.*—To evaluate the causes of laser programming errors in refractive surgery and outcomes in these cases.

*Methods.*—In this multicenter, retrospective chart review, 22 eyes of 18 patients who had incorrect data entered into the refractive laser computer system at the time of treatment were evaluated. Cases were analyzed to uncover the etiology of these errors, patient follow-up treatments, and final outcomes. The results were used to identify potential methods to avoid similar errors in the future.

*Results.*—Every patient experienced compromised uncorrected visual acuity requiring additional intervention, and 7 of 22 eyes (32%) lost corrected distance visual acuity (CDVA) of at least one line. Sixteen patients were suitable candidates for additional surgical correction to address these residual visual symptoms and six were not. Thirteen of 22 eyes (59%) received surgical follow-up treatment; nine eyes were treated with contact lenses. After follow-up treatment, six patients (27%) still had a loss of one line or more of CDVA. Three significant sources of error were identified: errors of cylinder conversion, data entry, and patient identification error.

*Conclusion.*—Twenty-seven percent of eyes with laser programming errors ultimately lost one or more lines of CDVA. Patients who underwent surgical revision had better outcomes than those who did not. Many of the mistakes identified were likely avoidable had preventive measures been taken, such as strict adherence to patient verification protocol or rigorous rechecking of treatment parameters (Table 1).

► In the 2 decades I have been performing refractive surgery and seeing patients in consultation with complications related to refractive surgery, I have run across the issue of medical errors several times. I have had a few near misses myself. Several I remember vividly. One was catching an error I made in cylinder conversion and another catching a typo the technician made in entering data into the computer. Both of these errors were found before laser ablation during my "preflight check" when I compared the computer screen with my chart. The third was a patient identification error, where a patient with a very similar name was

TABLE 1.—Patient Demographics

| Case | Age (y) | Gender | Eye | Preoperative CDVA | Procedure | Error Type | Notes |
|---|---|---|---|---|---|---|---|
| 1 | 49 | N/A | Unilateral | 20/20 | LASIK | Data Entry | Cycloplegic refraction used in place of manifest refraction |
| 2 | 38 | N/A | Unilateral | 20/20 | LASIK | Timeout | |
| 3 | 38 | Male | Unilateral | 20/20 | LASIK | Cylinder Conversion | |
| 4 | 40 | Female | Unilateral | 20/20 | LASIK | Cylinder Conversion | |
| 5a[a] | 29 | Female | Bilateral | 20/20 | PRK | Data Entry | Decimal point in wrong location |
| 5b[a] | 29 | Female | Bilateral | 20/20 | PRK | Data Entry | Decimal point in wrong location |
| 6 | 47 | N/A | Unilateral | 20/20 | LASIK | Data Entry | Patient's pupil size used for cylinder value |
| 7a[a] | 27 | N/A | Bilateral | 20/20 | PRK | Cylinder Conversion | |
| 7b[a] | 27 | N/A | Bilateral | 20/20 | PRK | Cylinder Conversion | |
| 8 | N/A | N/A | Unilateral | 20/20 | LASIK | Cylinder Conversion | |
| 9 | N/A | Male | Unilateral | 20/20 | PRK | Data Entry | Sphere sign inversion |
| 10 | 35 | Female | Unilateral | 20/20 | LASIK | Cylinder Conversion | |
| 11a[a] | 49 | Male | Bilateral | 20/20 | LASIK | Timeout | Patient responded to wrong name in waiting room |
| 11b[a] | 49 | Male | Bilateral | 20/20 | LASIK | Timeout | Patient responded to wrong name in waiting room |
| 12 | N/A | Male | Unilateral | 20/20 | LASIK | Timeout | Doctor called patient by the wrong name during time out |
| 13 | N/A | Female | Unilateral | 20/20 | LASIK | Data Entry | Original LASIK treatment used in re-treatment |
| 14 | 49 | Female | Unilateral | 20/20 | LASIK | Cylinder Conversion | |
| 15 | 54 | Female | Unilateral | 20/20 | LASIK | Cylinder Conversion | |
| 16[b] | 36 | Male | Unilateral | 20/20 | LASIK | Cylinder Conversion | Second cylinder conversion error occurred during revision of initial cylinder conversion error |
| 16[b] | 36 | Male | Unilateral | 20/30 | LASIK | Cylinder Conversion | |
| 17 | 36 | Male | Unilateral | 20/20 | LASIK | Data Entry | |
| 18 | 54 | Male | Unilateral | 20/20 | LASIK | Cylinder Conversion | |

CDVA = corrected distance visual acuity; N/A = data not available; data entry = errors associated with incorrect entry of refraction data into the laser system; timeout = efforts associated with failure to correctly or completely comply with proper timeout procedure; PRK = photorefractive keratectomy.

[a]Experienced bilateral errors.

[b]Experienced separate errors during two separate procedures in the same eye.

brought into the laser room for treatment. The error was discovered during the "timeout," and the correct treatment was performed. In consultation, I have seen a patient treated with a +3-diopter (D) ablation when she was a -3D myope and another patient treated for monovision in the wrong eye.

The authors of this study accumulated medical errors in 22 eyes of 18 patients and divided the errors into 3 types: cylinder conversion, data entry, and patient identification (Table 1). The most amazing example they report is a patient with a manifest refraction (MR) of −6.00 −2.00 × 180 who was treated with −8.00 +2.00 × 180 due to a cylinder conversion error, resulting in an MR of −1.00 +4.25 × 100. The surgeon attempted to correct the error but entered −1.00 +4.25 × 010 (instead of axis 100), thereby essentially doubling the patient's astigmatism.

Fortunately, most laser platforms allowed direct transfer of data to the laser, most commonly when custom wavefront treatments are being performed. However, when conventional treatments are being done, conversion and data input errors can still occur. Timeouts, to identify correct patient and eye, as mandated in operating rooms, should always be done.

Last, but not least, when an error occurs, the natural reaction is often to make it go away with as little fuss as possible. Some surgeons might want to enhance the patient without telling the patient exactly what occurred. Hiding such errors from patients is a BAD idea and frequently compounds the problem for the surgeon. I agree 100% with the authors who stated "We therefore strongly recommend the surgeon immediately inform the patient in the event of any error during surgery."

**C. J. Rapuano, MD**

## Pupil Size and LASIK: A Review

Myung D, Schallhorn S, Manche EE (Stanford Univ School of Medicine, Palo Alto, CA; Univ of California—San Francisco)
*J Refract Surg* 29:734-741, 2013

*Purpose.*—To provide a literature review on the evidence both for and against pupil size as an independent predictor of adverse visual outcomes after LASIK.

*Methods.*—Peer-reviewed publications on the effect of pupil size on LASIK outcomes since 2002 are reviewed. Particular attention was paid to the following attributes of each publication: type of study, number of patients or eyes, mean age, mean level of myopia, mean pupil size, testing conditions, ablation zone diameter, presence or absence of blend zones, and mean follow-up period.

*Results.*—Among the 19 studies examined, none correlates a persistent relationship between pupil size and night vision complaints (NVCs) beyond 3 months when LASIK was performed with a 6.0-mm optical zone or larger ablation. The studies that did explicitly determine a correlation either included some or all patients with ablation zones smaller than 6.0 mm or did not specify ablation diameter at all. Among the studies that had drawn more mixed conclusions, the studies either covered short

TABLE 1.—Possible Etiologies for Reduced Visual Performance After LASIK

| |
|---|
| Irregular astigmatism |
| Small optical zone diameter |
| Small flap diameter |
| Decentered flap |
| Flap irregularity, such as straie, buttonhole, or displaced flap |
| Decentered ablation |
| Induced higher-order aberrations |
| Irregular corneal wound healing |
| Ectasia |
| Interface haze or scarring |
| Residual refractive error |
| Inadequate Stiles-Crawford effect |
| Poor cortical adaptation |
| Poor tear film |
| Other ocular conditions, such as cataract or retinal pathology |

follow-up intervals (1 to 3 months) or showed a progressive improvement in NVCs over time in a relatively small patient cohort.

*Conclusions.*—As keratorefractive technology continues to evolve, the role of pupil size warrants further investigation; however, based on the literature reviewed herein, modern LASIK has negated the role of the low light pupil in predicting adverse visual outcomes after LASIK outside of the early postoperative period (Table 1).

▶ In the early days of photorefractive keratectomy and laser-assisted in situ keratomileusis (LASIK), increased pupil size was thought to be associated with night vision complaints, and it probably was. However, at that time, smaller optical/ablation zones, in the 4.5- to 5.5-mm diameter range, were commonly used. Since the transition to 6-mm diameter optical/ablation zones or larger, the effect of pupil size on night vision complaints after excimer laser vision correction has been much less clear. The authors reviewed 19 studies since 2002 and conclude that although the role of pupil size warrants further investigation, there is no good evidence of a persistent relationship between pupil size and night vision complaints beyond 3 months when LASIK was performed with a 6-mm diameter optical/ablation zone or larger. The authors list numerous other possible etiologies for decreased visual performance after LASIK (Table 1).

**C. J. Rapuano, MD**

## The Effect of Procedure Room Temperature and Humidity on LASIK Outcomes

Seider MI, McLeod SD, Porco TC, et al (Univ of California, San Francisco)
*Ophthalmology* 120:2204-2208, 2013

*Objective.*—To determine whether procedure room temperature or humidity during LASIK affect refractive outcomes in a large patient sample.

*Design.*—Retrospective cohort study.

*Participants.*—A total of 202 394 eyes of 105 712 patients aged 18 to 75 years who underwent LASIK at an Optical Express, Inc., location in their United Kingdom and Ireland centers from January 1, 2008, to June 30, 2011, who met inclusion criteria.

*Methods.*—Patient age, gender, flap creation technique, pre- and 1-month post-LASIK manifest refraction, and ambient temperature and humidity during LASIK were recorded. Effect size determination and univariate and multivariate analyses were performed to characterize the relationships between LASIK procedure room temperature and humidity and postoperative refractive outcome.

*Main Outcome Measures.*—One month post-LASIK manifest refraction.

*Results.*—No clinically significant effect of procedure room temperature or humidity was found on LASIK refractive outcomes. When considering all eyes in our population, an increase of 1°C during LASIK was associated with a 0.003 diopter (D) more hyperopic refraction 1 month postoperatively, and an increase in 1% humidity was associated with a 0.0004 more myopic refraction. These effect sizes were the same or similar when considering only myopic eyes, only hyperopic eyes, and subgroups of eyes stratified by age and preoperative refractive error.

*Conclusions.*—Neither procedure room temperature nor humidity during LASIK were found to have a clinically significant relationship with postoperative manifest refraction in our population.

▶ There are at least 2 good reasons to believe that room temperature and humidity could significantly affect refractive outcomes of LASIK surgery. One is that the excimer laser light beam passes through the air before it hits the cornea and could therefore be affected by the room temperature and humidity. High humidity could decrease the amount of excimer laser light energy getting to the cornea, potentially causing under correction. The second is that after the flap is lifted, the stromal bed hydration could also be affected by room temperature and humidity. High humidity could cause more water to be retained in the stromal bed, thus decreasing the effect of the excimer laser treatment.

This retrospective study looked at a huge number of patients, more than 200 000, 1 month after LASIK performed with the VISX Star S4 IR excimer laser in the United Kingdom and Ireland. Although the manufacturer recommends ambient room temperature to be between 15°C and 27°C and the humidity to be between 35% and 65%, no attempt was made to control humidity in the operating room. Procedures were performed within a temperature range of 15°C to 30°C and 20% to 80% relative humidity. Although no eyes were treated at less than 15°C, 414 eyes (0.2%) were treated at 27°C or higher; 42 657 eyes (21%) were treated at 35% or less relative humidity and 320 (0.2%) eyes were treated at 65% or greater relative humidity. They found no clinically significant effect of the room temperature and/or humidity on the refractive outcomes. They also evaluated the groups of eyes that were treated outside the manufacturer's recommendation and found no clinically significant effect of temperature or humidity on postoperative refractive error. Although I believe it is reasonable to follow the manufacturer's recommendations, it is nice to know that temperature and humidity probably do not have much effect on refractive outcomes after LASIK.

**C. J. Rapuano, MD**

**Topical cyclosporine A for postoperative photorefractive keratectomy and laser in situ keratomileusis**

Hessert D, Tanzer D, Brunstetter T, et al (Naval Hosp Bremerton, WA; Naval Med Ctr San Diego, CA)

*J Cataract Refract Surg* 39:539-547, 2013

*Purpose.*—To compare the stability and predictability of the refractive outcomes in eyes treated with photorefractive keratectomy (PRK) or laser in situ keratomileusis (LASIK) with and without postoperative use of topical cyclosporine A emulsion.

*Setting.*—Naval Medical Center San Diego Refractive Surgery Center, San Diego, California, USA.

*Design.*—Randomized clinical trial.

*Methods.*—Patients had PRK or LASIK and were randomized, pairwise, to a standard postoperative treatment regimen with or without the addition of topical cyclosporine A 0.05% emulsion twice daily for 3 months postoperatively. Visual acuity, mesopic contrast acuity, refractions, and ocular symptoms were assessed through the 3-month examination. Tear-film samples (cytokines and chemokines) were analyzed preoperatively and 1 week and 1 and 3 months postoperatively.

*Results.*—The PRK group comprised 70 patients and the LASIK group, 54 patients. The addition of topical cyclosporine A twice a day after PRK or LASIK did not confer special benefits in terms of achievement of target refraction, final uncorrected distance visual acuity (UDVA), or rate of visual recovery (all $P > .05$, multivariate analysis of variance [MANOVA]). There was no significant difference in tear-film composition based on measurement of matrix metalloproteinase-9, interleukin (IL)-6, or IL-8 recovery (all $P > .05$, MANOVA).

*Conclusion.*—The addition of topical cyclosporine A twice daily for 3 months after PRK or LASIK did not provide a significant benefit in the rate of visual recovery, final UDVA, or patient symptoms, nor did it significantly change measured inflammatory mediators (cytokines) present in the tear film.

▶ The results of this study that cyclosporine A was not beneficial in a young healthy population (mean age 27–32 years, range 21–47 years) were not a surprise to me. That is why I do not routinely prescribe cyclosporine A for all my refractive surgery patients preoperatively. I do find it helpful in patients with dry eye signs or symptoms preoperatively. For these patients, I often add cyclosporine A 0.05% twice a day and recheck them about 1 month later. If the signs and symptoms of dryness are much better, I feel comfortable proceeding with refractive surgery. If not, I continue the cyclosporine A and check them back in a few months. If the signs and symptoms do not resolve, I typically hold off on any refractive surgery.

It is well known that surface ablation and LASIK can make dry eye symptoms worse. Most of us believe that the worse the dry eyes are preoperatively, the more severe and long lasting the symptoms are likely to be postoperatively. Patients with post–refractive surgery dry eye can be absolutely miserable. The dryness induced poor vision and discomfort is compounded by the guilt that patients themselves feel knowing they sought out this surgery and paid a lot of money for it. I ask all patients about dry eye symptoms and check carefully for signs of ocular surface disease preoperatively. If present, I aggressively treat the dry eyes (and blepharitis if present) to decrease the risks of causing prolonged dry eye problems postoperatively.

**C. J. Rapuano, MD**

---

**LASIK Versus Photorefractive Keratectomy for High Myopic (> 3 Diopter) Astigmatism**

Katz T, Wagenfeld L, Galambos P, et al (Univ Med Ctr Hamburg-Eppendorf, Germany)

*J Refract Surg* 29:824-831, 2013

---

*Purpose.*—To compare the efficacy, safety, predictability, and vector analysis indices of LASIK and photorefractive keratectomy (PRK) for correction of high cylinder of greater than 3 diopters (D) in myopic eyes.

*Methods.*—The efficacy, safety, and predictability of LASIK or PRK performed in 114 consecutive randomly selected myopic eyes with an astigmatism of greater than 3 D were retrospectively analyzed at the 2- to 6-month follow-up visits. Vector analysis of the cylindrical correction was compared between the treatment groups.

*Results.*—A total of 57 eyes receiving PRK and 57 eyes receiving LASIK of 114 refractive surgery candidates were enrolled in the study. No statistically significant difference in efficacy [efficacy index = 0.76 (±0.32) for PRK vs 0.74 (±0.19) for LASIK (*P* = .82)], safety [safety index = 1.10 (±0.26) for PRK vs 1.01 (±0.17) for LASIK (*P* = .121)], or predictability [achieved astigmatism <1 D in 39% of PRK- and 54% of LASIK-treated eyes, and <2 D in 88% of PRK- and 89% of LASIK treated eyes (*P* = .218)] was demonstrated. Using Alpins vector analysis, the surgically induced astigmatism and difference vector were not significantly different between the surgery methods, whereas the correction index showed a slight and significant advantage of LASIK over PRK (1.25 for PRK and 1.06 for LASIK, *P* < .001).

*Conclusions.*—LASIK and PRK are comparably safe, effective, and predictable procedures for excimer laser correction of high astigmatism of greater than 3 D in myopic eyes. Predictability of the correction of the

TABLE 2.—Efficacy and Safety Index of LASIK and PRK Treatment

| Variable | PRK | LASIK | $P^a$ | Total |
|---|---|---|---|---|
| Efficacy | | | | |
| No. of eyes | 57 | 57 | .818 | 114 |
| Median (Q25-Q75) | 0.7 (0.55–0.92) | 0.73 (0.64–0.82) | | 0.73 (0.62–0.86) |
| Mean ± SD | 0.76 ± 0.32 | 0.74 ± 0.19 | | 0.19 ± 114 |
| Safety | | | | |
| No. of eyes | 57 | 57 | .121 | 114 |
| Median (Q25-Q75) | 1.01 (0.91–1.27) | 1.0 (0.92–1.07) | | 1.0 (0.92–1.12) |
| Mean ± SD | 1.1 ± 0.26 | 1.01 ± 0.17 | | 1.06 ± 0.22 |

PRK = photorefractive keratectomy; Q25 = 25th quartile; Q75 = 75th quartile; SD = standard deviation
[a]Mann–Whitney test.

cylindrical component is lower than that of the spherical equivalent (Table 2).

▶ Unfortunately, the results of refractive surgery in eyes with high degrees of astigmatism are just not as good as in eyes with lower degrees of astigmatism. This study compared laser-assisted in situ keratomileusis (LASIK) using a Moria M2 microkeratome and photorefractive keratectomy (PRK) with alcohol removal of the epithelium and intraoperative mitomycin C in eyes with greater than 3 diopters of myopic astigmatism. Patients were treated with the Allegretto 200/400 excimer laser using the "wavefront optimized" mode. The follow-up time was between 2 and 6 months. Overall, the refractive and safety results were very similar between LASIK and PRK (Table 2).

However, this study has numerous drawbacks. First, it was not randomized. Second, although more than 500 eyes were treated for myopic astigmatism greater than 3 diopters during the study period, only 114 were included in this study. One reason for that is only one eye was included when both eyes were treated; however, most eyes were excluded because of lack of adequate follow-up. Third, there was a large range of follow-up time. Also, the shorter end of that time period may not be quite long enough for the final results of PRK to be measured. All in all, it is nice to see that both PRK and LASIK are equally safe and reasonably effective for these higher degrees of myopic astigmatism.

**C. J. Rapuano, MD**

## Long-term Outcomes of Photorefractive Keratectomy for Low to High Myopia: 13 to 19 Years of Follow-Up

Vestergaard AH, Hjortdal JØ, Ivarsen A, et al (Odense Univ Hosp, Denmark; Aarhus Univ Hosp, Denmark)
*J Refract Surg* 29:312-319, 2013

*Purpose.*—To evaluate long-term outcomes after photorefractive keratectomy (PRK).

*Methods.*—A retrospective follow-up study of patients who received PRK at 5.0- to 6.5-mm optical zones, using the Summit broad beam excimer laser (Summit Technology, Inc., Waltham, MA) at Odense University Hospital, Odense, Denmark, between 1992 and 1998. One randomly selected eye of each patient was used in the statistical analyses. Retreated eyes were excluded.

*Results.*—One hundred sixty eyes were included. Mean follow-up time was 16 years (range: 13 to 19 years). Mean preoperative spherical equivalent was −4.84 ± 2.95 diopters (D) (range: −20.25 to −1.25 D). At last follow-up examination, achieved refraction was −1.00 ± 1.56 D (range: −10.75 to +1.00 D) from attempted refraction, and the change in mean refractive error from 6 months postoperatively was less than 1.00 D. Results from a subgroup of unilateral treated patients indicated that myopic progression was the main reason for the residual refractive error. For eyes with low myopia (n = 124), the proportion of eyes within ±1.0 D of attempted refraction was 72%, and for eyes with high myopia (−6.00 D or more, n = 36) it was 47%. Forty-five percent had uncorrected distance visual acuity of 20/20 or better at last follow-up examination. Three eyes (2%) lost two or more lines and 13 eyes (8%) gained two or more lines of corrected distance visual acuity. Fourteen percent had haze (grade 0.5 to 2). Eighty-one percent were satisfied with the surgery.

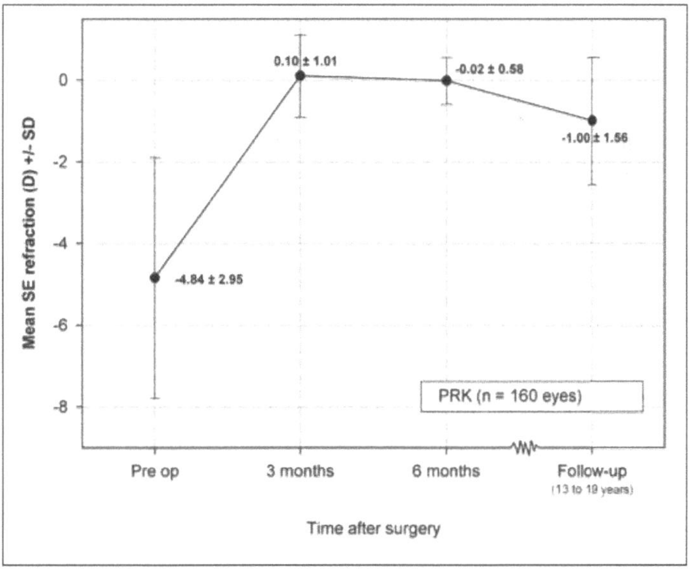


FIGURE 4.—Stability. Mean spherical equivalent (SE) ± standard deviation (SD) plotted as a function of time after photorefractive keratectomy (PRK) for eyes that completed the last follow-up examination. Preoperative (n = 160), 3 months (n = 150), 6 months (n = 126), and last follow-up (n = 160). Mean follow-up time was 16 years. (Reprinted from Vestergaard AH, Hjortdal JØ, Ivarsen A, et al. Long-term outcomes of photorefractive keratectomy for low to high myopia: 13 to 19 years of follow-up. *J Refract Surg*. 2013;29:312-319, with permission from SLACK Incorporated.)

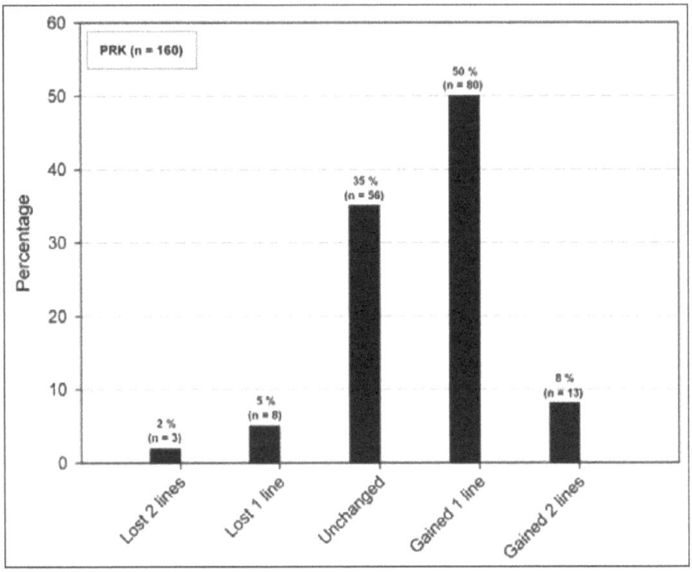


FIGURE 6.—Safety. The percentage of eyes in which there was a gain/loss of lines in corrected distance visual acuity at last follow-up examination including number of eyes (n). Mean follow-up time was 16 years after photorefractive keratectomy (PRK). (Reprinted from Vestergaard AH, Hjortdal JØ, Ivarsen A, et al. Long-term outcomes of photorefractive keratectomy for low to high myopia: 13 to 19 years of follow-up. *J Refract Surg*. 2013;29:312-319, with permission from SLACK Incorporated.)

*Conclusion.*—PRK for low degrees of myopia seemed safe and effective up to 19 years after surgery with conventional broad beam laser ablation. Refractive predictability was significantly lower and the occurrence of haze was higher in eyes with high myopia (Figs 4 and 6).

▶ The authors present one of the largest photorefractive keratectomy (PRK) studies with the longest follow-up. When looking at the results, we need to keep in mind that these surgeries were performed with 20-year-old technology. The Apex laser is no longer in use, and the Summit Technology company no longer exists. This laser was a broad-beam laser and used relatively small ablation zones of 5 to 6.5 mm diameter. Mitomycin C was not used in any eyes. Consequently, the results are not directly comparable to today's PRK. Additionally, only 160 patients of the 751 (21%) originally treated were examined for this study. This is not bad for a 13- to 19-year follow-up but still not great. However, there is still certainly useful information to be learned.

First, the procedure remained safe with only 2% of eyes losing 2 lines of best-corrected visual acuity and 8% of eyes gaining 2 lines of best-corrected visual acuity (Fig 6).

Second, although 22% of eyes had corneal haze 3 and 6 months postoperatively, that number was 14% at last follow-up. Only one-quarter of those were grade 2, and all of those were treated for myopia greater than −6 diopters (D).

Third, there were no eyes with postoperative ectasia.

Fourth, the refractions were fairly stable with mean regression to −1D at last follow-up (Fig 4).

Fifth, patient satisfaction remained fairly high. A total of 66.5% were very satisfied and another 14.6% were satisfied.

Pretty good stuff!

**C. J. Rapuano, MD**

---

### Visual Acuity Outcomes in Eyes With Flat Corneas After PRK

Varssano D, Waisbourd M, Minkev L, et al (Tel-Aviv Univ, Israel; Care Vision, Tel-Aviv, Israel; et al)
*J Refract Surg* 29:384-389, 2013

---

*Purpose.*—To evaluate the impact of corneal curvatures less than 35 diopters (D) after photorefractive keratectomy (PRK) on visual acuity outcomes.

*Methods.*—Visual acuity outcomes of 5,410 eyes that underwent PRK from January 2006 to November 2010 were retrospectively analyzed for the impact of postoperative corneal curvatures on visual outcomes. All procedures were performed on a single platform (Allegretto 200 Hz excimer laser; Alcon Laboratories, Inc., Irvine, CA). Main outcome measures were postoperative corrected distance visual acuity (CDVA) and loss of CDVA.

*Results.*—Corneas with a measured or a calculated postoperative flat meridian less than 35 D and those with a measured postoperative steep meridian less than 35 D had worse postoperative CDVA than corneas with meridians of either 35 D or more ($P \leq .021$). However, the preoperative CDVA was worse in the flatter curvatures in all comparisons performed ($P \leq .024$). Consequently, the measured or calculated meridian curvature had no effect on CDVA loss ($P \geq .074$).

*Conclusion.*—Postoperative corneal keratometry values (flat and steep meridians) less than 35 D did not have a predictive effect on the risk of losing visual acuity following myopic PRK performed on the Allegretto 200 Hz excimer laser (Table 1).

▶ These authors investigated an interesting, and somewhat controversial, question in refractive surgery. Do corneas with very flat keratometry readings after refractive surgery have worse acuity than corneas with steeper keratometry readings? I was the chairperson of the faculty responsible for the American Academy of Ophthalmology Basic and Clinical Science Course section 13 on Refractive Surgery for several years, and part of the faculty that wrote the first edition. During the writing of the first edition and subsequent revisions, our committee had numerous discussions regarding this particular question. Some committee members believed that flat corneas were associated with worse quality of vision, whereas others did not. The compromise that is in the text is "Excessive corneal flattening (flatter than approximately 34.00D) ... after refractive surgery may

TABLE 1.—Preoperative Corrected Distance Visual Acuity

| Meridian | <35 D No. | <35 D Mean ± SD logMAR (CDVA) | ≥ 35 D No. | ≥ 35 D Mean ± SD logMAR (CDVA) | P |
|---|---|---|---|---|---|
| Measured final flat meridian | 70 | 0.0452 ± 0.07234 (20/22.194) | 771 | 0.0068 ± 0.05978 (20/20.316) | .001 |
| Measured final steep meridian | 22 | 0.0388 ± 0.05157 (20/21.869) | 805 | 0.0093 ± 0.06068 (20/20.433) | .024 |
| Calculated final flat meridian | 45 | 0.0554 ± 0.07569 (20/22.721) | 4,539 | −0.0022 ± 0.06414 (20/19.899) | .001 |
| Calculated final steep meridian | 26 | 0.0666 ± 0.08131 (20/23.315) | 3,725 | 0.0005 ± 0.06735 (20/20.023) | .001 |

D = diopters; CDVA = corrected distance visual acuity; SD = standard deviation

increase the risk of poor quality vision." Why 34 diopters (D)? Because this was the consensus of the group. There were no data on the subject.

The results of this report are interesting. The author did not elaborate on why they chose a cutoff of 35D. I believe it is most likely because 35D is quite flat, and if their cutoff was lower, their numbers would have been too small for good statistical analysis. They concluded that the calculated final flat or steep keratometry values (which can be calculated preoperatively) do not predict loss of lines of best-corrected visual acuity. They did find, however, that best-corrected visual acuity was statistically significantly worse in eyes with keratometry readings less than 35D postoperatively (about 20/22 compared with about 20/20), but that difference was present preoperatively (Table 1).

They found that the magnitude of treatment was about 3D greater for eyes ending up with keratometry readings flatter than 35D than other eyes, and they still didn't lose more best-corrected visual acuity. Although Snellen best-corrected visual acuity is a useful measurement of vision, we all know it doesn't tell the whole story. It would be interesting to compare higher-order aberrations or contrast sensitivity in eyes with very flat (or steep for that matter) corneas. We also need to keep in mind that these results may or may not translate to other excimer laser platforms.

**C. J. Rapuano, MD**

**Photorefractive keratectomy in patients with suspected keratoconus: Five-year follow-up**

Guedj M, Saad A, Audureau E, et al (Rothschild Foundation, Paris, France)
*J Cataract Refract Surg* 39:66-73, 2013

*Purpose.*—To assess the long-range outcomes of photorefractive keratectomy (PRK) using functional and topographic criteria in myopic eyes with suspected keratoconus.

*Setting.*—Rothschild Foundation, Paris, France.

*Design.*—Retrospective interventional case series.

*Methods.*—Eyes of patients classified as keratoconus suspects or keratoconus by the Corneal Navigator software of the OPD-Scan II device were included. They were treated with myopic PRK using an EC-5000 excimer laser between 2004 and 2007. The main outcome measures were refractive stability, mean corneal keratometry, mean central pachymetry, mean thinnest point value, and the occurrence of postoperative complications such as corneal ectasia.

*Results.*—The study evaluated 62 eyes of 42 patients. The mean patient age was 34.6 years ± 15.1 (SD) and the mean spherical equivalent (SE), −3.96 ± 3.05 diopters (D). The mean central pachymetry was 529.4 ± 32.8 μm and the mean simulated keratometry, 45.75 ± 1.75 D. The percentage of similarity to keratoconus suspects or keratoconus was positive in all 62 eyes and exceeded a 50% similarity score in 30 eyes (48.4%). The mean follow-up was 4.8 ± 1.4 years. The mean magnitude of the SE was −0.53 ± 1.35 D over the follow-up. Two patients required glasses postoperatively because of significant myopic regression. No case of corneal ectasia was reported.

*Conclusion.*—Photorefractive keratectomy in eyes with suspected keratoconus based on a Placido neural network may be safe and effective for myopia and astigmatism in carefully selected patients.

▶ It is well accepted that laser-assisted in-situ keratomileusis can induce or exacerbate corneal ectasia in some eyes. Although corneal ectasia has been described after photorefractive keratectomy (PRK) in rare instances (about 10 patients in the literature), in many of these eyes the preoperative corneal topographies showed irregular inferior steepening, suggestive of early keratoconus. Although it is tempting to conclude that all eyes with irregular corneal topographies, therefore, shouldn't undergo PRK, more information is needed to correctly draw that conclusion.

The authors retrospectively analyzed data on all 330 eyes that underwent PRK at their institute in Paris from 2004 to 2007. Although not stated in the report, I presume that there was no slit lamp evidence of keratoconus in any of these eyes. They reanalyzed the preoperative Nidek OPD – Scan II topographies with new Corneal Navigator software trained to recognize specific corneal topographic patterns. Eyes with a keratoconus suspect or a keratoconus score of greater than 50% were included. Interestingly, the preoperative topographies of 62 of the 330 eyes (19%) that had undergone PRK were classified as keratoconus suspect or keratoconus. Mean age of these 62 patients was 35 years (no range was given). Mean thinnest pachymetry was 522 μ. Forty-seven patients were followed up for almost 5 years, and none of these eyes developed corneal ectasia.

The authors caution that their study only followed up with patients for 5 years and that ectasia could still develop in the future. They bring up the novel idea that they believe it is possible that the inflammation induced by the PRK procedure might actually strengthen the cornea by localized corneal crosslinking in the area of the ablation, which may actually halt the progression of keratoconus. This is an interesting theory. Although I am not going to start doing PRK on eyes with keratoconus, perhaps very slight inferior steepening on topography is not an absolute contraindication to surface ablation. Of course, many other factors come into play including the patient's age, family history of keratoconus, and corneal thickness.

**C. J. Rapuano, MD**

**Photorefractive keratectomy modification of postkeratoplasty anisometropic refractive errors**

Ward MS, Wandling GR, Goins KM, et al (Univ of Iowa Hosps and Clinics, Iowa City)
*Cornea* 32:273-279, 2013

*Purpose.*—To evaluate the efficacy, refractive predictability and stability, and complications of photorefractive keratectomy (PRK) with adjunctive mitomycin C (MMC) in patients with postkeratoplasty anisometropia.

*Methods.*—A retrospective review was carried out of all cases of PRK performed for postkeratoplasty anisometropia with the VISX Star S4 excimer laser with MMC between January 1, 2004, and December 31, 2008. The main outcome measures were best spectacle-corrected distance visual acuity (CDVA) and patient tolerance of full spectacle refractive correction. Secondary outcome measures were uncorrected distance visual acuity (UDVA), refractive accuracy and stability, and complications.

*Results.*—Twenty cases met the inclusion criteria. At 6 months, the spectacle CDVA had improved from a preoperative mean of 20/50 to 20/30 ($P = 0.01$). Ten eyes (50%) gained 2 or more lines of CDVA. Eighteen eyes (90%) had a CDVA of 20/40 or better. All 20 patients (100%) were subjectively satisfied with full binocular spectacle correction. There was an improvement in UDVA from a preoperative mean of 20/282 to 20/52 ($P < 0.001$). Thirteen patients (65%) had an UDVA of 20/40 or better. There was a reduction in the mean refractive spherical equivalent from −5.2 to −0.9 diopters (D), in myopia from −7.6 to −1.8 D, and in astigmatism from 4.9 to 2.0 D. No significant change in visual acuity or refractive error occurred between 3 and 12 months. No sight-threatening complications occurred. One eye (5%) lost 2 lines of CDVA.

*Conclusions.*—PRK with adjunctive MMC is an effective method of reducing postkeratoplasty anisometropia and providing satisfactory spectacle rehabilitation.

► Despite new and improved instrumentation and techniques, large and unpredictable refractive errors remain a persistent problem after penetrating keratoplasty (PK). Although soft and especially rigid gas-permeable contact lenses can successfully correct most of these refractive errors, many patients cannot or will not use them. Photorefractive keratectomy (PRK) was used to correct some of these large refractive errors years ago, but it was essentially abandoned because of a high incidence of visually significant corneal haze. Laser in situ keratomileusis (LASIK) was also tried but was less than optimal, as the LASIK procedure itself often changed the refraction and on occasion also affected the wound strength and integrity.

Newer excimer lasers with improved ablation profiles, combined with the use of mitomycin C (MMC), have significantly reduced the incidence of postoperative haze after routine PRK. These advances led the authors to perform PRK with MMC on eyes with significant post-PK anisometropia. They used a 6.5-mm diameter ablation with an 8.0-mm blend zone on a VISX excimer laser. They applied MMC 0.02% for 12 seconds. They report remarkably good results in 20 eyes at 1 year. Mean uncorrected vision improved from 20/282 to 20/52. Mean spherical equivalent improved from −5.2 diopters to −0.9 diopters (Fig 1 in the original article). Mean myopia improved from −7.6 diopters to −1.8 diopters. Mean refractive cylinder improved from 4.9 diopters to 2.0 diopters. Surprisingly, mean best-corrected visual acuity went from 20/50 to 20/30, suggesting some improvement in irregular astigmatism as well. Also importantly, no eyes developed anterior stromal haze. While the refractive results certainly aren't as good as in unoperated eyes, they are encouraging enough for me to try PRK in my (unfortunately not rare) patients with significant anisometropia after PK.

**C. J. Rapuano, MD**

---

**Randomized dose-response analysis of mitomycin-C to prevent haze after photorefractive keratectomy for high myopia**

Hofmeister EM, Bishop FM, Kaupp SE, et al (Naval Med Ctr, San Diego, CA)
*J Cataract Refract Surg* 39:1358-1365, 2013

---

*Purpose.*—To evaluate the safety and efficacy of mitomycin-C (MMC) 0.01% (0.1 mg/mL) in preventing haze formation after wavefront-guided photorefractive keratectomy (PRK) for higher myopia at 3 exposures.

*Setting.*—United States Navy Refractive Surgery Center, San Diego, California, USA.

*Design.*—Double-masked randomized prospective trial.

*Methods.*—Sixty-, 30-, and 15-second exposures of MMC 0.01% were compared in wavefront-guided PRK for higher myopia. One eye received MMC (surgical sponge) and the other a placebo. All eyes received a 4-month tapering postoperative topical steroid regimen. Endothelial cell densities, haze scores, high- and low-contrast acuities, and manifest refraction were measured preoperatively and 1, 3, 6, and 12 months postoperatively. Outcomes were analyzed as repeated measures over time.

*Results.*—The mean preoperative manifest refraction spherical equivalent was −5.98 diopters (D) (range −4.4 to −8.0 D). No eye developed more than trace haze. There was a significant difference in haze scores between MMC-treated eyes and untreated eyes at 1 and 3 months ($P = .034$) but no difference at 6 and 12 months. Endothelial cell densities decreased in the treated eyes and untreated eyes at all 3 exposures at 1 month but returned to baseline by 6 months. There was no difference in acuities or refractions with or without MMC.

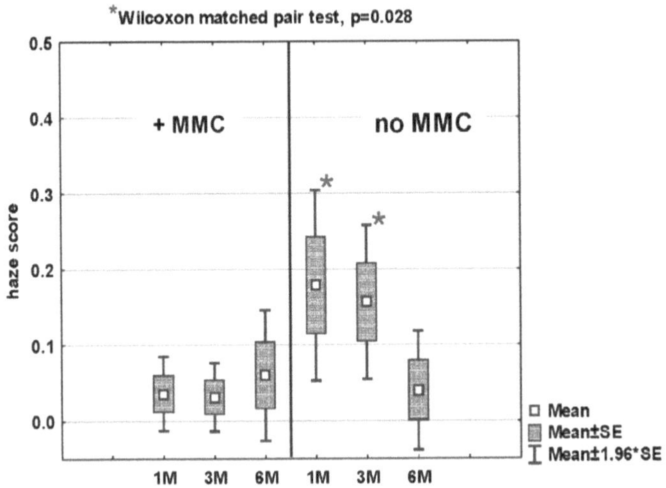


FIGURE 1.—Subjective haze scores rated by postoperative biomicroscopic examinations (MMC = mitomycin-C). (Reprinted from The Journal of Cardiac Failure. Hofmeister EM, Bishop FM, Kaupp SE, et al. Randomized dose-response analysis of mitomycin-C to prevent haze after photorefractive keratectomy for high myopia. *J Cataract Refract Surg*. 2013;39:1358-1365, Copyright 2013, with permission from ASCRS and ESCRS.)

*Conclusions.*—Mitomycin-C may not be needed to prevent haze after modern PRK with a 4-month steroid taper. There was no clinically significant difference in haze formation between MMC eyes and control eyes at the concentration and exposures used (Fig 1).

▶ Of the 3 main reasons for the rapid conversion of many refractive surgeons from photorefractive keratectomy to laser in situ keratomileusis in the late 1990s, namely pain, slower visual recovery, and haze, I always felt the visual effect of haze was the most important. The haze was difficult to treat and often prolonged, adversely affecting visual function, which is the very phenomenon the surgery was supposed to improve. Although the use of bandage soft contact lenses and topical nonsteroidal anti-inflammatory drops improved the pain significantly and visual recovery somewhat, I believe the use of mitomycin C (MMC) to decrease the risk of corneal haze was the most important factor in the resurgence of surface ablation in the mid-2000s. At least most of us thought it was the MMC. As Dr Hofmeister and coauthors note, the use of MMC coincided with improved laser technology, especially larger ablation zones with smoother laser profiles. Could it have been the laser changes alone that decreased haze, and the mitomycin C wasn't doing anything? I doubt it. MMC has been found to decrease the risk of haze/scar after other corneal procedures, including excimer laser phototherapeutic keratectomy, the laser profile of which hasn't changed since US Food and Drug Administration approval in 1995. But maybe the MMC isn't as important as many of us think.

In this study, the authors found that in 28 patients treated for moderately high myopia (−4.4 to −8.0 diopters), 0.01% MMC for 15 to 60 seconds seemed to have a small beneficial effect on haze at 1 and 3 months and no effect on haze at 6 and 12 months postoperatively. MMC was not found to have an effect on visual acuity or endothelial cell counts. This brings up the question of whether MMC is needed at all with current laser profiles. That is an important question for a much larger study to answer. Other parameters that could be examined are strength of MMC (most surgeons I know use 0.02%, whereas 0.01% was used in this study); the use of topical steroids, including their strength, frequency, and duration; and treating a broader spectrum of refractive errors. Although this study provides interesting and compelling data, given that haze can be extremely problematic for patients and is difficult to treat, I am not yet stopping the use of MMC after surface ablation until we have some larger confirmatory studies.

**C. J. Rapuano, MD**

**Short-time mitomycin-C application during photorefractive keratectomy in patients with low myopia**

Shojaei A, Ramezanzadeh M, Soleyman-Jahi S, et al (Basir Eye Ctr, Tehran, Iran; Baghiatollah Univ of Med Sciences, Tehran, Iran; Tehran Univ of Med Sciences, Iran)

*J Cataract Refract Surg* 39:197-203, 2013

*Purpose.*—To evaluate the safety and efficacy of 5 seconds of mitomycin-C (MMC) application during photorefractive keratectomy (PRK) for low myopia.

*Setting.*—Basir Eye Clinic, Tehran, Iran.

*Design.*—Prospective randomized sham-controlled double-masked clinical trial.

*Methods.*—Patients with low myopia and an ablation depth of less than 65 μm were recruited. One eye of each patient was included in the study and was randomly assigned to receive intraoperative topical MMC 0.02% for 5 seconds or a balanced salt solution in the same manner (control group). Corneal haze development during the 6 months after the PRK was the main outcome measure.

*Results.*—Of the 184 eligible patients (MMC = 93; control = 91), 152 (78 and 74, respectively) completed the follow-up. The postoperative haze grade was significantly lower in the MMC group ($P = .01$). The mean endothelial cell density was not significantly different between the MMC group and the control group preoperatively (2879.97 cells/mm$^2$ ± 298.04 [SD] versus 2819.69 ± 303.89 cells/mm$^2$; $P = .22$) or 6 months postoperatively (2878.79 ± 283.04 cells/mm$^2$ versus 2878.79 ± 283.04 cells/mm$^2$; $P = .25$). No notable ocular complication occurred throughout the study.

*Conclusion.*—Short-time application of MMC 0.02% was safe and effective in preventing haze formation in eyes having PRK with an ablation depth of less than 65 μm compared with matched controls up to 6 months (Table 4).

▶ Topical mitomycin C (MMC) is used routinely at the time of surface ablation in many eyes. Some surgeons use it only in eyes with moderately high degrees

TABLE 4.—Haze Development 3 Months and 6 Months After PRK

| | Number (%) | | | | | |
|---|---|---|---|---|---|---|
| | Haze at 3 Months | | | Haze at 6 Months | | |
| Group | Clear | Trace | 1+ | Clear | Trace | 1+ |
| MMC | 72 (97.3) | 2 (2.7) | 0 | 73 (98.6) | 1 (1.4) | 0 |
| Control | 63 (80.8) | 12 (15.4) | 3 (3.8) | 68 (87.2) | 9 (11.5) | 1 (1.3) |

MMC = mitomycin-C.

of myopia (eg, more than −4 to −6 diopters). Other surgeons use it in all eyes. Some surgeons use the same concentration and application time for all eyes they treat, whereas other surgeons modify the concentration or application time by degree of refractive error. I personally used to use MMC only for eyes with more than 6 diopters of myopia but over the last decade have been slowly decreasing that threshold to about 2 diopters of myopia. I use it in more eyes because I noted some haze even in eyes with relatively low levels of myopia and also because of the increasing body of literature on the safety of the use of prophylactic MMC during refractive surgery.

The authors performed a prospective, randomized study using MMC vs placebo for only 5 seconds (compared with the 12–30 seconds used by most surgeons to prophylactically decrease the risk of haze) in eyes with less than 4 diopters of spherical equivalent and less than 1.5 diopters of cylinder, eyes typically considered at low risk for haze. They evaluated refractive results, haze, and epithelial healing and numerous endothelial specular microscopy parameters at 6 months. Visual acuity, refractive, epithelial healing and all specular microscopy results were the same in both the MMC and control eyes. Although overall there wasn't much haze in either group, there was statistically significantly less haze in the MMC-treated eyes than the control eyes (Table 4). Whether this difference is clinically significant is unknown. This study emphasizes the fact that some haze develops in low myopes and that short-exposure MMC is effective at reducing that haze in a safe manner at least for 6 months. It would be nice to know whether the amount of haze was related to the degree of myopia even in this low myopia cohort.

**C. J. Rapuano, MD**

**The effects of mitomycin C on tear function after photorefractive keratectomy: a contralateral comparative study**

Farahi A, Hashemi H, Mehravaran S (Noor Eye Hosp, Tehran, Iran)

*J Refract Surg* 29:260-264, 2013

*Purpose.*—To assess the effects of adjuvant mitomycin C (MMC) on tear function tests after photorefractive keratectomy (PRK) for myopia.

*Methods.*—In this prospective, randomized, double-blind study, one eye of myopic patients undergoing PRK was randomly chosen for PRK and the other eye was treated with PRK plus the application of 0.02% MMC for

20 seconds onto the ablated stroma. All patients had corneal esthesiometry, fluorescein break-up time testing, fluorescein and Rose Bengal staining, and Schirmer testing with anesthesia, and they also completed a questionnaire preoperatively and at 1.5, 3, 6, and 12 months after surgery.

*Results.*—Twenty-seven patients with a mean age of 25 ± 3.27 years were enrolled. There were no statistically significant differences between the PRK and PRK+MMC groups regarding the symptoms and tear function tests preoperatively or at any postoperative follow-up visit. Preoperative and postoperative results in the total sample were also compared; statistically significantly different results were observed in fluorescein break-up time and dry eye symptoms at 1.5 months, which showed improvement thereafter. Corneal sensation was significantly lower at all postoperative follow-up visits compared with preoperative results.

*Conclusions.*—The intraoperative use of MMC during PRK did not induce tear deficiency, and it seems that MMC can be used safely when necessary.

▶ Although the number of patients is somewhat small at 27, the authors provide good evidence that mitomycin C does not adversely affect tear function, at least in the first year after photorefractive keratectomy. They only included eyes being treated for −4D because they treat all eyes with myopia greater than that with mitomycin C to prevent corneal haze. This study provides further evidence confirming the safety of topical mitomycin C at the time of surface ablation.

**C. J. Rapuano, MD**

---

**Systemic absorption of mitomycin-C when used in refractive surgery**

Crawford C, Ainbinder DJ, Davis R, et al (Fort Campbell Army Dept of Ophthalmology, KY; Madigan Army Med Ctr Dept of Ophthalmology, Tacoma, WA; et al)

*J Cataract Refract Surg* 39:193-196, 2013

---

*Purpose.*—To determine whether corneal topical application of mitomycin-C (MMC) results in measurable plasma levels of systemic absorption.

*Setting.*—Madigan Army Medical Center, Refractive Surgery Center, Fort Lewis, Washington, and Micro-Constants Laboratory, San Diego, California, USA.

*Design.*—Case-control study.

*Methods.*—The study comprised male and female active-duty soldiers having excimer laser photorefractive keratectomy with MMC. Patients who met inclusion criteria were asked to provide a blood sample immediately after being treated with MMC 0.2 mg/mL (0.02%) for 30 seconds. Human plasma samples were evaluated by liquid chromatography mass spectrometry to determine whether MMC was present.

*Results.*—Thirty samples were submitted for evaluation. There was zero detection of MMC in the submitted samples. The quantifiable limit was greater than 10.0 ng/mL. All samples were below this.

*Conclusions.*—In this study of 30 patients with topical application of MMC for refractive surgery, there was no measurable evidence of systemic absorption. Although systemic absorption has been found with use in larger quantities, it was not known whether MMC toxicity concerns could be extrapolated to the refractive surgery population. This information allows counseling of patients on the extremely low likelihood of systemic absorption or toxicity following current techniques for refractive surgery.

▶ Mitomycin C (MMC) is currently used to prevent haze prophylactically in patients undergoing surface ablation procedures and to prevent recurrence of haze/scar tissue or pathology, such as Salzmann's nodular degeneration, in eyes undergoing phototherapeutic keratectomy (PTK). Several, but not all, studies have confirmed the safety of MMC on eyes when used during refractive surgery and PTK. The systemic absorption of MMC during ocular use has not been studied.

The authors drew blood 30 minutes after performing PRK with MMC 0.02% for 30 seconds and irrigating the cornea with 5 mL of saline. There was a zero detection of MMC in the blood samples of the 30 patients tested. Although we have assumed that there would be minimal to no systemic absorption of MMC through an avascular structure such as the cornea, it is now nice to know that for sure. This is good information for surgeons and patients.

**C. J. Rapuano, MD**

---

**Posterior chamber phakic intraocular lens to correct myopia: Long-term follow-up**

Torun N, Bertelmann E, Klamann MKJ, et al (Univ Medicine Charité Berlin, Germany)

*J Cataract Refract Surg* 39:1023-1028, 2013

---

*Purpose.*—To evaluate the long-term safety and efficacy of a refractive phakic intraocular lens (pIOL) (PRL) to correct moderate to high myopia.

*Setting.*—Department of Ophthalmology, University Medicine Charité Berlin, Berlin, Germany.

*Design.*—Retrospective cohort study.

*Methods.*—Uncorrected (UDVA) and corrected (CDVA) distance visual acuities, refraction, intraocular pressure, endothelial cell loss, and adverse events were evaluated.

*Results.*—The study enrolled 53 eyes (mean spherical equivalent [SE] −12.17 diopters [D] ± 4.12 [SD]) of 29 patients. The mean age was 34.6 ± 9.2 years and the mean follow-up, 86 ± 21.2 months. The mean UDVA improved from 1.37 ± 0.28 logMAR preoperatively to 0.14 ± 0.19 logMAR at the last postoperative visit ($P < .05$). The mean CDVA improved from 0.10 ± 0.18 logMAR to −0.01 ± 0.09 logMAR ($P < .05$). The overall mean efficacy index and mean safety index were 0.9 and 1.21, respectively, at the last follow-up visit. The mean endothelial cell loss at the last follow-up was 6.4%. The complications were slight posterior chamber (PC) pIOL decentration (5 eyes, 9.4%), severe PC pIOL decentration resulting in pIOL removal (1 eye, 1.8%), glaucoma (4 eyes, 7.5%), clinically significant cortical lens opacification resulting in cataract surgery (4 eyes, 7.5%), clinically asymptomatic anterior subcapsular cataract formation (6 eyes, 11.3%), and retinal detachment (2 eyes, 3.8%).

*Conclusions.*—Posterior chamber phakic pIOL implantation to correct moderate to high myopia provided predictable and stable refractive results but with a high rate of serious complications over the long term.

▶ There is no doubt that phakic intraocular lenses (IOLs) can provide almost immediate, excellent-quality uncorrected vision in many eyes. There are numerous studies to support this. The issue is the complication rate—both short and long term. Endophthalmitis, although extremely rare, has been reported after phakic IOL implantation. Endophthalmitis is tragic, but I am much more concerned about long-term issues.

These authors report minimum 5-year follow-up on 53 eyes after phakic posterior chamber IOL implant to correct myopia. As expected, the refractive error and refractive stability results were very good. The 5-year endothelial cell loss rate was 5.7%. Physiologic endothelial cell loss is said to be 0.6% per year, or 3% over 5 years. Almost twice the rate of and endothelial cell loss is concerning; 7.5% developed significant enough lens opacities to require cataract surgery and another 11.3% have anterior subcapsular lens opacities that have not required cataract surgery—*yet*. Although many surgeons do not consider cataract a "major complication," note that one of these eyes developed a retinal detachment 3 months after the cataract surgery, and that *is* a major complication, especially in these highly myopic eyes.

**C. J. Rapuano, MD**

---

**Intraocular Pressure after Implantation of the Visian Implantable Collamer Lens With CentraFLOW Without Iridotomy**

Higueras-Esteban A, Ortiz-Gomariz A, Gutiérrez-Ortega R, et al (Universidad Europea de Madrid, Spain; et al)

*Am J Ophthalmol* 156:800-805, 2013

---

*Purpose.*—To compare the intraocular pressure (IOP) values during a 3-month period after implantation of the new Visian Implantable Collamer Lens (ICL; STAAR Surgical Company, Nidau, Switzerland) V4c design with CentraFLOW technology without iridotomy using a standard procedure followed by implantation of the conventional ICL V4b model.

*Design.*—Retrospective cohort study.

*Methods.*—This study included 17 eyes implanted with the ICL V4b model and 18 eyes implanted with the ICL V4c model. The mean preoperative spherical equivalent refractions were −7.48 ± 5.00 diopters and −8.66 ± 4.2 diopters, respectively. We compared the best-corrected distance visual acuity before surgery with the uncorrected distance visual acuity after surgery. The intraocular pressure (IOP) was measured 1 week, 1 month, and 3 months after surgery. The central vault at 3 months was measured using optical coherence tomography.

*Results.*—Three months after surgery, the mean uncorrected distance visual acuities were −0.09 ± 0.12 logarithm of the minimal angle of resolution units with the V4b and −0.07 ± 0.11 logarithm of the minimal angle of resolution units with the V4c. The mean distances between the ICL and the anterior crystalline lens surface were 557 ± 224 μm and 528 ± 268 μm for the V4b and V4c, respectively ($P = .73$). After 1 week and 1 month, the mean IOPs were 13.7 and 13.3 mm Hg and 14.7 and 15.1 mm Hg, respectively. There were no significant differences in IOP within or between groups during the follow-up period ($P > .05$, for all comparisons).

*Conclusions.*—The new ICL with the CentraFLOW design seems to provide similar results as its predecessors for the correction of moderate to high myopia and maintenance of safe IOP levels without iridotomy (Fig 1).

▶ There are currently 2 US Food and Drug Administration-approved phakic intraocular lenses (IOLs) available for use in United States. The Visian posterior chamber phakic IOL requires peripheral iridotomies either days to weeks before placement of the lens or during the same procedure. Needless to say, peripheral iridotomies are not only an additional surgical procedure but also have potential complications including hyphema, inflammation, vitreous hemorrhage, and, rarely, retinal detachment. Additionally, peripheral iridotomies may be too small to be effective or may close, increasing the risk of the pupillary block. A lens design that would eliminate the need for peripheral iridotomies would certainly be an advantage.

A new version of the Visian ICL was developed with a central hole in the optic to improve aqueous humor circulation. Fig 1 shows an optical coherence tomography of the original lens on top and the new lens with the central hole on the bottom. Interestingly, the article does not state the exact size of the hole. This study reports a retrospective review of 17 eyes with the original lens and 18 eyes with the new model with the central hole followed for 3 months. Eyes that had the original lens implanted had laser peripheral iridotomies performed 2 weeks before the surgery, whereas eyes with the new version of the lens did not have peripheral iridotomies. Intraocular pressure results were similar between the 2 groups. There were no episodes of pupillary block. The vault between the phakic IOL and the anterior crystalline lens surface were also basically the same between groups. The authors did note in their discussion that they recorded temporary halos in patients with the new lens design. They also noted that these halos decreased significantly 1 month after surgery and suggested that patients adapted to the new lens.

Eliminating the need for preoperative or intraoperative peripheral iridotomies is certainly an advantage. It is surprising that the article does not give us the exact

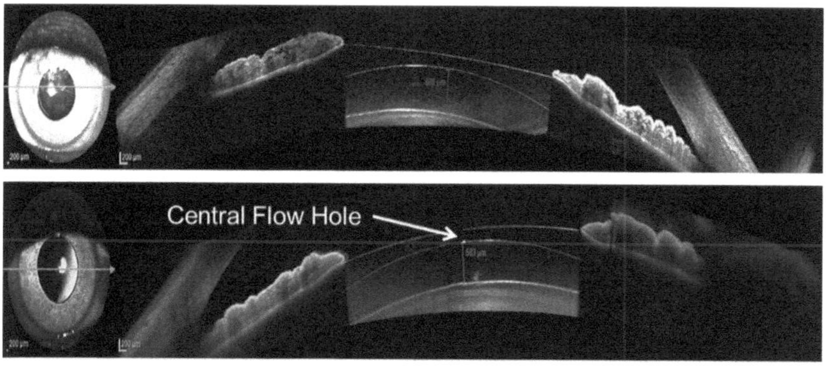


FIGURE 1.—Representative Spectralis anterior segment optical coherence tomography images of the distance between the Implantable Collamer Lens (ICL; STAAR Surgical Company) and the anterior lens surface (vault) for the ICL (Top) without a central hole and (Bottom) with CentraFLOW. (Reprinted from American Journal of Ophthalmology. Higueras-Esteban A, Ortiz-Gomariz A, Gutiérrez-Ortega R, et al. Intraocular pressure after implantation of the visian implantable collamer lens with CentraFlow without iridotomy. *Am J Ophthalmol.* 2013;156:800-805, with permission from Elsevier.)

size of the hole. An advantage to a larger hole is that is less likely to clog up and become nonfunctional, thus increasing the risk of pupillary block. A disadvantage to a larger hole is that it would be more likely to affect the quality of the vision. Longer-term follow-up is certainly needed to make sure that the hole remains patent and pupillary block or elevated intraocular pressure does not develop down the road. Additionally, better quality of vision analysis, including wavefront measurements, are required to compare the lenses with and without the central hole to determine the visual effect of the hole.

**C. J. Rapuano, MD**

---

**Anterior Segment Optical Coherence Tomography of Long-Term Phakic Angle-Supported Intraocular Lenses**

Alio JL, Abbouda A, Peña-Garcia P (Universidad Miguel Hernández, Alicante, Spain)

*Am J Ophthalmol* 156:894-901, 2013

---

*Purpose.*—To evaluate the long-term age-related anterior chamber changes by anterior segment optical coherence tomography (OCT) and the impact of such changes on the stability and behavior of angle-supported phakic intraocular lenses (IOLs).

*Design.*—A retrospective consecutive observational cohort study.

*Methods.*—A total of 23 eyes with high myopia implanted with an angle-supported phakic IOL between 1990 and 1996 at Vissum Corporación Oftalmológica de Alicante were included in the study. Patients were evaluated using OCT. Anterior chamber depth, anterior chamber width, crystalline lens rise, and the distance between phakic IOL and endothelium were measured.

TABLE 2.—Predictive Model of Endothelial Cell Count in Patients With Angle-Supported Phakic Intraocular Lenses

| | TI (y) | | | | | |
|---|---|---|---|---|---|---|
| Pre SE (D) | 15 | 20 | 25 | 30 | 35 | 40 |
| −10 | 2580 | 2334 | 2088 | 1842 | 1596 | 1350 |
| −15 | 2243 | 1997 | 1751 | 1505 | 1259 | 1013 |
| −20 | 1907 | 1661 | 1415 | 1169 | 923 | 677 |
| −25 | 1570 | 1324 | 1078 | 832 | 586 | 340 |
| −30 | 1233 | 987 | 741 | 495 | 249 | 3 |
| −35 | 895 | 649 | 403 | 157 | - | - |

D = diopters; Pre SE = preoperative spherical equivalent; TI = time implantation (in years).

Table shows the relationship between the preoperative spherical equivalent and the duration of implantation, providing an estimation of endothelial cell count. The values described in the table are predicted by linear regression model.

TABLE 3.—Predictive Model for Anterior Chamber Depth in Patients With Angle-Supported Phakic Intraocular Lenses

| | TI (y) | | | | |
|---|---|---|---|---|---|
| Pre SE (D) | 10 | 15 | 20 | 25 | 30 |
| −12 | −0.004 | −0.068 | −0.132 | −0.196 | −0.260 |
| −15 | −0.145 | −0.209 | −0.273 | −0.337 | −0.401 |
| −20 | −0.381 | −0.445 | −0.509 | −0.573 | −0.637 |
| −25 | −0.617 | −0.681 | −0.745 | −0.809 | −0.873 |
| −30 | −0.853 | −0.917 | −0.981 | −1.045 | −1.109 |

D = diopters; Pre SE = preoperative spherical equivalent; TI = time implantation (in years).

Table shows the relationship between the preoperative spherical equivalent and the duration of implantation providing an estimation of the reduction in mm of anterior chamber depth. The values described in the table are predicted by linear regression model.

*Results.*—Fifteen years after implantation, anterior chamber depth was 2.9 ± 0.3 mm, crystalline lens rise 748.18 ± 393.13 μm, and phakic IOL–endothelium distance 2.1 ± 0.30 mm. The predictive model showed that 30 years after implantation, endothelial cell count was less than 600 cells/mm$^2$ in patients with a preoperative spherical equivalent of −25 diopters (D). Twenty years after implantation, the safety zone of 1.5 mm between endothelium and the lens will not be respected in patients with a preoperative spherical equivalent of −20 D.

*Conclusions.*—The findings of this study could have an important influence on the decision about the indication to implant angle-supported phakic IOLs in young patients with a long postoperative life expectancy, as age-related changes in the anatomy of the anterior segment may create a long-term hazard for the implanted eye (Tables 2 and 3).

▶ There is currently no US Food and Drug Administration (FDA)-approved angle-supported phakic intraocular lens (IOL) in the United States. Issues with these lenses have included endothelial cell loss and cataract formation. This study looked at 23 eyes with high myopia (>10 diopters) that had angle-supported phakic IOLs (Baikoff ZB) placed at least 15 years ago (mean, 19.8 years). This number is a small fraction of the 208 eyes that had this type of lens placed during the same period. These 23 eyes had no further surgical procedure or ocular inflammation. In other words, they had some of the best outcomes of all of the eyes treated with this lens.

They found an increase in crystalline lens rise and a corresponding decrease in anterior chamber depth. They found a strong correlation between decreasing anterior chamber depth and decreased corneal endothelial cell density. Eyes with cataracts at the end of the study were also shown to have statistically significant increased crystalline lens rise with a trend toward decreased anterior chamber depth. They also found that the higher the myopia preoperatively, the greater chance of cataract formation. Consequently, the higher the myopia preoperatively, the lower the anterior chamber depth at the end of follow-up. Also, the higher the myopia preoperatively, the lower the endothelial cell density at the end of follow-up. They also found a significant correlation between the lower anterior chamber depth and the number of years of phakic IOL implantation, suggesting that the rapidity of cataract formation was not only related to the level of preoperative myopia but also to the presence of the phakic IOL. Table 2 shows a predictive model of endothelial cell count related to preoperative spherical equivalent and time after IOL implantation. Table 3 shows a predictive model for the progressive decrease in anterior chamber depth related to time after IOL implantation. Both of these models suggest that at least this model of phakic anterior chamber intraocular lens is not ideal for young patients with a long life expectancy, especially with higher degrees of myopia.

**C. J. Rapuano, MD**

---

**One-year safety and efficacy results of a hydrogel inlay to improve near vision in patients with emmetropic presbyopia**

Garza EB, Gomez S, Chayet A, et al (Laser Ocular hidalgo, Nuevo Leone, Mexico)

*J Refract Surg* 29:166-172, 2013

---

*Purpose.*—To conduct a feasibility study of the safety and efficacy of a corneal contouring inlay as a treatment for emmetropic presbyopia.

*Methods.*—The Raindrop corneal inlay (ReVision Optics, Inc., Lake Forest, CA) was implanted on the corneal stromal bed beneath a keratotomy flap in 20 nondominant eyes of 20 patients. The implant is designed to cause a change in the curvature of the overlying cornea, with a subsequent multifocal change in refractive power. Efficacy outcome was defined as at least 75% of eyes with uncorrected near visual acuity of 0.3 logMAR (20/40 Snellen) or better at 6 months. Main safety outcomes were retention of preoperative best-corrected distance visual acuity and reports of adverse events. Other outcome measures included contrast sensitivity; near, intermediate, and distance visual acuities; patient satisfaction; spectacle use; and complications.

*Results.*—All implanted eyes achieved uncorrected near visual acuity of 0.3 logMAR (20/40 Snellen) or better by the 1-week postoperative examination and remained so throughout the 1-year follow-up period, also averaging less than 0.1 logMAR (20/25 Snellen) monocularly and binocularly throughout that period. Mean binocular uncorrected distance visual acuity remained within 0.02 logMAR of the preoperative mean throughout the study. One patient who was dissatisfied with the resulting vision underwent explantation. At 1 year, 16 of 19 patients seldom or never wore glasses and all 19 were satisfied or very satisfied with their overall vision.

*Conclusions.*—The hydrogel corneal inlay improved uncorrected near and intermediate visual acuity in patients with emmetropic presbyopia, with high patient satisfaction and little effect on distance visual acuity.

▶ Now that we are successful in treating up to moderately high degrees of myopia and up to moderate degrees of hyperopia and astigmatism with corneal refractive surgery, the next frontier is correcting presbyopia. Multifocal ablations resulted in fairly good uncorrected near and distance visual acuity but often with a significant compromise in quality of vision, and they are not commonly performed. Corneal inlays have become a popular method for treating presbyopia. The Kamra inlay (creating a pinhole effect to increase depth of focus) has shown good results with a few years of follow-up.

These authors report good results in a small number of patients undergoing a different type of corneal inlay to treat presbyopia. The raindrop inlay is made of a clear hydrogel material and has a diameter of 2 mm and a central thickness of 32 μ. It is placed in the nondominant eye under an 8-mm, 150-μ corneal flap to increase the corneal curvature centrally to improve near vision. Inclusion criteria required the patients to wear a contact lens to correct for near vision in the nondominant eye for at least 5 days to make sure they were happy with monovision.

The procedure was performed in 20 eyes of 20 patients. In one eye, the inlay shifted position and had to be replaced one month after the original surgery. One patient was unhappy with his postoperative distance vision, especially with regard to playing tennis, and had the inlay removed. The results in the remaining 19 patients were quite good. At one year, 16 of the 19 patients reported that they seldom, if ever, used corrective lenses, compared with one patient preoperatively. Eighteen of the 19 patients were satisfied or very satisfied with the near and intermediate vision, and 19 of the 19 patients were satisfied with their distance vision and their overall visual outcomes. This is a promising technique, although more patients with a longer follow-up are needed.

**C. J. Rapuano, MD**

# 3 Glaucoma

**Inadvertent Implantation of Aqueous Tube Shunts in Glaucomatous Eyes With Unrecognized Intraocular Neoplasms: Report of 5 Cases**

Kaliki S, Eagle RC Jr, Grossniklaus HE, et al (Thomas Jefferson Univ, Philadelphia, PA; Emory Univ, Atlanta, GA; et al)

*JAMA Ophthalmol* 131:925-928, 2013

*Background.*—Glaucoma can develop secondarily to intraocular tumors, which may remain undetected. In the treatment of this glaucoma, drainage devices or aqueous tube shunts may be used to control intraocular pressure when the condition has not responded to medical or laser therapy. The inadvertent implantation of an aqueous tube shunt in eyes with tumor-related glaucoma is probably rare or underreported, but cases have occurred and may be related to extraocular tumor extension.

*Case Reports.*—Five patients from three institutions had aqueous tube shunts placed in glaucomatous eyes harboring unrecognized intraocular neoplasms. Histopathologic examination confirmed the presence of the intraocular tumors, with two patients having medulloepithelioma and three having uveal melanoma. Extraocular tumor extension occurred in four patients. The secondary glaucoma was misdiagnosed as neovascular glaucoma in one case, trauma-related glaucoma in two cases, uveitic glaucoma in one case, and iridocorneal endothelial syndrome in one case. The mean duration of the misdiagnosis was 65 months, with a range of 3 to 108 months. The mean time between aqueous shunt surgery and extraocular tumor extension was 23 months, with a range of 3 to 48 months.

*Discussion.*—Various intraocular tumors can produce elevated intraocular pressure. Children with a subluxed or cataractous lens and normal posterior fundus should be suspected to have an occult ciliary body medulloepithelioma, as was noted in two of the patients reported. It is not uncommon to have these conditions misdiagnosed and mismanaged, as occurred in this series. Melanoma, specifically diffuse iris melanoma, that invades the angle can also cause elevated intraocular pressure, but should be considered in patients who develop unilateral glaucoma and iris heterochromia. Careful evaluation can identify this entity, differentiating it from iridocorneal endothelial syndrome-n-associated glaucoma. The inadvertent evisceration of unsuspected choroidal melanoma has been reported, but the correct diagnosis may be established through clinical examination and imaging studies such as B-scan ultrasonography and magnetic resonance imaging. Glaucoma-filtering surgery and extraocular tumor extension may be related. Tumors of the anterior segment have greater access to the tube shunt than those in the posterior segment. Extraocular tumor extension occurred in four of the five cases reported, indicating that the aqueous tube shunt provides a means for tumor extension, especially for anterior segment neoplasms.

*Conclusions.*—Eyes that have glaucoma should be carefully assessed to determine if an occult intraocular tumor is present before inserting a tube shunt to reduce intraocular pressure. If a tumor is suspected, shunt surgery should be delayed until an ocular oncology consultation can be obtained and intraocular neoplasm can be ruled out.

▶ Transscleral filtration of aqueous may provide an avenue for extraocular tumor extension. Four of the 5 cases reported in this series involved extraocular tumor extension. Tumor cells were documented in the tube reservoir in 3 of the 5 cases. Unfortunately, diagnosis of intraocular neoplasm may not be straightforward, so a high degree of suspicion should be maintained. In particular, unilateral intractable glaucoma merits suspicion.

Intraocular surgery is not absolutely contraindicated in all eyes with intraocular tumors, but extreme caution must be exercised. Transscleral cyclophotocoagulation may be an option for glaucoma refractory to medical management in eyes with an intraocular tumor, but data on the specific risks and efficacy in this context is lacking.

Although likely underreported, filtering surgery in eyes with unrecognized tumor is presumably rare. This article is a reminder that rare and dangerous causes of glaucoma occur, and thorough evaluation before glaucoma surgery is important.

**S. Fudemberg, MD, FACS**

---

**From Clinical Examination of the Optic Disc to Clinical Assessment of the Optic Nerve Head: A Paradigm Change**

Chauhan BC, Burgoyne CF (Dalhousie Univ, Halifax, Nova Scotia, Canada; Devers Eye Inst, Portland, OR)

*Am J Ophthalmol* 156:218-227, 2013

---

*Purpose.*—To review and interpret the anatomy of the optic nerve head (ONH) detected with spectral-domain optical coherence tomography (SD OCT) pertaining to the clinical examination of the optic disc and to propose that a paradigm change for clinical assessment of the ONH is necessary.

*Design.*—Perspective.

*Methods.*—Presently, the clinician evaluates neuroretinal rim health according to the appearance of the optic disc, the clinically visible surface of the ONH. Recent anatomic findings with SD OCT have challenged the basis and accuracy of current rim evaluation. We demonstrate why incorporation of SD OCT imaging of the ONH into the clinical examination of the disc is required.

*Results.*—Disc margin-based rim evaluation lacks a solid anatomic basis and results in variably inaccurate measurements for 2 reasons. First, the clinically visible disc margin is an unreliable outer border of rim tissue because of clinically and photographically invisible extensions of Bruch's membrane. Second, rim tissue orientation is not considered in width measurements. We propose alternative anatomically and geometrically accurate SD OCT-based approaches for rim assessment that have enhanced detection of glaucoma. We also argue for new data acquisition and analysis strategies with SD OCT that account for the large interindividual variability in the angle between the fovea and ONH.

*Conclusions.*—We propose a 4-point paradigm change for clinical assessment of the ONH that is anchored to the eye-specific anatomy and geometry of the ONH and fovea. Our approach is designed to enhance the accuracy and consistency of rim width, as well as of peripapillary and macular intraretinal thickness measurements.

▶ The limitation of end points through which we measure progression is among the most fundamental problems in glaucoma care. Visual fields provide a functional end point, but are subjective and notoriously variable. Furthermore, defining progression on a visual field may be difficult. Even the seminal trials in glaucoma could not create a universally applicable standard for visual field progression. Worse, significant glaucoma progression must occur before a visual field defect appears, so visual fields miss early glaucoma progression. Clinical optic nerve evaluation is a structural test that may help identify rim loss before development of a visual field defect, but this is still subjective. Also, changes occur in the optic nerve during glaucoma progression that cannot be clinically appreciated.

Optic nerve analyzers hold tremendous potential to provide structural end points for glaucoma progression that are objective and highly sensitive. Currently, use of these tests may be frustrating. Studies show that the resolution and reproducibility of spectral-domain optical coherence tomography (OCT) are high, but patient cooperation, technician skill, and media issues contribute to fluctuation that confounds confident interpretation of OCT results. Also, the structural characteristics measured by optic nerve analyzers are inherently variable even among normal subjects. Ultimately, we should strive to create a meaningful evidence-based standard to correlate microns of retinal nerve fiber layer thinning with clinically significant glaucoma progression and then visual disability.

**S. Fudemberg, MD, FACS**

**Anterior Chamber Bleeding After Laser Peripheral Iridotomy**

Golan S, Levkovitch-Verbin H, Shemesh G, et al (Tel Aviv Univ, Israel)

*JAMA Ophthalmol* 131:626-629, 2013

*Importance.*—To our knowledge, this is the first study to describe the correlation of anterior chamber bleeding after laser peripheral iridotomy (LPI) and antiplatelet therapy.

*Objective.*—To determine the incidence and amount of anterior chamber bleeding after laser peripheral iridotomy in patients whose condition is suggestive of primary angle-closure glaucoma (PACS) who continued their antiplatelet or anticoagulant treatment before undergoing LPI compared with when they discontinued treatment.

*Design and Setting.*—A prospective controlled trial.

*Patients.*—Patients with suspected bilateral primary angleclosure and no other ocular disease who take antiplatelet or anticoagulant medications regularly (from January 2010-October 2011) were enrolled.

*Main Outcome and Measure.*—The incidence of anterior chamber bleeding with and without antiplatelet and anticoagulant therapy.

*Results.*—A total of 104 patients (208 eyes) participated in the study. Thirty-six eyes (34.6%) in the treated and untreated arms bled. The amount of bleeding did not differ significantly when the patient was on or off antiplatelet or anticoagulant treatment, nor did the immediate post-procedure mean intraocular pressure ($P = .13$). The type of antiplatelet or anticoagulant, total laser energy, age, sex, or color of irides were not risk factors for increased bleeding ($P = .156$ for all parameters).

*Conclusions.*—No indication was noted for discontinuing these medications before a high-powered pulsed laser peripheral iridotomy.

▶ Oral anticoagulants are more commonly being used to reduce the risk of serious cardiovascular events. For surgeons, the risk of bleeding in anticoagulated patients must be balanced against the chance that holding anticoagulation therapy may precipitate a stroke or myocardial infarction. The risk of laser peripheral iridotomy (LPI) procedures is generally low. Mild bleeding occurs relatively often (reportedly in about 40% of LPIs) but rarely leads to clinically significant complications like persistently elevated intraocular pressure and decreased vision. However, in worst-case scenarios, profound bleeding after an LPI may pose vision-threatening problems and require surgical evacuation. Strategies such as use of argon laser pretreatment and holding anticoagulants may reduce the risk of bleeding, but are they necessary?

This study is well designed and indicates that withholding anticoagulation before neodymium-doped yttrium aluminum garnet (Nd:YAG) laser iridotomy alone (no argon pretreatment) does not statistically significantly alter the risk of bleeding. Given that significant bleeding is a rare event, further study of this issue is needed, but the results are reassuring. Additionally, the danger of withholding anticoagulation varies based on the reason it was initiated, and the potential for serious or even life-threatening complications related to stopping anticoagulation should always be remembered.

**S. Fudemberg, MD, FACS**

**Clinical Results of Ab Interno Trabeculotomy Using the Trabectome for Open-Angle Glaucoma: The Mayo Clinic Series in Rochester, Minnesota**

Ahuja Y, Ma Khin Pyi S, Malihi M, et al (Mayo Clinic, Rochester, MN; Mayo Med School, Rochester, MN)

*Am J Ophthalmol* 156:927-935.e2, 2013

*Purpose.*—To determine outcomes of ab interno trabeculotomy for treatment of open-angle glaucoma (OAG).

*Design.*—Retrospective interventional single-surgeon, single-center case series.

*Methods.*—Data were collected from 246 patients undergoing ab interno trabeculotomy between September 1, 2006, and December 1, 2010, with 3 months' follow-up or longer. Kaplan-Meier analysis was performed using Criteria A (postoperative intraocular pressure [IOP] ≤21 mm Hg or ≥20% reduction from preoperative IOP) and Criteria B (IOP ≤18 mm Hg and ≥20% reduction in IOP). Failure included increased glaucoma medications or subsequent surgery. Failure risk factors were identified using Cox proportional hazards ratio (HR).

*Results.*—Of 88 cases of ab interno trabeculotomy-only and 158 cases of ab interno trabeculotomy with cataract extraction, the retention rate was 70% for 1 year and 62% for 2 years. Preoperative mean IOP was 21.6 ± 8.6 mm Hg; the number of glaucoma medications was 3.1 ± 1.1. At 24 months postoperatively, mean IOP was reduced 29% to 15.3 ± 4.6 mm Hg ($P < 0.001$) and the number of glaucoma medications was reduced 38% to 1.9 ± 1.3 ($P < 0.001$) with a success rate of 62% (95% CI, 56%–68%) using Criteria A and 22% (95% CI, 16%–29%) using Criteria B. Failure risk factors using Criteria A included primary OAG (HR 3.14, $P < 0.01$, 95% CI, 1.91–5.17) and past argon laser trabeculoplasty (HR 1.81, $P < 0.01$, 95% CI, 1.18–2.77). Using Criteria B, the HR for pseudoexfoliative glaucoma was 0.43 ($P < 0.01$, 95% CI 0.27–0.67). Of the cases, 66 (26.8%) required subsequent surgery on an average of 10 months (2 days to 3.2 years) after ab interno trabeculotomy.

*Conclusions.*—For criteria involving IOP ≤18 mm Hg, the 24-month survival of ab interno trabeculotomy is low. This surgery is appropriate for patients requiring a target IOP of 21 mm Hg or above (Table 2).

▶ Trabectome is one the microincisional glaucoma surgeries (MIGS) with which we now have years of experience. Although MIGS procedures have fewer side effects than traditional filtering surgeries, like trabeculectomy and tube shunts, they generally don't work as well to lower intraocular pressure

TABLE 2.—Mean Intraocular Pressure of the Operative Eye Before and After Undergoing Ab Interno Trabeculotomy for Open-Angle Glaucoma

| | Mean IOP (mm Hg) ± SD | | |
|---|---|---|---|
| | All Cases | Trabeculotomyonly Cases | Trabeculotomy with CE Cases |
| Baseline | 21.6 ± 8.6 | 25.9 ± 8.9 | 19.3 ± 7.4 |
| n | 246 | 88 | 158 |
| 1 week | 15.7 ± 7.4 | 16.1 ± 7.1 | 15.5 ± 7.6 |
| % reduction, *P*[a] | 27.4, *<0.001* | 37.8, *<0.001* | 19.6, *<0.001* |
| n | 242 | 87 | 155 |
| 1 month | 16.2 ± 7.1 | 19.4 ± 8.1 | 14.4 ± 5.8 |
| % reduction, *P* | 25.2, *<0.001* | 25.1, *<0.001* | 25.1, *<0.001* |
| n | 243 | 86 | 157 |
| 3 months | 15.8 ± 6.0 | 17.5 ± 6.2 | 14.8 ± 5.6 |
| % reduction, *P* | 27.0, *<0.001* | 32.6, *<0.001* | 23.0, *<0.001* |
| n | 218 | 81 | 137 |
| 6 months | 15.6 ± 5.5 | 17.4 ± 6.4 | 14.8 ± 4.8 |
| % reduction, *P* | 27.7, *<0.001* | 32.9, *<0.001* | 23.1, *<0.001* |
| n | 186 | 60 | 126 |
| 12 months | 15.1 ± 4.4 | 16.5 ± 5.6 | 14.6 ± 3.7 |
| % reduction, *P* | 30.1, *<0.001* | 36.4, *<0.001* | 24.3, *<0.001* |
| n | 152 | 44 | 108 |
| 18 months | 14.7 ± 4.6 | 16.8 ± 6.3 | 14.0 ± 3.7 |
| % reduction, *P* | 32.1, *<0.001* | 35.1, *<0.001* | 27.2, *<0.001* |
| n | 111 | 27 | 84 |
| 24 months | 15.3 ± 4.6 | 16.8 ± 2.8 | 14.9 ± 4.9 |
| % reduction, *P* | 29.1, *<0.001* | 35.1, *<0.001* | 22.8, *0.10* |
| N | 69 | 17 | 52 |
| 30 months | 15.1 ± 4.7 | 15.5 ± 5.3 | 15.0 ± 4.6 |
| % reduction, *P* | 30.2, *0.002* | 40.0, *0.02* | 22.2, *0.08* |
| N | 50 | 11 | 39 |
| 36 months | 15.0 ± 5.9 | 13.5 ± 2.9 | 15.3 ± 6.3 |
| % reduction, *P* | 30.6, *0.04* | 47.9, *0.005* | 20.4, *0.26* |
| N | 37 | 6 | 31 |
| 42 months | 13.1 ± 3.6 | 15.2 ± 3.6 | 12.3 ± 3.4 |
| % reduction, *P* | 39.1, *0.09* | 41.4, *0.14* | 36.3, *0.26* |
| N | 16 | 5 | 11 |
| 48 months | 12.0 ± 2.6 | 13.0 | 11.8 ± 3.0 |
| % reduction, *P* | 44.5, *0.36* | 49.8 | 39.0, *0.47* |
| n | 5 | 1 | 4 |

CE = cataract extraction; IOP = intraocular pressure; SD = standard deviation.
[a]Percent reduction and *P* values compare mean IOP at each visit to baseline using the generalized estimating equation models.

(IOP). The trabectome is no exception, as demonstrated by the results of this study. By 2 years, most patients did not achieve IOP less than 18 with IOP reduction of 20% or more. There are conflicting reports on long-term success with Trabectome. Like for many of the current MIGS procedures, refining the list of good candidates for the procedure will affect the rates of success and complications.

**S. Fudemberg, MD, FACS**

**Initial central scotomas *vs* peripheral scotomas in normal-tension glaucoma: clinical characteristics and progression rates**

Cho H-K, Lee J, Lee M, et al (Sungkyunkwan Univ School of Medicine, Seoul, Korea; Kong Eye Ctr, Seoul, Korea; Dankook Univ School of Medicine, Cheonan, Korea)

*Eye* 28:303-311, 2014

*Purpose.*—To investigate clinical characteristics and progression rates of the initial central scotomas (ICS) compared with the initial peripheral scotomas (IPS) in normal-tension glaucoma (NTG) patients.

*Methods.*—Among NTG patients showing a single hemifield defect and who performed more than five reliable standard visual field (VF) tests, medical records of ICS (involvement of ≥3 adjacent points with $P < 5\%$ within the central 12° of fixation and one point with a $P < 0.01$ within the central 6° of fixation) ($n = 32$) or IPS (no VF abnormality within the central 6° of fixation) ($n = 34$) were retrospectively analyzed. The changes of mean thresholds from 10 zones of the glaucoma hemifield test, central 6° and 12° zones, peripheral zones other than central 6° and 12°, and the entire hemifield were inspected. To calculate the progression rates, linear mixed-effect model was employed.

*Results.*—There were no significant differences between the two groups in age, gender, ocular factors including baseline/mean treated intraocular pressure, and systemic factors including systolic or diastolic blood pressure/perfusion pressure, mean ocular perfusion pressure (all $P > 0.05$). There were no significant differences in baseline mean deviation and pattern standard deviation ($P > 0.05$) between the two groups, but VF index was significantly lower in ICS group than in IPS group ($P = 0.001$). The progression rates between the two groups were not significantly different in all zones we investigated (all $P > 0.05$).

*Conclusions.*—Newly diagnosed cases of NTG with ICS may not differ from those with IPS in clinical characteristics and progression rates under treatment (Fig 1, Table 1).

▶ Open-angle glaucoma is classically associated with visual field defects that start peripherally and only affect the central vision in advanced disease. However, early central visual field defects may occur, especially in low-tension glaucoma. Given that paracentral defects may be more visually significant for the patient, it is critical to identify these defects and their association with glaucoma. Low-tension glaucoma patients may be tricky to detect, and cases with initial visual field defect in the central area are particularly insidious. Although complete loss of neuroretinal rim in an area should be needed to justify a visual field defect, these cases sometimes involve notching with only moderate cupping that does not clearly involve complete neuroretinal rim loss. Presentation of central defects on a 24° (or greater) visual field may be subtle. Notched nerves in the presence of average intraocular pressure deserve extra attention.

This study is a retrospective comparison of patients with initial central scotomas versus initial peripheral scotomas in open-angle glaucoma. No statistically

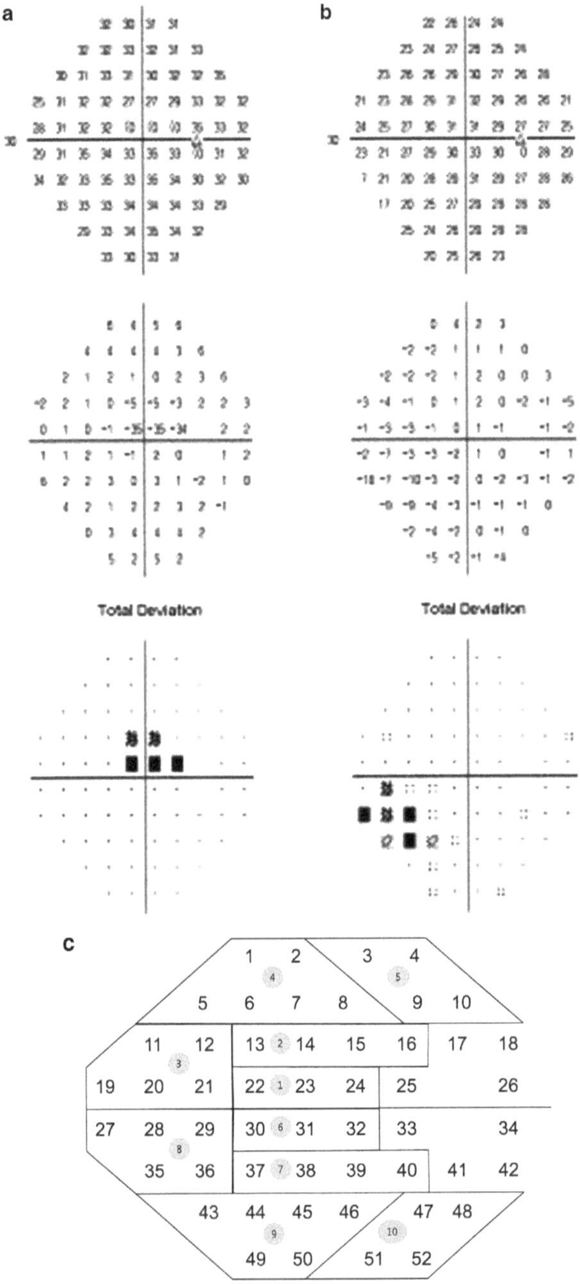


FIGURE 1.—Examples of initial central scotomas (a) and initial peripheral scotomas (b) on the Humphrey 30-2 Swedish interactive threshold algorithm total deviation plot evaluated in the study. Diagram showing the definition of 10 zones of the glaucoma hemifield test and 52 points (c). (Reprinted from Cho H-K, Lee J, Lee M, et al. Initial central scotomas *vs* peripheral scotomas in normal-tension glaucoma: clinical characteristics and progression rates. *Eye*. 2014;28:303-311, with permission from Macmillan Publishers Limited.)

TABLE 1.—Comparison of Clinical Characteristics of Normaltension Glaucoma Patients with Initial Central or Peripheral Visual Field Defects

| Characteristics (mean ± SD) | Initial Central Scotomas (N = 32) | Initial Peripheral Scotomas (N = 34) | *P*-Value |
|---|---|---|---|
| Follow-up period (yr) | 7.19 ± 2.53 | 7.47 ± 2.06 | 0.626[a] |
| Demographic factors | | | |
| Age(yrs) | 49.87 ± 11.60 | 48.50 ± 14.76 | 0.677[a] |
| Gender, female | 18 (56.3%) | 19 (55.8%) | 0.976[b] |
| Family history of glaucoma | 2 (6.3%) | 3 (8.8%) | 1.000[c] |
| Systemic factors | | | |
| Diabetes mellitus | 3 | 3 | 1.000[c] |
| Hypertension | 4 | 6 | 0.734[b] |
| Migraine | 4 | 3 | 0.705[c] |
| Orthostatic hypotension | 4 | 5 | 1.000[c] |
| Peripheral vascular disease | 2 | 0 | 0.231[c] |
| Ocular factors | | | |
| Spherical equivalent(D) | −1.79 ± 1.78 | −1.68 ± 2.37 | 0.834[a] |
| CCT(um) | 526.26 ± 32.96 | 529.83 ± 38.28 | 0.697[a] |
| Disc hemorrhage | 6 (18.8%) | 7 (20.6%) | 0.851[b] |
| β-zone PPA | 27 (84.4%) | 31 (91.2%) | 0.469[c] |
| Baseline IOP | 17.03 ± 3.21 | 17.62 ± 2.87 | 0.436[a] |
| Post-therapeutic mean IOP | 14.85 ± 2.04 | 15.21 ± 2.15 | 0.495[a] |

*Abbreviations:* CCT, central corneal thickness; D, diopters; IOP, intraocular pressure; m, month; PPA, peripapillary atrophy; SD, standard deviation; VF, visual field; yr, year.
[a]Independent t-test.
[b]$\chi^2$-test.
[c]Fisher exact test.

significant differences were determined between clinical characteristics, including mean ocular perfusion pressure. The rate of progression was not statistically significantly different either. It remains unclear why most patients develop peripheral field defects early in glaucoma while others get early paracentral defects.

**S. Fudemberg, MD, FACS**

## Three-Month Randomized Trial of Fixed-Combination Brinzolamide, 1%, and Brimonidine, 0.2%

Katz G, DuBiner H, Samples J, et al (Huron Ophthalmology, Ypsilanti, MI; Clayton Eye Ctr, Morrow, GA; Glaucoma Consultants of Colorado, Parker; et al)
*JAMA Ophthalmol* 131:724-730, 2013

*Importance.*—This study evaluates the contribution of the individual components of an investigational non–β-antagonist fixed combination of brinzolamide, 1%, and brimonidine, 0.2%. This study and its sister study provide the first randomized data showing the intraocular pressure (IOP)-lowering activity and the toxicity profile of this novel topical antihypertensive fixed combination.

*Objective.*—To compare IOP-lowering efficacy of fixed-combination brinzolamide, 1%, and brimonidine, 0.2%, with that of its components in patients with open-angle glaucoma or ocular hypertension.

*Design.*—In this phase 3, double-masked, parallel-group, multicenter study, eligible patients were randomized 1:1:1 to treatment with fixed-combination brinzolamide, 1%, and brimonidine, 0.2%; brinzolamide, 1%; or brimonidine, 0.2%, 3 times daily for 3 months.

*Setting.*—Sixty-six academic and private practice study sites throughout the United States.

*Participants.*—A total of 660 adults with a clinical diagnosis of open-angle glaucoma or ocular hypertension from a referred sample were enrolled. Thirty-four patients discontinued participation due to treatment-related nonserious adverse events.

*Intervention.*—Topical administration of study medication (fixed-combination brinzolamide, 1%, and brimonidine, 0.2%; brinzolamide, 1%; or brimonidine, 0.2%) 1 drop 3 times daily for 3 months.

*Main Outcomes and Measures.*—Mean IOP at the 3-month visit at all time points (8 AM, 10 AM, 3 PM, and 5 PM).

*Results.*—A total of 660 patients were enrolled. Baseline mean IOP values were similar among treatment groups at all 4 time points. At 3 months, the mean IOP of the brinzolamide-brimonidine group (16.3-19.8 mm Hg) was significantly lower than that of either the brinzolamide group (19.3-20.9 mm Hg; $P \leq .002$) or the brimonidine group (17.9-22.5 mm Hg; $P < .001$) across all time points. One of 10 serious adverse events (chest pain, brinzolamide group) was judged as treatment related. A total of 129 patients experienced at least 1 treatment-related adverse effect (brinzolamide-brimonidine, 22.9%; brinzolamide, 18.6%; and brimonidine, 17.3%; $P = .31$), most of which were ocular.

*Conclusions and Relevance.*—This registrational study provides evidence that the fixed combination of brinzolamide, 1%, and brimonidine, 0.2%, can safely and effectively lower IOP in patients with open-angle glaucoma or ocular hypertension, showing significantly superior IOP-lowering activity compared with either brinzolamide or brimonidine monotherapy while providing a safety profile consistent with that of its individual components.

*Trial Registration.*—clinicaltrials.gov Identifier: NCT01297517.

▶ The release of a new fixed-combination topical medication for lowering intraocular pressure (IOP) that doesn't include a β-blocker is big news. Although highly effective and used successfully for many years in glaucoma management, β-blockers pose serious potential risks. These risks include constriction of reactive airways, bradycardia, depression, fatigue, confusion, and memory loss. Impotence is also a potential adverse effect, as it affects quality of life and is likely underreported. The Centers for Disease Control (CDC) report that about half of Americans carry at least one of the key risk factors for heart disease (hypertension, high low-density lipoprotein cholesterol, smoking). Also according to the CDC, more than 15 million Americans report having chronic obstructive pulmonary disease (COPD) diagnosed, and more than 50% of adults with low pulmonary function were not aware they had COPD.[1-4] Fortunately, serious adverse events with β-blockers are uncommon, but the at-risk population for these side effects is likely to increase.

Fixed-combination medications spare patients from the hassle of managing 2 separate bottles of medication. Individual medications may run out at different times requiring more trips to the pharmacy for refills (or more periods during which one of the medications is not used). Individual medications must be administered with sufficient wait time between them, which complicates the process for patients or leads to dilution of the medicine effect when drops are used back to back. Financial burdens with multiple copays may be a problem as well, although drug costs may be frustratingly variable and confusing.

The fixed-combination brinzolamide 1% and brimonidine 0.2% (Simbrinza, Alcon, Fort Worth, TX) offers another weapon for treating glaucoma. However, combination medications may adopt the side-effect profile of both the component drugs. This study compares the combination with its components and indicates that it works well, but treatment-related adverse events were slightly higher for the fixed combination. Nonetheless, many patients on the combination would otherwise be on the components anyway.

**S. Fudemberg, MD, FACS**

*References*

1. CDC. Million hearts: strategies to reduce the prevalence of leading cardiovascular disease risk factors—United States, 2011. *MMWR Morb Mortal Wkly Rep*. 2011; 60:1248-1251.
2. Hoyert DL, Xu JQ. Deaths: preliminary data for 2011. *Natl Vital Stat Rep*. 2012; 61:1-65.
3. National Center for Health Statistics. 2012. Hyattsville, MD.
4. Centers for Disease Control and Prevention. Chronic obstructive pulmonary disease among adults—United States, 2011. *MMWR Morb Mortal Wkly Rep*. 2012;61:938-943.

## Alteration of Travel Patterns With Vision Loss From Glaucoma and Macular Degeneration

Curriero FC, Pinchoff J, van Landingham SW, et al (Johns Hopkins Bloomberg School of Public Health, Baltimore, MD; Johns Hopkins School of Medicine, Baltimore, MD; et al)

*JAMA Ophthalmol* 131:1420-1426, 2013

*Importance.*—The distance patients can travel outside the home influences how much of the world they can sample and to what extent they can live independently. Recent technological advances have allowed travel outside the home to be directly measured in patients' real-world routines.

*Objective.*—To determine whether decreased visual acuity (VA) from age-related macular degeneration (AMD) and visual field (VF) loss from glaucoma are associated with restricted travel patterns in older adults.

*Design.*—Cross-sectional study.

*Setting.*—Patients were recruited from an eye clinic, while travel patterns were recorded during their real-world routines using a cellular tracking device.

TABLE 1.—Descriptive Characteristics for the Study Population Stratified by the Control, Glaucoma, and AMD Classifications

| Variable | Control (n = 59) | Glaucoma (n = 74) | AMD (n = 60) |
|---|---|---|---|
| Acuity, mean (SD), logMAR | 0.07 (0.12) | 0.25 (0.33) | 0.44 (0.32) |
| Acuity, Snellen | 20/23 | 20/36 | 20/55 |
| Better-eye VF MD, mean (SD) | 0.10 (1.34) | −10.63 (7.43) | NA |
| Age, mean (SD), y | 69.6 (5.2) | 70.5 (5.3) | 74.4 (5.0) |
| Male, % | 40.7 | 44.6 | 41.8 |
| African American, % | 20.3 | 33.8 | 1.8 |
| Married, %[a] | 71.2 | 68.9 | 70.0 |
| Employed (yes vs no), % | 39.0 | 44.6 | 21.8 |
| Driving status (yes vs no), %[b] | 89.9 | 77.2 | 75.7 |
| Education, mean (SD), y | 15.3 (2.8) | 14.9 (2.7) | 14.9 (2.1) |
| Population/sq mile, mean (SD)[c] | 4.3 (5.2) | 5.0 (6.4) | 3.4 (5.3) |
| Weekday (yes vs no), %[d] | 68.1 | 66.3 | 61.8 |

*Abbreviations*: AMD, age-related macular degeneration; MD, mean deviation; NA, not available; VF, visual field.
[a]Married also included those living together vs not married.
[b]Any self-reported driving in the prior 3 months.
[c]Population per squaremile in units of 1000 people.
[d]Weekday variable summarized over all 1048 person tracking days.

*Participants.*—Sixty-one control subjects with normal vision, 84 subjects with glaucoma with bilateral VF loss, and 65 subjects with AMD with bilateral or severe unilateral loss of VA had their location tracked every 15 minutes between 7 AM and 11 PM for 7 days using a tracking device.

*Main Outcomes and Measures.*—Average daily excursion size (defined as maximum distance away from home) and average daily excursion span (defined as maximum span of travel) were defined for each individual. The effects of vision loss on travel patterns were evaluated after controlling for individual and geographic factors.

*Results.*—In multivariable models comparing subjects with AMD and control subjects, average excursion size and span decreased by approximately one-quarter mile for each line of better-eye VA loss ($P \leq .03$ for both). Similar but not statistically significant associations were observed between average daily excursion size and span for severity of better-eye VF loss in subjects with glaucoma and control subjects. Being married or living with someone and younger age were associated with more distant travel, while less-distant travel was noted for older individuals, African Americans, and those living in more densely populated regions.

*Conclusions and Relevance.*—Age-related macular degeneration-related loss of VA, but not glaucoma-related loss of VF, is associated with restriction of travel to more nearby locations. This constriction of life space may impact quality of life and restrict access to services (Table 1).

▶ The authors of this study utilized cellular tracking to monitor the position of patients with visual impairment from glaucoma and age-related macular degeneration. Measuring position offers an objective, although indirect, measure of visual disability. Interestingly, loss of central acuity from macular degeneration was associated with decreased average maximum distance from home and average maximum excursion span. However, visual field loss from glaucoma was not associated with the same restrictions in travel. It stands to reason that reduced mobility affects quality of life and even access to care.

Although reducing intraocular pressure in patients with glaucoma to prevent vision loss is the basic objective of glaucoma care, the real purpose of caring for patients with glaucoma is to avoid visual disability and maximize quality of life. Not all vision loss is disabling, and treatment for glaucoma in the absence of vision loss (preperimetric glaucoma) may negatively affect quality of life. Medication side effects and cost could decrease quality of life in glaucoma patients who are otherwise asymptomatic. Complications of surgery could cause visual disability in patients whose glaucoma has not yet caused vision loss. Every step taken toward understanding disability from glaucoma (or glaucoma care) helps us approach the ultimate goal of minimizing it.

**S. Fudemberg, MD, FACS**

**Assessment of the Quality of Glaucoma Referral Letters Based on a Survey of Glaucoma Specialists and a Glaucoma Guideline**

Cheng J, Beltran-Agullo L, Trope GE, et al (Univ of Toronto, Ontario, Canada)

*Ophthalmology* 121:126-133, 2014

*Objective.*—To assess the quality of glaucoma referral letters and to report on the results of a survey of glaucoma specialists about referral letter content.

*Design.*—Cross-sectional study.

*Participants.*—A survey of 135 glaucoma specialists and audit of 200 consecutive referral letters to a tertiary glaucoma unit.

*Methods.*—An online questionnaire was sent to members of the Canadian and American Glaucoma Societies asking what they considered the most important data to be included in a glaucoma referral. Consecutive referral letters to a tertiary glaucoma unit were assessed for legibility

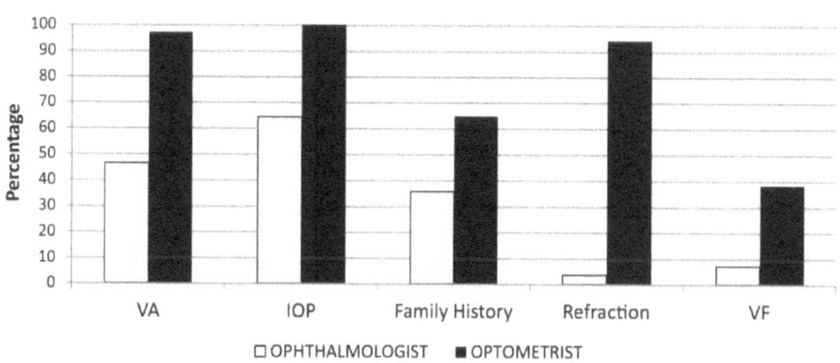


FIGURE 2.—Percentage of referrals from ophthalmologists and optometrists that included visual acuity (VA), intraocular pressure (IOP), family history, refraction, and visual fields (VFs) in referral letters requesting the diagnosis of glaucoma. All 5 information items have statistically significant differences between ophthalmologists and optometrists. (Reprinted from Cheng J, Beltran-Agullo L, Trope GE, et al. Assessment of the quality of glaucoma referral letters based on a survey of glaucoma specialists and a glaucoma guideline. *Ophthalmology.* 2014;121:126-133, Copyright 2014, with permission from by the American Academy of Ophthalmology.)

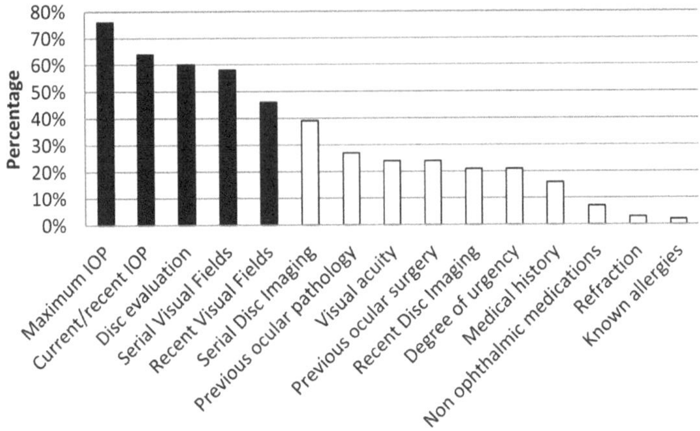


FIGURE 3.—Survey results for the top 5 clinical information items to be included in a referral letter for the diagnosis of glaucoma. The top 5 answers are in *black*, and the remaining are in *white*. IOP = intraocular pressure. (Reprinted from Cheng J, Beltran-Agullo L, Trope GE, et al. Assessment of the quality of glaucoma referral letters based on a survey of glaucoma specialists and a glaucoma guideline. *Ophthalmology*. 2014;121:126-133, Copyright 2014, with permission from by the American Academy of Ophthalmology.)

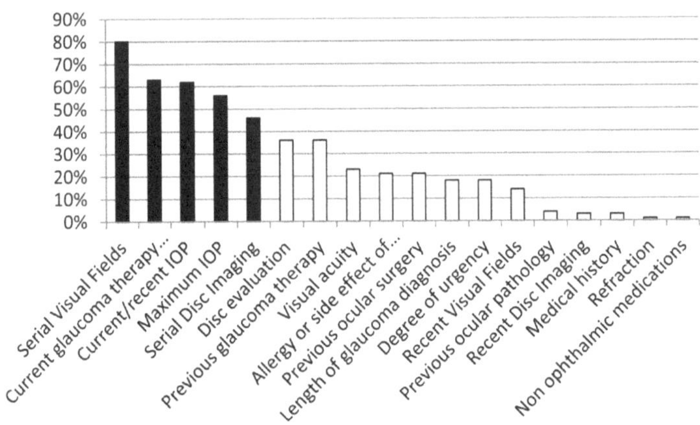


FIGURE 4.—Survey results for the top 5 information items to be included in a referral letter for unstable glaucoma (progression or surgery). The top 5 answers are in black, and the remaining are in white. IOP = intraocular pressure. (Reprinted from Cheng J, Beltran-Agullo L, Trope GE, et al. Assessment of the quality of glaucoma referral letters based on a survey of glaucoma specialists and a glaucoma guideline. *Ophthalmology*. 2014;121:126-133, Copyright 2014, with permission from by the American Academy of Ophthalmology.)

and content on the basis of the survey results and information items in current guidelines.

*Main Outcome Measures.*—Survey outcome and proportion of included content items in referral letters.

*Results.*—The survey revealed that the top 5 most important data that glaucoma specialists would like to be included in a referral letter for

TABLE 1.—Source and Reason for Referral

| Referral Source | Diagnosis of Glaucoma | Assessment for Progression or Surgery | Narrow Angle Assessment | Transfer of Care | Second Opinion | Other Acute, Uncontrolled IOP after Surgery | Cataract Assessment | Total |
|---|---|---|---|---|---|---|---|---|
| Ophthalmologist | 28 (14) | 41 (20.5) | 3 (1.5) | 5 (2.5) | 7 (3.5) | 8 (4) | 0 (0) | 92 (46) |
| Optometrist | 34 (17) | 8 (4) | 31 (15.5) | 8 (4) | 2 (1) | 0 (0) | 1 (0.5) | 84 (42) |
| Family physician | 8 (4) | 1 (0.5) | 0 (0) | 6 (3) | 4 (2) | 0 (0) | 1 (0.5) | 20 (10) |
| Other | 3 (1.5) | 0 (0) | 0 (0) | 1 (0.5) | 0 (0) | 0 (0) | 0 (0) | 4 (2) |
| Total | 73 (36.5) | 50 (25) | 34 (17) | 20 (10) | 13 (7.5) | 8 (4) | 2 (1) | 200 (100) |

IOP = intraocular pressure. Data are n (%).

progressive glaucoma were serial visual fields (VFs), current glaucoma therapy, current intraocular pressure (IOP), maximum IOP, and serial disc imaging. These items often were omitted in the referral letters audited. A total of 200 referral letters were assessed, 46% from ophthalmologists, 42% from optometrists, 10% from family practitioners, and 2% from other sources. Reasons for referral were diagnosis of glaucoma (37%), unstable glaucoma (25%), angle assessment (17%), and others (21%). Some 26% of the referral letters were deemed illegible (18% from ophthalmologists vs. 6% from optometrists; $P < 0.01$). Degree of urgency was mentioned in 27% of referrals. Optometrists were more likely than ophthalmologists to provide visual acuity (VA), IOP, refraction, and VFs ($P < 0.01$ for each). Some 24% of referrals for progression included more than 10 of the 14 information points suggested by the Canadian glaucoma guidelines, and 34% included fewer than 8 of the 14 points.

*Conclusions.*—Referral letters frequently did not include important information, with 34% of referral letters deemed substandard. Optometrist referrals were better than ophthalmologist referrals in terms of content and legibility. A checklist of clinical details for referring physicians is suggested, which includes maximum and current IOP, disc evaluation, serial VFs, and serial disc imaging (Figs 2-4, Table 1).

▶ Communication of information among different facilities and members of the health care system is fraught with barriers. Lack of uniformity in medical record systems precludes easy flow and interpretation of data. Efforts to protect privacy are essential but add steps to the process of transferring information. Busy clinical schedules make conversations among practitioners difficult. These and other obstacles may lead to duplication of services and problems with triaging patients when care is transferred to a specialist.

This study examines the referral letter by surveying glaucoma specialists about desired information and assessing referral letters for legibility and content. Table 1 describes the referred patients, and Figs 3 and 4 show specialists desired information. Table 2 in the original article shows that referral letters often lack the basic information specialists want.

Ultimately, better organization of the referral process and medical records would help patients, referring doctors, and specialists.

**S. Fudemberg, MD, FACS**

---

## The Ahmed Versus Baerveldt Study: Three-Year Treatment Outcomes

Christakis PG, Tsai JC, Kalenak JW, et al (Univ of Toronto Faculty of Medicine, Canada; Yale School of Medicine, New Haven, CT; Drs. Massaro & Kalenak SC, Milwaukee, WI; et al)

*Ophthalmology* 120:2232-2240, 2013

---

*Objective.*—To compare 2 commonly used aqueous drainage devices for the treatment of refractory glaucoma.

TABLE 3.—Reasons for Failure during Three Years of Follow-up

| | Ahmed (n = 124) | Baerveldt (n = 114) |
|---|---|---|
| Success | 61 (49%) | 75 (66%) |
| Complete* | 5 (4%) | 13 (11%) |
| Failure† | 63 (51%) | 39 (34%) |
| High IOP (>18 mm Hg for consecutive visits) | 50 (40%) | 21 (18%) |
| Requiring additional glaucoma surgery | 14 (11%) | 7 (6%) |
| Volatile IOP or inadequate reduction‡ | 9 (7%) | 8 (7%) |
| Progression to NLP | 2 (2%) | 4 (4%) |
| Devastating complications | 2 (2%) | 6 (5%) |

IOP = intraocular pressure; NLP = no light perception.
*$P = 0.047$ (Fisher exact test).
†$P = 0.013$ (Fisher exact test).
‡Consecutive visits in which IOP >18 or <5 mm Hg or <20% reduction from baseline.

TABLE 5.—Postoperative Complications during 3 Years of Follow-up

| | Ahmed (n = 124) | Baerveldt (n = 114) | *P* Value* |
|---|---|---|---|
| Shallow anterior chamber | 18 (15%) | 19 (17%) | 0.72 |
| Choroidal effusion | 16 (13%) | 16 (14%) | 0.85 |
| Persistent Iritis | 7 (6%) | 11 (10%) | 0.33 |
| Persistent corneal edema | 9 (7%) | 16 (14%) | 0.095 |
| Encapsulated bleb | 14 (11%) | 3 (3%) | 0.011 |
| Tube complications† | 18 (15%) | 18 (16%) | 0.86 |
| Cataract progression‡ | 7 (6%) | 10 (9%) | 0.45 |
| Motility disorder | 7 (6%) | 3 (3%) | 0.34 |
| Persistent hyphema | 4 (3%) | 6 (5%) | 0.53 |
| No light perception | 5 (4%) | 6 (5%) | 0.76 |
| Malignant glaucoma | 2 (2%) | 2 (2%) | 1.00 |
| Suprachoroidal hemorrhage | 0 (0%) | 3 (3%) | 0.11 |
| Retinal/choroidal detachment | 1 (1%) | 3 (3%) | 0.35 |
| Endophthalmitis/episcleritis | 2 (2%) | 0 (0%) | 0.50 |
| Patients with complications | 64 (52%) | 71 (62%) | 0.12 |

*Fisher exact test.
†Includes tube obstruction, malposition, and erosion.
‡Corrected for the number of phakic patients.

*Design.*—International, multicenter, randomized trial.

*Participants.*—Patients aged 18 years or older with uncontrolled or high-risk glaucoma refractory to maximum medical therapy, many of whom had failed trabeculoplasty and trabeculectomy.

*Methods.*—Eligible patients were randomized to an Ahmed-FP7 valve implant (New World Medical, Inc., Rancho Cucamonga, CA) or a Baerveldt-350 implant (Abbott Medical Optics, Inc., Santa Ana, CA) using a standardized surgical technique.

*Main Outcome Measures.*—The primary outcome was failure, defined as intraocular pressure (IOP) outside of the target range (5–18 mm Hg, with

≥20% reduction from baseline) for 2 consecutive visits after 3 months, vision-threatening complications, de novo glaucoma procedures, or loss of light perception. Secondary outcome measures include IOP, medication use, visual acuity, complications, and interventions.

*Results.*—A total of 238 patients were enrolled and randomized; 124 received the Ahmed implant and 114 received the Baerveldt implant. Baseline characteristics were similar in both groups. Half the study group had secondary glaucoma, and 37% had previously failed trabeculectomy. The mean preoperative IOP was 31.4 ± 10.8 mm Hg on 3.1 ± 1.0 glaucoma medications. Median baseline Snellen visual acuity was 20/100. At 3 years, the cumulative probability of failure was 51% in the Ahmed group and 34% in the Baerveldt group ($P = 0.03$). Mean IOP was 15.7 ± 4.8 mm Hg in the Ahmed group (49% reduction) and 14.4 ± 5.1 mm Hg in the Baerveldt group (55% reduction; $P = 0.09$). Mean number of glaucoma medications was 1.8 ± 1.4 in the Ahmed group (42% reduction) and 1.1 ± 1.3 in the Baerveldt group (65% reduction; $P = 0.002$). There was a moderate but similar decrease in visual acuity in both groups ($P < 0.001$). The 2 groups had similar complication rates (52% Ahmed, 62% Baerveldt; $P = 0.12$); however, the Baerveldt group had a higher rate of hypotony-related vision-threatening complications (0% Ahmed, 6% Baerveldt; $P = 0.005$). More interventions were required in the Baerveldt group, although the difference did not reach statistical significance (38% Ahmed, 50% Baerveldt; $P = 0.07$). Most complications were transient, and most interventions were slit-lamp procedures.

*Conclusions.*—Both devices were effective in reducing IOP and glaucoma medications. The Baerveldt group had a lower failure rate and required fewer medications than the Ahmed group after 3 years, but it experienced more hypotony-related vision-threatening complications (Tables 3 and 5).

▶ Both Ahmed and Baerveldt tubes have benefits and limitations. The Ahmed tube shunt includes a valve mechanism at the plate that should limit early hypotony. The Baerveldt shunt has no valve and generally requires steps to minimize early hypotony but has a larger plate that may ultimately yield lower intraocular pressure (IOP).

There are multiple strategies to address early postoperative IOP with Baerveldt shunts. Often, Baerveldt shunts are tied with a dissolvable ligature during surgical implantation (such as 8-0 vicryl), and then venting slits are placed in the tube to allow some aqueous flow during the early postoperative period. Sometimes, an orphan trabeculectomy may be used to lower IOP before release of the dissolvable ligature instead of venting slits. Additionally, a ripcord suture or Latina suture (such as a 4-0 nylon) may be placed into the tube before ligation of a Baerveldt tube and buried underneath the conjunctiva. If elevated IOP is problematic before release of the ligature, a small conjunctival incision at the slit lamp over the ripcord suture permits its removal to allow flow through the tube.

Unfortunately, the early IOP-lowering effect of both shunts may be imprecise. Hypotony and flat chamber may occur despite the Ahmed shunt's valve. A ligature may prove ineffective, or venting slits may yield overfiltration and early hypotony.

Venting slits on a Baerveldt are typically effective for a few weeks but may not be effective at all. A hypertensive phase may occur a few weeks into to the postoperative period with Ahmed shunts. The relatively new Ahmed M4 model (the M4 became clinically available after enrollment for this trial) may mitigate the hypertensive phase. When the dissolvable ligature on a Baerveldt releases, hypotony and flat chamber may be a problem. The Baerveldt 350 shunt has been thought to provide better long-term IOP control. These issues, as well as many others, must be considered when selecting a tube for an individual patient.

The Ahmed Versus Baerveldt Study and The Ahmed Baerveldt Comparison Study are very well-designed, randomized, controlled, prospective clinical trials to elucidate the benefits and limitations of these shunts. This article shows 3-year treatment outcomes of The Ahmed Versus Baerveldt Study. The Baerveldt tube achieved statistically significantly more success with fewer medications than the Ahmed but with more vision-threatening hypotony related complications.

Both shunts achieved impressive results because success required an average of 40% IOP lowering to reach a relatively stringent target of IOP ≤18 mm Hg. However, the failure rates are also impressive. Probability of failure was 51% for Ahmeds and 34% for Baerveldts. Failure rates at a target of ≤14 mm Hg were described as exceptionally high. Unfortunately, complete success was 4% for Ahmeds and 11% for Baerveldts. It's important to keep in mind that tube shunt surgery is typically performed in refractory cases of glaucoma, which affects results.

The outcome of glaucoma filtration surgery, including trabeculectomy, is checkered by failure but remains our most effective surgical treatment for glaucoma.

**S. Fudemberg, MD, FACS**

---

## The effect of steep Trendelenburg positioning on intraocular pressure and visual function during robotic-assisted radical prostatectomy

Hoshikawa Y, Tsutsumi N, Ohkoshi K, et al (St Luke's International Hosp, Tokyo, Japan; et al)
*Br J Ophthalmol* 98:305-308, 2014

---

*Background.*—To evaluate intraocular pressure (IOP) changes in patients undergoing robotic-assisted radical prostatectomy and to evaluate complications from increased IOP.

*Methods.*—Thirty-one eyes scheduled for robotic prostatectomy were included. Perioperative IOP measurements were performed as follows: prior to induction of anaesthesia while supine and awake (T1); immediately post-induction while supine (T2); every hour from 0 to 5 h while anaesthetised in a steep Trendelenburg position (T3–T8); prior to awakening while supine (T9); and 30 min after awakening while supine (T10). A complete ophthalmic examination including visual acuity and retinal nerve fibre layer thickness (RNFL) was performed at enrolment and 1 month postoperatively.

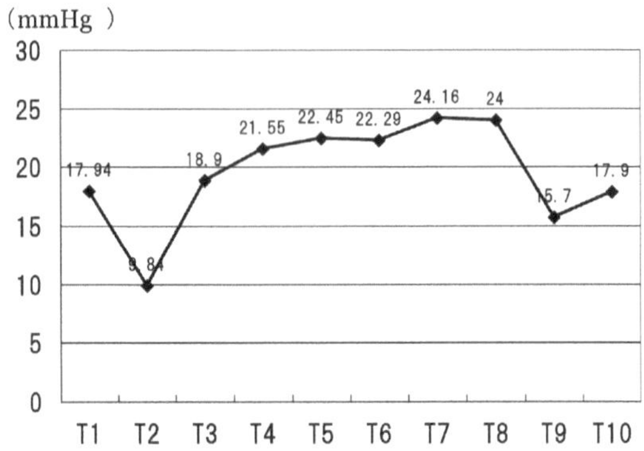


**FIGURE 1.**—Scatter plot of mean intraocular pressure (IOP) at each time point. IOP increases time dependently after steep Trendelenburg positioning (T3–T8). (Reprinted from Hoshikawa Y, Tsutsumi N, Ohkoshi K, et al. The effect of steep Trendelenburg positioning on intraocular pressure and visual function during robotic-assisted radical prostatectomy. *Br J Ophthalmol.* 2014;98:305-308, with permission from the BMJ Publishing Group Ltd.)

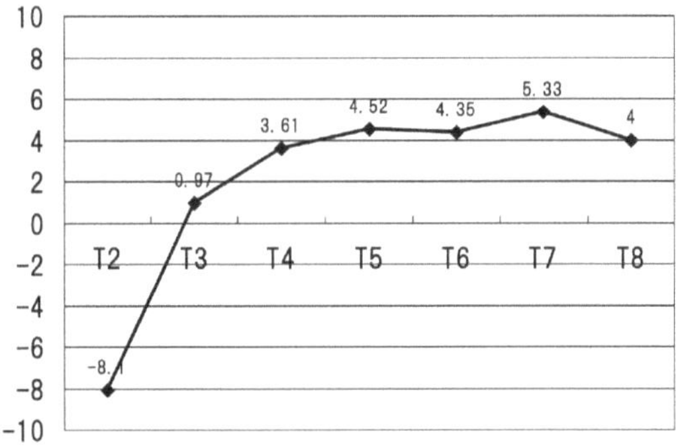


**FIGURE 2.**—Mean change from baseline IOP (T1). IOP increases time dependently after steep Trendelenburg positioning (T3–T8). (Reprinted from Hoshikawa Y, Tsutsumi N, Ohkoshi K, et al. The effect of steep Trendelenburg positioning on intraocular pressure and visual function during robotic-assisted radical prostatectomy. *Br J Ophthalmol.* 2014;98:305-308, with permission from the BMJ Publishing Group Ltd.)

*Results.*—Average IOP (mm Hg) for each time point was as follows: T1 = 18.0, T2 = 9.8, T3 = 18.9, T4 = 21.6, T5 = 22.5, T6 = 22.3, T7 = 24.2, T8 = 24.0, T9 = 15.7 and T10 = 17.9. The proportion of eyes with intraoperative IOP ≥30 mm Hg were as follows: T3 = 0%, T4 = 3.23%, T5 = 9.68%, T6 = 6.45%, T7 = 22.22%, and T8 = 25%. Maximum IOP was 36 mm Hg. Mean visual acuity (logarithm of the minimal angle of resolution) and RNFL showed no statistically significant difference before and after operation and no other ocular complications were found at final examination.

*Conclusions.*—While IOP increased in a time-dependent fashion in anesthaetised patients undergoing robotic-assisted radical prostatectomy in a steep Trendelenburg position, visual function showed no significant change postoperatively and no complications were seen. Steep Trendelenburg positioning during time-limited procedures appears to pose little or no risk from IOP increases in patients without pre-existing ocular disease (Figs 1 and 2).

▶ Robotic-assisted radical prostatectomy is a relatively new surgical technique to treat prostate cancer. The technique involves placing the anesthetized patient in steep Trendelenburg position so gravity will pull the abdominal viscera away from the pelvic cavity. Insufflation of the peritoneal cavity with carbon dioxide is also used to maintain the working field. This results in elevated intraocular pressure (IOP). As the robotic-assisted technique gains popularity, the risk of vision loss in glaucoma patients receives increasing attention in the urology and anesthesiology communities. Patients with glaucoma may now require clearance from an ophthalmologist to undergo this procedure.

This report provides important information about the effect of robotic prostatectomy on IOP. Time points were labeled as T1 to T10:

T1, before induction while supine and awake; T2, immediately postinduction while supine; T3 to 8, every hour while anesthetized in steep Trendelenburg; T9, before awakening while supine; and T10, 30 minutes after awakening while supine.

Figs 1 and 2 show mean IOP at each time point and mean change in IOP from baseline, respectively. They indicate that IOP increases time dependently after steep Trendelenburg positioning. Maximum IOP reached 36 mm Hg, and the proportion of eyes with IOP at least 30 mm Hg increased from 0% at T3 to 25% at T8.

This study strongly shows that IOP increases during robotic prostatectomy. There are no clear guidelines about the risk of vision loss with periods of IOP elevation. Therefore, it is difficult to weigh the risk of vision loss from glaucoma as a result of this technique against the potential benefits of its use. Nonetheless, consideration of the risk is appropriate, particularly for patients with advanced glaucoma.

**S. Fudemberg, MD, FACS**

# 4 Cornea

## Preoperative Graft Thickness Measurements Do Not Influence Final BSCVA or Speed of Vision Recovery After Descemet Stripping Automated Endothelial Keratoplasty

Phillips PM, Phillips LJ, Maloney CM (Sightline Ophthalmic Associates, Sewickley, PA)
*Cornea* 32:1423-1427, 2013

*Purpose.*—To evaluate the influence of preoperative graft thickness (GT) on final visual acuity and speed of vision recovery after Descemet stripping automated endothelial keratoplasty (DSAEK).

*Methods.*—The best spectacle-corrected acuity (BSCVA) was measured after DSAEK was performed at 1, 3, 6, 12, and 24 months. A regression analysis was performed to determine whether GT predicted the BSCVA across each time gate. The time to achieve the "1-year maximum BSCVA" was determined to assess the "speed" of recovery for all eyes that had data at 1, 3, 6, and 12 months. Additionally, the final BSCVA was compared between 2 distinct groups of "thin" (<125-μm) versus "thick" (>165-μm) tissue.

*Results.*—There were 144 eyes evaluated. No significant correlations were found between the GT and the BSCVA at any of the time gates: 1, 3, 6, 12, or 24 months. Speed of vision recovery was not affected by the GT. The average GT values of the eyes that achieved BSCVA by 1, 3, 6 months and 1 year were not significantly different and were 154.7, 141.3, 149, and 150.1 μm, respectively. No difference was found between the BSCVA of "thick" versus "thin" tissues at any of the time gates: 1, 3, 6, or 12 months.

*Conclusions.*—Preoperative GT measurements were not correlated with the BSCVA after the DSAEK was performed at 1, 6, 12, or 24 months postoperatively and do not determine the speed of vision recovery. Additionally, no difference was found in postoperative vision outcomes when directly comparing tissues at either end of the GT spectrum of this study.

▶ With the advent of Descemet membrane endothelial keratoplasty (DMEK), associated with faster visual recovery with improved refractive results, there is a trend toward performing thin and ultrathin Descemet stripping endothelial keratoplasty (DSEK), in hopes of mirroring some of the DMEK success without the difficulties and complications. Thin endothelial grafts have their own inherent issues, including being more difficult to cut, increased tissue wastage from eyebanks, and slightly more difficulty with intraoperative manipulation.

There have been a few studies both supporting and refuting preoperative and postoperative thinness leading to improved visual acuity. In this study, 144 eyes undergoing DSEK were evaluated, comparing preoperative thickness with postoperative visual results over several visits. No difference was found in visual outcomes and speed of visual recovery at any time point.

In this study, thin endothelial grafts were defined as donors less than 125 μm. Only 3 grafts could be considered ultrathin, measuring less than 100 μm. Theoretically, ultrathin grafts may have some benefits in terms of faster visual recovery with improved visual outcomes compared with thin grafts; additional studies specifically focusing on this subset of corneal grafts would be beneficial.

Because of concerns regarding potential corneal tissue waste associated with cutting very thin corneas, the authors conclude that demanding thinner corneal preparation is not warranted at this time. Although these results do support that, as mentioned above, additional data on ultrathin grafts may alter that recommendation. Although our local eye bank does supply thin/ultrathin endothelial grafts, we currently cut our own corneal tissue in most cases. Until we have further evidence supporting thinner endothelial grafts, we will likely continue to do so.

**P. K. Nagra, MD**

### The Steroids for Corneal Ulcers Trial (SCUT): Secondary 12-Month Clinical Outcomes of a Randomized Controlled Trial

Srinivasan M, for the Steroids for Corneal Ulcers Trial Group (Aravind Eye Care System, Madurai, India; et al)

*Am J Ophthalmol* 157:327-333.e3, 2014

*Purpose.*—To determine whether topical corticosteroids as adjunctive therapy for bacterial keratitis improves long-term clinical outcomes.

*Design.*—Randomized, placebo-controlled, double-masked clinical trial.

*Methods.*—This multicenter trial compared 1.0% prednisolone sodium phosphate to placebo in the treatment of bacterial keratitis among 500 patients with culture-positive ulcers receiving 48 hours of moxifloxacin before randomization. The primary endpoint was 3 months from enrollment, and 399 patients were evaluated at 12 months. The outcomes examined were best spectacle-corrected visual acuity (BSCVA) and scar size at 12 months. Based on previous results, regression models with adjustments for baseline status and/or causative organism were used for analysis.

*Results.*—No significant differences in clinical outcomes by treatment group were seen with the prespecified regression models (BSCVA: −0.04 logMAR, 95% CI, −0.12 to 0.05, $P=.39$; scar size: 0.03 mm, 95% CI, −0.12 to 0.18, $P=.69$). A regression model including a *Nocardia*-treatment arm interaction found corticosteroid use associated with a mean 1-line improvement in BSCVA at 12 months among patients with non-*Nocardia* ulcers (−0.10 logMAR, 95% CI, −0.19 to −0.02, $P=.02$). No significant difference was observed in 12-month BSCVA for *Nocardia* ulcers (0.18 logMAR, 95% CI, −0.04 to 0.41, $P=.16$). Corticosteroids were associated with larger mean scar size at 12 months among *Nocardia* ulcers (0.47 mm, 95% CI, 0.06-0.88, $P = .02$) and no significant difference was identified by treatment for scar size for non-*Nocardia* ulcers (−0.06 mm, 95% CI, −0.21 to 0.10, $P = .46$).

*Conclusions.*—Adjunctive topical corticosteroid therapy may be associated with improved long-term clinical outcomes in bacterial corneal ulcers not caused by *Nocardia* species.

▶ The SCUT trial,[1] published in early 2012, found no benefit of corticosteroids for corneal ulcers at 3 months. However, subgroup analysis found that severe ulcers may benefit from the addition of steroids, whereas ulcers caused by *Nocardia* species fared worse with steroids.

The Corneal Ulcers Trial Group followed these patients for 12 months from enrollment and present their findings in this article. They found that steroid use was associated with a 1-line improvement in best spectacle-corrected visual acuity at 12 months in patients with non-*Nocardia* ulcers. In patients with *Nocardia* ulcers, a larger mean scar size was found at 12 months compared with non-*Nocardia* ulcers. The authors conclude that corticosteroids may improve long-term outcomes in ulcers not caused by *Nocardia*.

These study results underscore the importance of microbiology testing in corneal ulcers. Given the difference in outcome based on the microbe identified, performing cultures and having positive results may be important in considering the use of steroids, especially for patients with atypical-appearing or nonresponding infections. These results have directly affected our practice patterns; we typically avoid early steroid use in patients with *Nocardia*. With non-*Nocardia* ulcers, on the other hand, we are less hesitant to start steroids earlier.

**P. K. Nagra, MD**

*Reference*

1. Srinivasan M, Mascarenhas J, Rajaraman R, et al. Corticosteroids for bacterial keratitis: the Steroids for Corneal Ulcers Trial (SCUT). *Arch Ophthalmol.* 2012; 130:143-150.

---

**Topical 0.03% tacrolimus preventing rejection in high-risk corneal transplantation: a cohort study**

Magalhaes OA, Marinho DR, Kwitko S (Clinical Hosp of Porto Alegre, Brazil)
*Br J Ophthalmol* 97:1395-1398, 2013

---

*Background/Aims.*—The present study aims to identify the rate of rejection and safety of 0.03% tacrolimus eye drops associated with 1% prednisolone in a topical formulation, comparing them with the use of 1% prednisolone eye drops alone in patients with high-risk corneal transplantation.

*Methods.*—Retrospective cohort study with 72 patients (72 eyes) who underwent more than one penetrating keratoplasty (PK) in the same eye or had severe chemical burn between 2004 and 2011 in the department of cornea and external disease of the Clinical Hospital of Porto Alegre, Brazil. We compared the records of 36 patients that performed unilateral PK and received only 1% prednisolone eye drops between May 2004 and July 2008, with 36 patients that received 0.03% tacrolimus eye drops in addition to 1% prednisolone between August 2008 and August 2011.

*Results.*—The mean follow-up of the group exposed to tacrolimus was 23.1 months and 24.0 in the prednisolone alone group. The demographics, intraoperative and initial indications for first PK were similar between groups, as well as the number of regrafts performed. Intraocular pressure (IOP) was not statistically different among groups. Regarding irreversible rejections, topical tacrolimus showed greater protection: only seven grafts (19.4%) lost transparency against 16 (44.4%) in the 1% prednisolone alone group ($p < 0.05$).

*Conclusions.*—Topical 0.03% tacrolimus was effective in preventing irreversible rejection in patients with high-risk corneal transplantation without increasing IOP.

▶ Although corneal transplantation is a highly successful procedure, allograft rejection remains a risk, especially among some groups, including repeat grafts, vascularized corneas, chemical burns, and underlying autoimmune disease. The mainstay of prevention of corneal graft rejection is topical steroids. Topical steroids are beneficial but not always successful in preventing rejection, and they also carry inherent risks, including elevated intraocular pressure and cataract formation in phakic patients.

This study evaluated topical tacrolimus, used in conjunction with topical prednisolone 1% in the prevention of high-risk corneal transplant rejection. In this retrospective cohort study comparing prednisolone alone vs prednisolone plus topical tacrolimus, the combination of tacrolimus and prednisolone resulted in significantly less irreversible rejection. Fewer rejection episodes overall were also noted in the tacrolimus group, although this was not statistically significant. Among the 36 patients using tacrolimus, the treatment was well tolerated; no elevation in intraocular pressure was noted in any patients in either group.

Limitations of this study include its small size and retrospective design. Nonetheless, its findings are noteworthy, suggesting we may consider adding tacrolimus to our armamentarium in the management of high-risk corneal transplants. I look forward to additional studies, especially a larger, randomized trial to further establish the efficacy and safety of this treatment.

**P. K. Nagra, MD**

### Deep Anterior Lamellar Keratoplasty versus Penetrating Keratoplasty for Macular Corneal Dystrophy: A Randomized Trial

Sogutlu Sari E, Kubaloglu A, Unal M, et al (Balıkesir Univ, Turkey; Kartal Training and Res Hosp, Istanbul, Turkey; Akdeniz Univ Med Faculty, Antalya, Turkey; et al)
*Am J Ophthalmol* 156:267-274, 2013

*Purpose.*—To compare outcomes of big-bubble deep anterior lamellar keratoplasty (DALK) and penetrating keratoplasty (PK) for macular corneal dystrophy.

*Design.*—Prospective, randomized, interventional case series.

*Methods.*—

*Setting:* Single hospital.

*Patients:* Eighty-two eyes of 54 patients requiring keratoplasty for the treatment of macular corneal dystrophy without endothelial involvement were included.

*Main Outcome Measures:* Operative complications, uncorrected visual acuity, best-corrected visual acuity, contrast sensitivity function, higher-order aberrations, and endothelial cell density were evaluated.

*Results.*—The DALK and PK group consisted of 35 and 41 eyes, respectively. Best-corrected visual acuity after surgery was 20/40 or better 68.5% and 70.7% of the eyes in the DALK and PK groups, respectively ($P > .05$). No statistically significant differences between groups were found in contrast sensitivity function with and without glare for any spatial frequency ($P > .05$). Significantly higher levels of higher-order aberrations were found in the DALK group ($P < .01$). In both groups, a progressive and statistically significant reduction in endothelial cell density was found ($P < .01$). At the last follow-up, the mean endothelial cell loss was 18.1% and 26.9% in DALK and PK groups, respectively ($P = .03$). Graft rejection episodes were seen in 5 eyes (12.1%) in the PK group, and regrafting was necessary in 3 eyes (7.3%). Recurrence of the disease was documented in 5.7% and 4.8% of the eyes in the DALK and PK groups, respectively.

*Conclusions.*—Deep anterior lamellar keratoplasty with the big-bubble technique provided comparable visual and optical results as PK and resulted in less endothelial damage, as well as eliminating endothelial rejection in macular corneal dystrophy. Deep anterior lamellar keratoplasty surgery is a viable option for macular corneal dystrophy without endothelial involvement.

▶ Deep anterior lamellar keratoplasty (DALK) has several advantages over penetrating keratoplasty, including lower risk of graft rejection, less endothelial cell loss, and decreased surgical risk associated with no open-sky time. DALK traditionally has been considered a reasonable and possibly preferred treatment option for conditions such as keratoconus and anterior scars. However, in other conditions, such as macular dystrophy in which there is deep stromal and possible endothelial cell involvement, penetrating keratoplasty (PK) was considered a preferred treatment. Concerns with DALK for macular dystrophy included interface opacification, faster recurrence, and higher rate of endothelial cell loss due to a possible weak or fragile state of the endothelium/Descemet's membrane.

The authors of this study performed a prospective, randomized trial evaluating DALK vs PK for macular dystrophy. Eighty-two eyes of 54 patients were included, with 35 DALK eyes and 41 PK eyes. They found DALK was comparable with PK in visual results, with less endothelial cell loss and no endothelial rejection.

The "big-bubble technique" was performed successfully in 27 eyes; the remaining 8 eyes required manual stromal dissection. Visual outcomes were superior in patients who underwent big-bubble DALK compared with the manual dissection, as would be expected due to interface haze, noted in all manually dissected patients. Interface haze may be more prominent in macular patients compared with patients with more superficial pathology or keratoconus, due to the deep stromal haze noted in this dystrophy.

There was no difference in recurrence of macular dystrophy, with 2 eyes in the DALK group and 2 eyes in the PK group noted to have recurrences at 30 months of follow-up. Further studies with a longer follow-up time would be interesting to see if there was a difference between these procedures.

Overall, based on the results of this study, Descemet's-baring DALK is comparable with PK in visual outcomes, and in fact may be the preferred approach for macular dystrophy given the additional benefits of decreased endothelial cell loss and rejection.

**P. K. Nagra, MD**

---

**Descemet's Stripping Automated Endothelial Keratoplasty: Three-Year Graft and Endothelial Cell Survival Compared with Penetrating Keratoplasty**

Price MO, Gorovoy M, Price FW Jr, et al (Cornea Res Foundation of America, Indianapolis, IN; Gorovoy Eye Specialists, Fort Myers, FL; Price Vision Group, Indianapolis, IN; et al)

*Ophthalmology* 120:246-251, 2013

---

*Purpose.*—To assess 3-year outcomes of Descemet's stripping automated endothelial keratoplasty (DSAEK) in comparison with penetrating keratoplasty (PKP) from the Cornea Donor Study (CDS).

*Design.*—Prospective, multicenter, nonrandomized clinical trial.

*Participants.*—A total of 173 subjects undergoing DSAEK for a moderate risk condition (principally Fuchs' dystrophy or pseudophakic corneal edema) compared with 1101 subjects undergoing PKP from the CDS.

*Methods.*—The DSAEK procedures were performed by 2 experienced surgeons using the same donor and similar recipient criteria as for the CDS PKP procedures, performed by 68 surgeons. Graft success was assessed by Kaplan-Meier survival analysis. Central endothelial cell density (ECD) was determined from baseline donor and postoperative central endothelial images by the reading center used in the CDS Specular Microscopy Ancillary Study.

*Main Outcome Measures.*—Graft clarity and ECD.

*Results.*—The donor and recipient demographics were comparable in the DSAEK and PKP groups, except that the proportion of Fuchs' dystrophy cases was higher in the DSAEK cohort. The 3-year survival rate did not differ significantly between DSAEK and PKP procedures performed for either Fuchs' dystrophy (96% for both; $P = 0.81$) or non-Fuchs' cases (86% vs. 84%, respectively; $P = 0.41$). Principal causes of graft failure or regraft within 3 years after DSAEK and PKP were immunologic graft rejection (0.6% vs. 3.1%), endothelial decompensation in the absence of documented rejection (1.7% vs 2.1%), unsatisfactory visual or refractive outcome (1.7% vs. 0.5%), and infection (0% vs. 1.1%), respectively. The 3-year predicted probability of a rejection episode was 9% with DSAEK versus 20% with PKP ($P = 0.0005$). The median 3-year cell loss for DSAEK and PKP was 46% and 51%, respectively ($P = 0.33$), in Fuchs' dystrophy cases and 59% and 61%, respectively ($P = 0.70$), in the non-Fuchs' cases. At 3 years, use of a smaller DSAEK insertion incision was associated with significantly higher cell loss (60% vs. 33% for 3.2- and 5.0-mm incisions, respectively; $P = 0.0007$), but not with a significant difference in graft survival ($P = 0.45$).

*Conclusions.*—The graft success rate and endothelial cell loss were comparable at 3 years for DSAEK and PKP procedures. A 5-mm DSAEK incision width was associated with significantly less cell loss than a 3.2-mm incision (Fig 1).

▶ The benefits of Descemet stripping automated endothelial keratoplasty (DSAEK) over penetrating keratoplasty (PK) have become well established over the past decade in the cornea literature, including faster visual recovery with improved refractive visual outcomes. Other factors, such as graft failure rates and endothelial cell count loss, have been more difficult to compare between the 2 procedures.

This study prospectively evaluated 173 patients undergoing DSEAK and compared the results to a similar group of 1101 patients from the Cornea Donor Study (CDS) who underwent PK. Although the incidence of graft rejection may be lower in the DSAEK eyes, with a predicted 9% probability of rejection in DSAEK compared with 20% for PK in the cohort from the CDS, the authors found that overall graft survival was similar. At 3 years, the graft survival in both groups was 96% for Fuchs patients and 86% versus 84% in non-Fuchs patients.

In addition, this study found the median cell loss at 3 years was 46% and 51% for DSAEK and PK, respectively. However, small-incision DSAEK (3.2 compared with 5.0 mm) did have statistically significant higher cell loss compared with PK but without a significant difference in graft survival. Given the additional trauma expected in transplanting the endothelial graft through a smaller incision, this finding is not surprising.

Fig 1 shows the median endothelial cell density over time. As the figure demonstrates, DSAEK eyes had a higher rate of cell loss at 1 year (36% vs 18%,

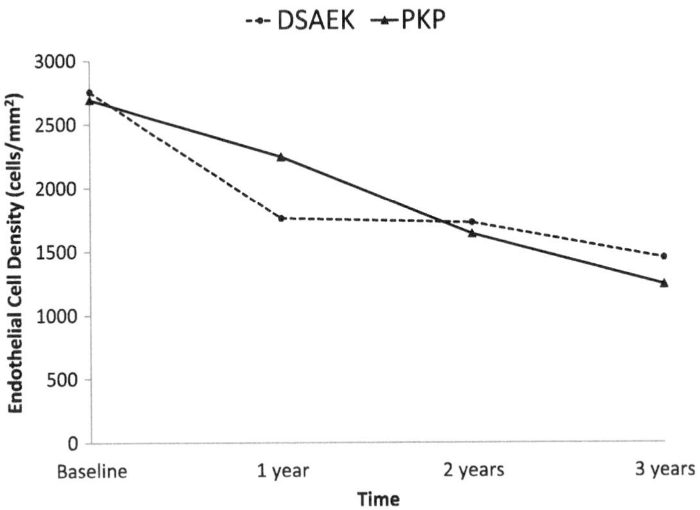


FIGURE 1.—Median endothelial cell density as a function of time for subjects treated with Descemet's stripping automated endothelial keratoplasty (DSAEK) or with penetrating keratoplasty (PKP) in the Specular Microscopy Ancillary Study of the Cornea Donor Study. (Reprinted from Price MO, Gorovoy M, Price FW Jr, et al. Descemet's stripping automated endothelial keratoplasty: three-year graft and endothelial cell survival compared with penetrating keratoplasty. *Ophthalmology.* 2013;120:246-251, Copyright 2013, with permission from the American Academy of Ophthalmology.)

$P < .0001$). There was no significant difference in cell loss at years 2 and 3. The trajectory in the figure suggests PK eyes may have a slow, steady decline, whereas the DSAEK eyes, having a larger initial decline, appear to plateau at 3 years. It would be interesting to follow these data to see what trends develop over several more years.

Although the number of DSAEK patients in the study is noteworthy, follow-up data on many fewer were reported, with only 104 eyes (of 173 eyes measured at baseline) having endothelial cell counts at 1 year and only 66 eyes with cell counts recorded at 3 years. Clearly, additional data are needed to determine the longer-term prognosis for endothelial cell loss. Nonetheless, given concerns regarding endothelial cell damage associated with DSAEK, the results are encouraging.

**P. K. Nagra, MD**

---

**Incidence of Endophthalmitis after Corneal Transplant or Cataract Surgery in a Medicare Population**

Du D, Wagoner A, Barone SB, et al (Ctr for Biologics Evaluation and Res, Rockville, MD; Acumen, LLC, Berkeley, CA; et al)
*Ophthalmology* 121:290-298, 2014

---

*Objective.*—To estimate the incidence of infectious endophthalmitis after corneal transplant or cataract surgery, to evaluate the trend of endophthalmitis during the study period, and to assess demographic risk factors for endophthalmitis after surgeries.

*Design.*—A retrospective population-based cohort study.

*Participants and Controls.*—Study cohorts were derived from the Medicare claims databases, 2006 to 2011. Patients were continuously enrolled in Medicare Part A, Part B, and Part D. Patients undergoing corneal transplant or cataract surgery were identified using International Classification of Diseases, Ninth Revision, Clinical Modification (ICD-9-CM) procedure codes.

*Methods.*—Endophthalmitis was defined in 3 different ways: (1) using ICD-9-CM codes (sensitive definition), (2) combining ICD-9-CM codes with Current Procedural Terminology, Fourth Edition (CPT-4) codes (specific definition), or (3) combining ICD-9-CM codes with antifungal prescriptions for endophthalmitis caused by fungal infection. Demographic risk factors for endophthalmitis were examined using multivariate Cox models.

*Main Outcome Measures.*—Incidence rates of endophthalmitis were calculated and compared for each definition of endophthalmitis at 6-week and 6-month intervals after corneal transplant or cataract surgery.

*Results.*—The infectious endophthalmitis incidence rates ranged from 0.11% to 1.05% in the corneal transplant cohort, 0.06% to 0.20% in the cataract surgery cohort, and 0.16% to 0.68% in the concurrent surgery cohort, depending on the definition and time interval after surgery. Compared with the cataract surgery cohort, the corneal transplant cohort had a higher adjusted hazard ratio (HR) of endophthalmitis within the 6-week postoperative interval (HR, 2.744; 95% confidence interval [CI], 1.544–4.880 in the sensitive definition and HR, 2.792; 95% CI, 1.146–6.802 in the specific definition) and within the 6-month postoperative interval (HR, 4.607; 95% CI, 3.144–6.752 for the sensitive definition and HR, 4.385; 95% CI, 2.245–8.566 for the specific definition).

*Conclusions.*—It is possible to monitor the trend of infectious endophthalmitis after corneal transplant or cataract surgery through examining Medicare claims databases as long as a consistent definition of endophthalmitis is used. The annual incidence of endophthalmitis was stable over time during the study period for both corneal transplant and cataract surgery procedures; however, there was a wider year-to-year variation for the corneal transplant cohort.

► One of the most worrisome complications of intraocular surgery is endophthalmitis. This study evaluated the incidence of endophthalmitis after corneal transplantation and cataract surgery, looking at Medicare claims from 2006 to 2011. The authors assessed the incidence from millions of these surgeries over this period based on ICD-9 codes for endophthalmitis, procedure codes for vitrectromy or intraocular injection of medications, and prescription for antifungal medication (to attempt to distinguish fungal endophthalmitis, as there is no ICD-9 code specifically for this entity).

The incidence rates for endophthalmitis in corneal transplants were 3 times higher than those after cataract surgery at 6 weeks and 5 times higher at 6 months. The annual incidence was stable during the study period although more variation was noted in the corneal transplant cohort with higher rates noted in 2010.

The authors acknowledge several limitations of this study, including reliance on ICD-9 codes and associated unknown coding accuracy, with the study limited to Medicare beneficiaries and difficulty tracking fungal endophthalmitis. Although this Medicare patient population may more accurately represent the cataract patient population, there are large subsets of patients undergoing corneal transplantation that may be missed, specifically younger patients with keratoconus or corneal scars.

Nonetheless, this very large study provides noteworthy results regarding the higher risk of endophthalmitis in corneal transplant compared with cataract surgery. The results also lead to many additional questions, such as were the rates different among Descemet's stripping endothelial keratoplasty, penetrating keratoplasty and deep anterior lamellar keratoplasty patients, what were the culture results, were donor rims cultured and were the same organisms identified in this host, and, most importantly, what can be done to decrease the risk of endophthalmitis?

**P. K. Nagra, MD**

**Corneal Cross-Linking as a Treatment for Keratoconus: Four-Year Morphologic and Clinical Outcomes with Respect to Patient Age**

Vinciguerra R, Romano MR, Camesasca FI, et al (Humanitas Clinical and Res Ctr, Rozzano, Italy; et al)

*Ophthalmology* 120:908-916, 2013

*Purpose.*—To report the 4-year outcomes of corneal cross-linking (CXL) for progressive keratoconus in a population of different age groups.

*Design.*—Retrospective, single-center, nonrandomized clinical study.

*Participants.*—Four hundred consecutive eyes treated with CXL for progressive keratoconus from April 2006 through April 2010.

*Intervention.*—After removal of the epithelium, the cornea was irrigated for 30 minutes with a solution of 0.1% riboflavin and 20% dextran, followed by irradiation with an ultraviolet A light of 3 mW/cm$^2$ for 30 minutes.

*Main Outcome Measures.*—Best-corrected visual acuity (BCVA), sphere and cylinder refraction, corneal topography, Scheimpflug tomography, and aberrometry were assessed at baseline and at 1, 6, 12, 24, 36, and 48 months after CXL treatment. The compiled data were stratified according to age (group A, younger than 18 years; group B, 18–29 years; group C, 30–39 years; and group D, older than 40 years).

*Results.*—Comparative analysis included 400 eyes of 301 patients. Functional results showed a significant increase in BCVA in group A by a mean reduction of −0.11 logarithm of the minimum angle of resolution (logMAR) after 12 months, in group B by a mean reduction of −0.31 logMAR after 36 months, in group C by a mean reduction of −0.33 logMAR after 36 months, and in group D by a mean reduction of −0.26 logMAR after 36 months. Morphologic results showed an analogous regularization of corneal shape with a significant reduction of opposite sector index by a mean value of −0.53 at 12 months in group A, −1.14 at 36 months in group B, −1.10 at 36 months in group C, and −0.55 at 12 months for group D. Optical quality improvement was demonstrated by a mean significant reduction of coma −1.52 μm after 12 months in group A, −1.58 μm after 24 months in group B, −2.57 μm after 36 months for group C, and −0.25 μm after 36 months in group D.

*Conclusions.*—Outcomes stratified by age indicate the efficacy of corneal CXL in stabilizing the progression of ectatic disease in all age groups and improving the functional and morphologic parameters in select groups. Results indicated better functional and morphologic results in the population between 18 and 39 years of age.

▶ Collagen cross-linking (CCL) is a promising new technique used to stabilize or slow the progression of keratoconus. The optimal patient population for this procedure, which was developed in Europe a little more than decade ago, is still being evaluated; however, many cornea specialists agree that this procedure should be recommended for patients showing signs of progressive keratoconus.

The authors of this retrospective study evaluated their outcomes in 400 patients who underwent CCL for progressive keratoconus over a 4-year interval. The patients were stratified into 4 different groups based on their age: less than 18 years, 18 to 29 years, 30 to 39 years, and older than 40 years. They found stabilization in all age groups, although the best visual/functional results and structural/morphologic results were noted in the 18- to 29-year group and the 30- to 39-year group.

Because the youngest patients with keratoconus may be the most likely to progress, theoretically, these patients may benefit most from CCL. This study found patients between 18 and 39 years of age had better functional and morphologic results than patients less than 18. Of note, there were fewest patients in the less-than-18 age group, and data beyond 2 years was not evaluated for this group because the numbers were too small. The authors hypothesize the reason more improvement was not seen with this youngest group was because keratoconus is a more aggressive disease in this patient population. CCL in this more aggressive disease state may produce the observed reduced efficacy compared with older patients with less-aggressive disease.

The main goal of cross-linking is stabilization, and this was achieved in all age groups. As I counsel my patients, although we hope for improvement in visual functioning after this procedure, it is a secondary goal and unfortunately not always realized. This study suggests this may be particularly true for the youngest and oldest patients we treat with keratoconus.

**P. K. Nagra, MD**

## Anatomic and Visual Outcomes of Descemetopexy in Post-Cataract Surgery Descemet's Membrane Detachment

Jain R, Murthy SI, Basu S, et al (L V Prasad Eye Inst, Hyderabad, India)
*Ophthalmology* 120:1366-1372, 2013

*Objective.*—To study the anatomic and visual outcomes of descemetopexy in Descemet's membrane detachment (DMD) after cataract surgery.

*Design.*—Retrospective case series.

*Participants.*—Clinical notes of 60 patients who underwent DMD after cataract surgery between 2007 and 2011.

*Methods.*—Descemetopexy was performed with air or 14% isoexpansile perfluoropropane ($C_3F_8$).

*Main Outcome Measures.*—Anatomical (reattachment rates) and functional results (best-corrected visual acuity) were studied. Secondary outcome measures were assessment of surgical complications and association of various factors with final visual outcome.

*Results.*—The mean age of the patients was 64.3 ± 8.3 years, and the male: female ratio was 21:39. At 1 month, the mean logarithm of the minimum angle of resolution (logMAR) interval visual acuity (IVA) improved from 1.27 ± 0.8 to 0.42 ± 0.49 ($P < 0.001$). Five patients (8.3%) obtained 20/20 vision, and 37 of 60 patients (61.6%) achieved IVA of ≥20/40. Ninety-five percent (57/60) of patients had successful reattachment of the Descemet's membrane (DM) after the intervention. Multiple linear regression analysis showed that patients with a cataract score of 5 (estimate = 0.38; $P = 0.014$), with a cataract score of 4 with compromised visibility due to a corneal opacity (estimate = 0.45; $P = 0.039$), and prolonged duration between cataract surgery and descemetopexy (estimate = 0.012; $P = 0.007$) were associated with a significantly poorer final visual outcome. No association of final visual outcome was observed with age; sex; eye treated; cataract scores 2, 3, and 4; preoperative visual acuity; and involvement of the visual axis ($P > 0.5$). The eyes in which air was used for descemetopexy (estimate = −0.2; $P = 0.009$) had statistically significantly better final visual outcomes. Three patients (5%) had treatment failures and required subsequent endothelial transplantation. Pupillary block was observed in the early postoperative period in 7 patients (11.66%) in whom $C_3F_8$ had been used and was not seen with air ($P = 0.02$).

*Conclusions.*—This study suggests that DMD after cataract surgery can be treated effectively and good visual outcomes can be expected if the patient is treated in time with anterior chamber injection of gas. Air has advantages of better efficacy than $C_3F_8$ without the risk of pupillary block and thus should be preferred.

▶ Descemet's membrane detachment (DMD) is a known complication of cataract surgery. However, the management of this condition (ie, when to intervene, the gas of choice for descemetopexy) and the long-term prognosis of these patients have not been clearly defined.

The authors present the largest case series to date of patients undergoing descemetopexy after postcataract extraction DM detachment. The authors treated 60 patients with detachments, mostly women, with positive outcomes. Only 3 patients (5%) did not respond to treatment and required endothelial keratoplasty. They found 100% air and $C_3F_8$ had similar success rates, but $C_3F_8$ was associated with a higher complication rate (pupillary block seen in 11.66%), thus, 100% air may be the gas of choice for this procedure. The average duration to intervention was 11.46 ± 13 days, and the authors found the final visual acuity was adversely affected by prolonged duration.

One of the major limitations of this study is its retrospective nature. One of the main questions remains: When should we observe for spontaneous resolution vs when should we intervene? Only patients who underwent descemetopexy were included in this study; no data are available regarding how many patients did not require treatment. Further, they found that delay in intervention was associated with worse visual outcome, but there were no clearly defined criteria for when or why descemetopexy was performed.

Further, the primary measures were studied at 1 month. Although 1 month may be sufficient time for patients with healthy endothelial cells to have complete resolution of corneal edema, it may not be enough time for patients with compromised endothelial cell function. Similarly, they noted patients with denser cataracts had worse visual results at 1 month, perhaps related to increased trauma to their endothelial cells during cataract extraction. Outcomes measured at 3 months may be interesting to note, especially in patients with larger detachments, preexisting endothelial cell dysfunction, or more advanced cataracts.

In spite of these limitations, this report adds to our current understanding of the management of DM detachment. We look forward to additional work expanding on these data and especially focusing on when DM detachment can be observed and which require intervention.

**P. K. Nagra, MD**

---

**Rheumatoid Arthritis–Associated Corneal Ulceration: Mortality and Graft Survival**

Stylianides A, Jones MNA, Stewart RMK, et al (Royal Liverpool Univ Hosp, UK; NHS Blood and Transplant, Bristol, UK; et al)

*Ophthalmology* 120:682-686, 2013

---

*Purpose.*—To investigate mortality and graft survival in patients undergoing penetrating keratoplasty (PKP) for rheumatoid arthritis-associated corneal ulceration (RACU), Fuchs' endothelial dystrophy (FED), and pseudophakic bullous keratopathy (PBK).

*Design.*—Case-control study.

*Participants and Controls.*—Patients listed on the UK Transplant Registry who had undergone a PKP for RACU, FED, or PBK between January 4, 1999, and January 4, 2006. Comparative standardized mortality ratios (SMRs) and causes of death were obtained from the Office for National Statistics.

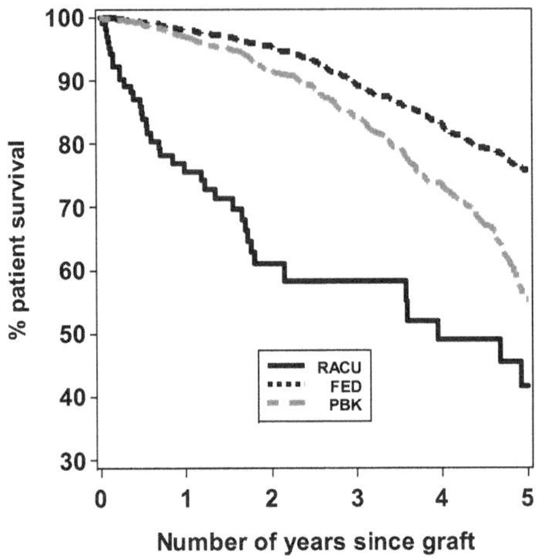


FIGURE 1.—Patient survival for the first penetrating keratoplasty (PKP) for rheumatoid arthritis-associated corneal ulceration (RACU) (*bottom solid line*, n = 106), Fuchs' endothelial dystrophy (FED) (*top broken line*, n = 1700), and pseudophakic bullous keratopathy (PBK) (*middle broken line*, n = 1846). Five-year patient survival rates were 42% (95% confidence interval [CI], 26–56) for RACU, 55% (95% CI, 50–60) for PBK, and 76% (95% CI, 72–78) for FED ($P < 0.0001$). (Reprinted from Ophthalmology. Stylianides A, Jones MNA, Stewart RMK, et al. Rheumatoid arthritis-associated corneal ulceration: mortality and graft survival. *Ophthalmology*. 2013;120:682-686, Copyright 2013, with permission from the American Academy of Ophthalmology.)

*Methods.*—Outcome data were collected from the UK Ocular Tissue National Transplant database and supplementary questionnaires at transplantation and at 1, 2, and 5 years. Institutional review board approval for the National Health Service Blood and Transplant to undertake the study was obtained.

*Main Outcome Measures.*—Mortality and graft survival.

*Results.*—A total of 3665 patients were included: RACU (117), PBK (1701), and FED (1847). Five-year survival of patients with RACU was 42% (95% confidence interval [CI], 26–56) compared with 76% (95% CI, 72–78) for FED and 55% for PBK (95% CI, 50–60; $P < 0.01$). The SMRs for female and male patients with RACU were 43.5 (95% CI, 19.5–63.3) and 12.2 (95% CI, 7.1–19.5), respectively, in comparison with 1.84 and 1.45 for patients with RA, respectively ($P < 0.01$). There were no significant differences in the causes of death among patients with RACU, FED, or PBK ($P > 0.9$), with infection the most common cause. The 5-year graft survival rate was 48% (95% CI, 32–62) for RACU, 59% (95% CI, 56–62) for PBK, and 84% (95% CI, 82–86) for FED ($P < 0.01$).

*Conclusions.*—Mortality and ocular morbidity were significantly increased in patients with RACU. Accelerated immunosenescence should be considered in the differential diagnosis of patients presenting with RACU, and a multidisciplinary approach to management is required (Fig 1).

▶ Rheumatoid arthritis-associated corneal ulceration (RACU) is an uncommon diagnosis for penetrating keratoplasty. Often, patients with RACU present with peripheral corneal melts, typically not amenable to central penetrating keratoplasty, although patch grafts, eccentric grafts, or crescentic grafts may be used, with the primary goal of preserving the eye. It is not surprising, therefore, that these corneal grafts do not do as well as grafts performed for Fuchs' endothelial dystrophy or pseudophakic bullous keratopathy (PBK), as this study confirmed. Interestingly, the main cause of graft failure for patients with RACU was infection, compared with endothelial failure, as was seen in patients with Fuchs' and PBK.

The authors of this study also evaluated mortality in patients with these conditions who required penetrating keratoplasty. As would be expected, patients with RACU had a higher mortality rate. The difference was very significant, with patients with RACU found to be 16 times more likely to die within 5 years of their corneal transplants compared with patients with Fuchs'. Patients with PBK were 1.6 times more likely to die in the same period than their Fuchs' counterparts. As Fig 1 displays, most of the deaths in patients with RACU (85%) occurred within the first 2 years, with only 5 deaths (12%) occurring between years 3 and 5. These findings underscore the severity of the underlying disease and overall poorer systemic health in patients with RACU compared with patients with Fuchs' and PBK.

Although this study had noteworthy findings regarding increased rate of graft failure as well as mortality in patients with RACU, as discussed above, additional studies are required to determine the association between corneal ulceration and systemic vasculitis in patients with rheumatoid arthritis, to further our understanding of the pathology as well as potentially improve our management of this condition. Based on what is evident from this study, as the authors suggest, given the high mortality rate noted in patients with RACU requiring corneal transplantation, multidisciplinary treatment of these patients is critical.

**P. K. Nagra, MD**

---

### Corneal Changes in Neurosurgically Induced Neurotrophic Keratitis

Lambiase A, Sacchetti M, Mastropasqua A, et al (Univ of Rome, Italy; Ospedale San Raffaele di Milano, Italy)
*JAMA Ophthalmol* 131:1547-1553, 2013

---

*Importance.*—Neurotrophic keratitis (NK) represents a sight-threatening complication after trigeminal impairment. To our knowledge, the duration for which trigeminal injury may affect corneal structures and function has not been investigated previously.

*Objective.*—To describe the long-term clinical, morphological, and functional outcomes of NK after neurosurgical trigeminal damage.

*Design, Setting, and Participants.*—Observational case series performed at a corneal and ocular surface diseases referral center in 2010. Eight consecutive patients with monolateral NK from 1 to 19 years after neurosurgery and 20 age- and sex-matched healthy participants were included.

*Main Outcomes and Measures.*—Complete eye examination, tear film function tests, corneal staining, and Cochet-Bonnet esthesiometry were performed. The number and density of corneal nerves, number of hyperreflective keratocytes, and corneal epithelial, endothelial, and keratocyte cell densities were evaluated by in vivo slit scanning confocal microscopy. Clinical and morphological data were compared with the contralateral unaffected eyes and with the eyes of healthy control participants.

*Results.*—All patients showed superficial punctate keratitis and dry eye in the NK eye and a healthy contralateral eye. Decreased corneal sensitivity was observed in all affected eyes (mean [SD], 2.0 [1.9] mm in the affected eyes vs 5.8 [0.3] mm in the contralateral unaffected eyes; $P = .01$) and was related to decreased subbasal nerve length ($P = .04$; $R = 0.895$). Corneal epithelial and endothelial cell densities were significantly decreased and the number of hyperreflective keratocytes was significantly increased in NK eyes compared with contralateral unaffected eyes and with the eyes of healthy participants. A longer duration of NK was associated with lower endothelial cell density ($P = .046$; $R = -0.715$).

*Conclusions and Relevance.*—Corneal morphology and function were impaired even years after neurosurgical trigeminal damage, suggesting that assessment of tear film and corneal sensitivity as well as in vivo confocal microscopy examination should be performed in all patients with trigeminal impairment.

▶ This study investigated 8 consecutive patients with neurotrophic keratitis after neurosurgery in an attempt to evaluate clinical characteristics, including confocal microscopy and functional outcomes. All of these patients shared a history of prior corneal ulceration secondary to their neurotrophia. Half of the patients required tarsorrhaphy placement in their treatment. Although not a very attractive treatment in many ways, we find that tarsorrhaphy does remain an important way to treat patients after surgical trauma in whom no significant recovery of sensation is expected. Three of the remaining 4 patients were treated with a contact lens. The type of lens was not specified, but one does have concerns about the risk of infection with soft contact lens use in these patients with a poor surface and lack of feeling. The PROSE lens, which is a large scleral lens, may provide a reasonable alternative to tarsorrhaphy. The availability, while expanding, is still limited.

The most interesting finding from the confocal microscopy data is that the endothelial cell counts were reduced when compared with the patients' contralateral eye and controls. This has not previously been shown and should be evaluated further. One does wonder to what extent the patient suffered endothelial damage from the prior infectious/inflammatory ulceration. If the reduction of corneal sensation does indeed lead to reduced endothelial density, in the absence of other factors, this is clinically important. This would put patients at even higher risk for corneal decompensation than previously thought.

**K. M. Hammersmith, MD**

**Dry eye disease, dry eye symptoms and depression: the Beijing eye study**
Labbé A, Wang YX, Jie Y, et al (Beijing Tongren Hosp, China; et al)
*Br J Ophthalmol* 97:1399-1403, 2013

*Aim.*—To investigate the association between dry eye symptoms and depression in an adult population.

*Methods.*—In this population-based cross-sectional study, a random sample of 1957 subjects from the Beijing Eye Study was examined for dry eye disease (DED) in 2006. All patients completed an interviewer-assisted questionnaire on dry eye symptoms and underwent measurement of tear break-up time (TBUT), slit-lamp evaluation of corneal staining and meibomian gland dysfunction (MGD), and the Schirmer test. In 2011, 1456 subjects from this sample were evaluated for depression using a depression scale. The association between depression symptoms and dry eye clinical tests was evaluated.

*Results.*—Definite depression was more prevalent in patients with DED than in subjects without DED (13.7±0.4% vs 8.6±0.3%, $p$=0.02). The depression score was correlated with dry eye symptoms (correlation coefficient r=0.07; $p$=0.013) but not with TBUT ($p$=0.18), the Schirmer test ($p$=0.37), corneal staining ($p$=0.30) and MGD evaluation ($p$=0.93). In multivariate regression analysis, the risk of definite depression remained significantly associated with dry eye symptoms ($p$=0.028) after adjusting for lower cognitive status ($p$=0.01), rural region of habitation ($p$=0.023) and lower body weight ($p$=0.05).

*Conclusions.*—In an older population from Beijing, depression was associated with DED and in particular with dry eye symptoms (Table 4).

▶ This is an interesting article, assessing the association between dry eye disease (DED) and depression. Using the Beijing Eye Study, almost 2000 patients were randomly selected in 2006 to have a clinical evaluation for DED. Those patients were also asked a short (3-point) questionnaire to assess for dry eye symptoms. Of those 2000 patients, 1450 were assessed for depression in 2011. The authors found definite depression was more prevalent in patients diagnosed with DED than those without DED. Most interesting was that there was no association among the signs of DED (Schirmer, tear break-up time, corneal staining) but significant association between the symptoms of DED and depression. Thus, the patients who were symptomatic from DED had a higher incidence of definite depression. The study is plagued by the fact that the clinical examination was performed 5 years before the depression evaluation although they did repeat the symptom questionnaire in 2011, and the results were similar to those in 2006. The study also did not assess the use of systemic medications, particularly antidepressants. The issue of the effects of antidepressants on dry eye is a frequent clinical question. Antidepressants may worsen dry eyes, or they may help with associated depression and interpretation of dry eye symptomatology. In my clinical practice, I feel more individuals are helped than harmed by

TABLE 4.—Multivariate Logistic Regression Analysis Between Definite Depression, Demographics and Dry Eye Parameters

| Parameters | OR | Significance | 95% CI Lower | 95% CI Upper |
|---|---|---|---|---|
| Age | 0.99 | *p*=0.57 | 0.96 | 1.02 |
| Female gender | 1.19 | *p*=0.55 | 0.67 | 2.12 |
| Rural residence | **0.45** | ***p*=0.023*** | **0.22** | **0.89** |
| Level of education | 1.28 | *p*=0.09 | 0.96 | 1.7 |
| Gross income | 1 | *p*=0.35 | 0.99 | 1 |
| Body height | 0.99 | *p*=0.89 | 0.96 | 1.03 |
| Body weight | **0.98** | ***p*=0.05*** | **0.96** | **1** |
| Cognitive evaluation | **0.93** | ***p*=0.01*** | **0.87** | **0.98** |
| BCVA | 0.64 | *p*=0.42 | 0.22 | 1.87 |
| DED | 1.11 | *p*=0.77 | 0.55 | 2.25 |
| DES | **1.14** | ***p*=0.028*** | **1.01** | **1.27** |

The dependent variable was the presence of definite depression. Significant values are shown in bold.
BCVA, best corrected visual acuity; DED, dry eye disease; DES, dry eye symptoms.
**p* Values <0.05 were considered significant.

antidepressants with regard to quality of life and DED. This area is certainly in need of more objective data.

**K. M. Hammersmith, MD**

# 5 Retina

## Long-term Outcomes in Ranibizumab-Treated Patients With Retinal Vein Occlusion; The Role of Progression of Retinal Nonperfusion

Sophie R, Hafiz G, Scott AW, et al (The Johns Hopkins Univ School of Medicine, Baltimore, MD)

*Am J Ophthalmol* 156:693-705.e11, 2013

*Purpose.*—To determine the percentage of ranibizumab-treated patients with retinal vein occlusion (RVO) who had resolution of edema for at least 6 months after the last injection, along with factors and outcomes that correlate with resolution.

*Design.*—Post hoc analysis of open-label clinical trial.

*Methods.*—Twenty patients with branch RVO (BRVO) and 20 with central RVO (CRVO) received ranibizumab monthly for 3 months and as needed for recurrent/persistent macular edema, no more frequently than every 2 months. Patients still requiring injections after month 40 received scatter and grid laser photocoagulation to try to reduce the need for injections. Main outcome measures included the percentage of patients who had resolution of edema, change in best-corrected visual acuity (BCVA) from baseline, and change in area of retinal nonperfusion in central subfields.

*Results.*—Nine patients with BRVO (45%) had edema resolution from injections alone after a mean of 20.2 months, 4 resolved after addition of laser, 4 were unresolved through 72 months, and 3 exited prior to resolution. Five patients with CRVO (25%) resolved from injections alone after a mean of 14.0 months, 8 remained unresolved through 72 months despite addition of laser, and 7 exited prior to resolution. For BRVO or CRVO, there was a negative correlation between posterior retinal nonperfusion area and BCVA at months 18, 24, and 36 ($P < .05$).

*Conclusions.*—In patients with RVO, infrequent ranibizumab injections to control edema may not be sufficient to prevent progression of retinal nonperfusion, which may contribute to loss of visual gains.

► Management of macular edema in the setting of a retinal vein occlusion can be challenging. Most recently, intravitreal ranibizumab has been successful to some degree. However, there is a subset of patients that require long-term injections beyond 2 to 3 years. The progression of nonperfusion in both branch retinal vein occlusions (BRVO) and central retinal vein occlusions (CRVO) has been reported widely. The relationship between the macular edema and nonperfusion remains unclear. The study investigators explored the role of nonperfusion on the management of macular edema and visual outcomes. Over the first 3 years, nearly

65% of patients with a BRVO or CRVO showed progression of nonperfusion. Consequently, some patients suffered a decline in visual acuity. When laser was applied to areas of nonperfusion, the results were mixed. In the BRVO arm, the macular edema resolved in 45% of patients with injections alone. Laser resolved the macular edema that was previously unresolved with injections in 20% of patients. However, 20% also did not respond to laser, and the macular edema persisted. In the CRVO arm, the macular edema resolved in 25% of patients with injections alone. In this case, laser did not seem to help resolve additional cases of macular edema. Approximately, 40% of patients were reported to have unresolved macular edema at 72 months despite injections and laser. Unfortunately, retinal vein occlusions represent a large spectrum of severity. Intravitreal injections seem to resolve macular edema in some cases, whereas other cases are recalcitrant despite this combination therapy.

**O. P. Gupta, MD**

**Tubulointerstitial Nephritis and Uveitis Syndrome in Children: A Prospective Multicenter Study**

Saarela V, Nuutinen M, Ala-Houhala M, et al (Oulu Univ Hosp, Finland; Tampere Univ Hosp, Finland; et al)

*Ophthalmology* 120:1476-1481, 2013

*Purpose.*—To evaluate the occurrence and characteristics of uveitis related to tubulointerstitial nephritis (TIN) in children.

*Design.*—Prospective, observational, multicenter, partly placebo-controlled treatment trial.

*Participants.*—Nineteen children with a biopsy-proven TIN.

*Methods.*—Patients were treated with prednisone or followed without treatment. In addition to the nephrologic evaluations, the prospective follow-up included structured ophthalmological examinations at the onset of TIN and at 3 and 6 months after the diagnosis.

*Main Outcome Measures.*—Occurrence, clinical features, and outcome of uveitis.

*Results.*—Some 84% (16/19) of the patients had uveitis, 83% (5/6) in the nontreatment group and 82% (9/11) in the prednisone-treated group. The remaining 2 patients, originally in the nontreatment group, were switched to the prednisone group after 2 weeks. Both of them developed uveitis. Altogether, 3 patients developed uveitis during prednisone treatment and 2 patients showed worsening of uveitis despite the systemic corticosteroid. Some 50% (8/16) of the patients with uveitis presented with no ocular symptoms; 88% (14/16) of the patients had a chronic course of uveitis. Two patients were diagnosed with uveitis before nephritis; nephritis and uveitis were diagnosed within 1 week from each other in 7 patients, and uveitis developed 1 to 6 months after the diagnosis of TIN in 7 patients.

*Conclusions.*—There was no statistically significant difference in the occurrence of uveitis in patients with TIN in the prednisone and nontreatment groups. In this study, the occurrence of uveitis associated with TIN was considerably higher than previously reported. Uveitis related to TIN may develop late and is often asymptomatic. The ophthalmological follow-up of all patients with TIN is warranted for at least 12 months starting with 3-month intervals.

▶ Tubulointerstitial nephritis (TIN) is an inflammatory disease of the kidneys with nearly half the cases associated with uveitis. The highest incidence of uveitis associated with TIN occurs in patients less than 20 years old. This evaluated the occurrence and characteristics of uveitis in these patients. The incidence of uveitis was similar between groups treated with prednisone compared with those that were followed conservatively. The overall incidence was approximately 82% to 84%. In addition, these patients were often asymptomatic. The onset of uveitis can be the presenting symptom of TIN or develop up to 6 months after the diagnosis is made. Currently, most patients are being treated with methotrexate. The authors recommend initially performing an ophthalmologic screening every 3 months followed by at least a yearly examination.

**O. P. Gupta, MD**

---

**A Prospective Randomized Trial of Intravitreal Bevacizumab Versus Ranibizumab for the Management of Diabetic Macular Edema**

Nepomuceno AB, Takaki E, Paes de Almeida FP, et al (Univ of São Paulo, Ribeirão Preto, Brazil; et al)

*Am J Ophthalmol* 156:502-510.e2, 2013

---

*Purpose.*—To compare visual acuity and spectral-domain optical coherence tomography (SDOCT) outcomes associated with intravitreal (IV) bevacizumab vs IV ranibizumab for the management of diabetic macular edema (DME).

*Design.*—Prospective randomized trial.

*Methods.*—Forty-eight patients (63 eyes) with center-involved DME were randomly assigned to receive 1.5 mg (0.06 cc) IV bevacizumab or 0.5 mg (0.05 cc) IV ranibizumab at baseline and monthly if central subfield thickness was greater than 275 μm.

*Results.*—Forty-five patients (60 eyes) completed 48 weeks of follow-up. At baseline, mean ± standard error best-corrected visual acuity (BCVA) (logMAR) was 0.60 (20/80) ± 0.05 in the IV bevacizumab group and 0.63 (20/85) ± 0.05 in the IV ranibizumab group. A significant improvement in mean BCVA was observed in both groups at all study visits ($P < .05$); this improvement was significantly greater in the IV ranibizumab group compared with the IV bevacizumab group at weeks 8 ($P = .032$) and 32 ($P = .042$). A significant reduction in mean central subfield thickness was observed in both groups at all study visits compared with baseline ($P < .05$), with no significant difference in the magnitude of macular thickness reduction between groups. The mean number of injections was significantly higher ($P$ =.005) in the IV bevacizumab group (9.84) than in the IV ranibizumab group (7.67).

*Conclusions.*—IV bevacizumab and IV ranibizumab are associated with similar effects on central subfield thickness in patients with DME through 1 year of follow-up. IV ranibizumab is associated with greater improvement in BCVA at some study visits, and the mean number of injections is higher in the IV bevacizumab group.

▶ In the CATT trial, bevacizumab and ranibizumab were found to have similar outcomes in patients treated for neovascular age-related macular degeneration. However, in other retinal conditions that have a relatively higher vascular endothelial growth factor (VEGF) load, there is an interesting debate on the superiority of anti-VEGF agents. This study compared bevacizumab with ranibizumab for the management of diabetic macular edema. Eyes were randomly assigned to either medication and were eligible to receive monthly injections based on retreatment criteria. Focal laser photocoagulation was available at the 3-month time point as a rescue therapy. The improvement in visual acuity was significantly greater in the ranibizumab arm compared with the bevacizumab arm at the 48-week endpoint. In addition, the mean number of injections was higher in the bevacizumab arm compared with the ranibizumab arm. A significantly higher number of eyes met the criteria for rescue therapy in the bevacizumab arm compared with the ranibizumab arm. Although this study is limited because of its small sample size, it is a well-designed, prospective, randomized trial. Given the fact that ranibizumab has a higher affinity to VEGF, diabetic macular edema might respond differently to these 2 agents. Currently, larger studies are ongoing to help substantiate these findings.

**O. P. Gupta, MD**

---

**Mineralocorticoid receptor antagonism in the treatment of chronic central serous chorioretinopathy: a pilot study**

Bousquet E, Beydoun T, Zhao M, et al (Univ Rene Descartes Sorbonne Paris Cité, France)

*Retina* 33:2096-2102, 2013

---

*Purpose.*—Based on experimental data showing that central serous chorioretinopathy could result from overactivation of mineralocorticoid receptor pathway in choroid vessels, the authors studied eplerenone, a mineralocorticoid receptor antagonist, as a potential treatment for chronic central serous chorioretinopathy.

*Methods.*—This nonrandomized pilot study included 13 patients with central serous chorioretinopathy of at least 4-month duration, treated with 25 mg/day of oral eplerenone for a week followed by 50 mg/day for 1 or 3 months. The primary outcome measure was the changes in central macular thickness recorded by optical coherence tomography, and the secondary outcomes included changes in foveal subretinal fluid (SRF) measured by OCT, in best-corrected visual acuity (BCVA) and the percentage of eyes achieving complete resolution of subretinal fluid during the treatment period.

*Results.*—Central macular thickness decreased significantly from 352 ± 139 $\mu$m at baseline to 246 ± 113 $\mu$m and 189 ± 99 $\mu$m at 1 and 3 months under eplerenone treatment ($P < 0.05$ and $P < 0.01$, respectively). At 3 months, the subretinal fluid significantly decreased compared with baseline subretinal fluid ($P < 0.01$) and best-corrected visual acuity significantly improved compared with baseline best-corrected visual acuity ($P < 0.001$).

*Conclusion.*—Eplerenone treatment was associated with a significant reduction in central macular thickness, subretinal fluid level, and an improvement in visual acuity. Randomized controlled trials are needed to confirm these encouraging results.

▶ The management of chronic central serous chorioretinopathy (CSCR) is challenging. Several local and systemic treatments have been described with varied success. Most of the treatments have focused on the angiogenic or mineralocorticoid pathways of CSCR. Eplerenone is an oral medication that has been used for the treatment of hypertension and congestive heart failure. It is a diuretic but specifically acts as a mineralocorticoid receptor antagonist. Therefore, based on experimental data that CSCR results from an overactivation of the mineralocorticoid receptor pathway in choroidal vessels, the authors explored its use for the CSCR in this nonrandomized pilot study. Thirteen patients were included for at least 4 months and were treated with eplerenone, 25 mg/d for 1 week then 50 mg/d for 1 to 3 months. A reduction of mean central thickness on optical coherence tomography as well as subretinal fluid was noted. An improvement in visual acuity was also noted. However, some patients experienced a dramatic response, whereas other patients had virtually no response. This might reflect the variety of mechanisms that could result in what we clinically diagnose as CSCR. This is a small cohort study, and a larger analysis needs to be performed to determine the efficacy.

**O. P. Gupta, MD**

## Spontaneous Vitreous Hemorrhage in Children

Sudhalkar A, Chhablani J, Jalali S, et al (L.V. Prasad Eye Inst, Hyderabad, India; et al)

*Am J Ophthalmol* 156:1267-1271.e2, 2013

*Purpose.*—To determine the clinical profile, causes, and outcomes of "spontaneous" vitreous hemorrhage in children (<18 years).

*Design.*—Retrospective computer-assisted chart review.

*Methods.*—Charts of 124 eyes of 76 children who presented with nontraumatic, nonsurgical vitreous hemorrhage between 2002 and 2012 were reviewed. All children underwent an appropriate ocular and systemic examination. Data collected included demographics, visual acuity, cause of "spontaneous" vitreous hemorrhage, ocular and systemic findings at presentation and at last follow-up, investigations, management details, and visual outcomes.

*Results.*—The median age was 153.45 ± 56.19 months. There were 39 female and 37 male patients. Forty-eight patients had bilateral vitreous hemorrhage. The most common presenting complaints were diminished vision (96.45%) and behavioral changes (87.24%). The mean baseline BCVA in logMAR was 2.25 ± 1.11. The most common causes included vasculitis (34.6%) and hematologic disorders (27.4%). Patients were given medical therapy (topical and/or systemic) or underwent laser photocoagulation (29%) and/or surgery (55.6%). Twenty-nine eyes (23.3%) did not require any intervention. The mean number of surgeries was 1.89 ± 1.45 (range 1-4 surgeries). The mean final visual acuity was 0.76 ± 0.58 logMAR and was significantly better than the baseline ($P < .001$). The best anatomic and visual outcomes were seen in vasculitis, whereas congenital disorders such as retinoschisis had the worst.

*Conclusions.*—Spontaneous pediatric vitreous hemorrhage has a diverse etiology, vasculitis being the most common cause in our series. A comprehensive evaluation (systemic and ocular) is required to ensure that vision and life-threatening conditions are not missed.

▶ Spontaneous vitreous hemorrhage in children continues to be a common presentation to pediatric ophthalmologists and retinal specialists alike. The authors explored etiologies and outcomes, including trauma and retinopathy of prematurity, in patients that present with no known risk factors. Almost 40% of the time it can present bilaterally. The most presenting symptom in verbal patients was decreased vision. Behavioral changes were most common in nonverbal patients. Vasculitis, hematologic disorders, ocular tumors/vascular malformations, familial exudative vitreoretinopathy, retinal tear/detachment, and diabetic retinopathy were among the most frequent causes. Most cases required surgery, whereas about a quarter of patients did not require any intervention. The ultimate visual outcome was dependent on the underlying etiology. Although this report did not present significantly new data, it does provide a great review and systematic approach to evaluating these patients.

**O. P. Gupta, MD**

---

**Macular Edema After Cataract Surgery in Eyes Without Preoperative Central-Involved Diabetic Macular Edema**

Diabetic Retinopathy Clinical Research Network Authors/Writing Committee (Paducah Retinal Ctr, KY; Jaeb Ctr for Health Res, Tampa, FL; Wilmer Ophthalmological Inst, Baltimore, MD; et al)

*JAMA Ophthalmol* 131:870-879, 2013

---

*Importance.*—The incidence of development or worsening of macular edema (ME) is variable in eyes without diabetic ME (DME) undergoing cataract surgery.

*Objective.*—To estimate the incidence of central-involved ME 16 weeks following cataract surgery in eyes with diabetic retinopathy without definite central-involved DME preoperatively.

*Design, Setting, and Participants.*—In a multicenter, prospective, observational study, 293 participants with diabetic retinopathy without definite central subfield thickening on optical coherence tomography (OCT) underwent cataract surgery.

*Exposure.*—Cataract extraction surgery performed within 28 days of enrollment of eyes without DME in individuals with diabetes mellitus.

*Main Outcomes and Measures.*—Development of central-involved ME defined as the following: (1) OCT central subfield thickness of 250 μm or greater (time-domain OCT) or 310 μm or greater (spectral-domain OCT) with at least a 1-step increase in logOCT central subfield thickness preoperatively to the 16-week visit; (2) at least a 2-step increase in logOCT central subfield thickness preoperatively to the 16-week visit; or (3) nontopical treatment for ME received before the 16-week visit with either of the OCT criteria met at the time of treatment.

*Results.*—The median participant age was 65 years. The median visual acuity letter score was 69 letters (Snellen equivalent 20/40). Forty-four percent of eyes had a history of treatment for DME. Sixteen weeks postoperatively, central-involved ME was noted in 0% (95% CI, 0%-20%) of 17 eyes with no preoperative DME. Of eyes with non-central-involved DME, 10% (95% CI, 5%-18%) of 97 eyes without central-involved DME and 12% (95% CI, 7%-19%) of 147 eyes with possible central-involved DME at baseline progressed to central-involved ME. History of DME treatment was significantly associated with central-involved ME development ($P < .001$).

*Conclusions and Relevance.*—In eyes with diabetic retinopathy without concurrent central-involved DME, presence of non-central-involved DME immediately prior to cataract surgery or history of DME treatment may increase the risk of developing central-involved ME 16 weeks after cataract extraction.

▶ Risk stratifying patients with diabetic retinopathy in the preoperative assessment for cataract surgery can be challenging. The authors evaluated the incidence of central-involving diabetic macular edema (DME) 16 weeks after cataract surgery. In eyes without DME preoperatively, the postoperative risk of ME was 0%. In eyes with noncentral DME preoperatively, 10% progressed to central-involving ME. In eyes with possible central-involving DME preoperatively, 12% progressed to become central-involving ME. In addition, patients with a history of DME treatment had a 21% incidence of ME after cataract surgery at the 16-week endpoint. More than 85% of the eyes had a visual acuity of 20/40 or better. On the other hand, visual acuity loss of at least 10 letters occurred in about 4% of patients. Recognizing these high-risk patients and high-risk characteristics are key to optimizing outcomes.

**O. P. Gupta, MD**

**SAVE (Super-dose Anti-VEGF) Trial: 2.0 mg Ranibizumab for Recalcitrant Neovascular Age-Related Macular Degeneration: 1-Year Results**

Wykoff CC, SAVE Study Group (Methodist Hosp, Houston, TX)

*Ophthalmic Surg Lasers Imaging Retina* 44:121-126, 2013

*Objectives.*—To assess durability of visual and anatomic gains with 2.0 mg ranibizumab in recalcitrant neovascular age-related macular degeneration (AMD).

*Methods.*—Phase I-II trial of 88 patients with recalcitrant neovascular AMD treated as needed every 4 (cohort A) or 6 weeks (cohort B) following three monthly doses. ETDRS refraction and spectral-domain OCT–guided as-needed re-treatments.

*Results.*—Seventy-nine patients completed the 12-month endpoint and were given 11.6 (cohort A) and 8.6 (cohort B) mean treatments. Mean best corrected visual acuity gains of 4.1 letters following three monthly doses were sustained for 12 months for both cohorts. Anatomic improvements were sustained for 12 months for cohort A, but not for cohort B; cohort B demonstrated a gradual increase in mean central retinal thickness ($P = .03$).

*Conclusion.*—Visual and anatomic gains achieved with 2.0 mg ranibizumab in recalcitrant neovascular AMD were sustained for 1 year with monthly treatment. In comparison, anatomic gains were diminished with less than monthly treatment.

► As we move further along in the age of intravitreal injections for neovascular age-related macular degeneration, it has become increasingly clear that heterogeneity exists in the response to treatment. This study highlights a unique treatment for recalcitrant patients who were receiving a more standard regimen. At the higher dose of ranibizumab, the authors noted an improved visual and anatomic outcome. This was a well-designed prospective study of a small number of patients. The other issue is regarding practical application. Most likely there will not be another product issued for this clinical scenario. Practitioners will most likely use an increased volume of the standard concentration. This is not the product used in the study. The study used a more concentrated product with the standard volume of injection (0.05 mL). The increased volume is not ideal because of increased intraocular pressure as well as progression of glaucoma in patients with high risk.

**O. P. Gupta, MD**

**Impact of the Revised American Academy of Ophthalmology Guidelines Regarding Hydroxychloroquine Screening on Actual Practice**

Browning DJ (Charlotte Eye, Ear, Nose, and Throat Associates, Charlotte, NC)

*Am J Ophthalmol* 155:418-428, 2013

*Purpose.*—To determine the impact of the revised academy guidelines on screening for hydroxychloroquine retinopathy.

*Design.*—Retrospective, observational cohort study.

*Methods.*—

*Setting:* Private practice of 29 doctors.

*Study Population:* Total of 183 patients for follow-up and 36 patients for baseline screening.

*Observation Procedure:* Review of charts, 10-2 visual fields (VFs), multifocal electroretinograms (mfERG), and spectral-domain optical coherence tomography (SD-OCT) images before and after the revised guidelines.

*Main Outcome Measure:* Rates of use of ancillary tests and clinical intervention, costs of screening, follow-up schedules, and comparative sensitivity of tests.

*Results.*—New hydroxychloroquine toxicity was found in 2 of 183 returning patients (1.1%). Dosing above 6.5 mg/kg/d was found in 28 of 219 patients (12.8%), an underestimate because patient height, weight, and daily dose were not determined in 77 (35.1%), 84 (38.4%), and 59 (26.9%), respectively. In 10 of the 28 (35.7%), the dose was reduced, in 2 (7.1%) hydroxychloroquine was stopped, but in 16 (57.1%) no action was taken. The cost of screening rose 40%/patient after the revised guidelines. Fundus autofluorescence (FAF) imaging was not used. No toxicity was detected by adding mfERG or SD-OCT. In no case was a 5-year period free of follow-up recommended after baseline screening in a low-risk patient.

*Conclusions.*—Detection of toxic daily dosing is a cost-effective way to reduce hydroxychloroquine toxicity, but height, weight, and daily dose were commonly not checked. The revised guidelines, emphasizing mfERG, SD-OCT, or FAF, raised screening cost without improving case detection. The recommended 5-year screening-free interval for low-risk patients after baseline examination was ignored.

▶ The revised guidelines for hydroxychloroquine screening were published in 2011. The recommendations outlined the importance of multifocal electroretinogram as the gold standard. Fundus autofluorescence and spectral-domain optical coherence tomography have replaced other tests that were conventionally obtained. Although Humphrey visual fields are still ordered, color plate testing is no longer necessary. Since the guidelines were introduced, this article reported new toxicity was discovered in existing patients that had been previously screened with older criteria. Nevertheless, the adherence to these new guidelines still was poor.

**O. P. Gupta, MD**

**Non-responders to treatment with antagonists of vascular endothelial growth factor in age-related macular degeneration**

Krebs I, Glittenberg C, Ansari-Shahrezaei S, et al (The Ludwig Boltzmann Inst for Retinology and Biomicroscopic Laser Surgery, Vienna, Austria; et al)

*Br J Ophthalmol* 97:1443-1446, 2013

*Purpose.*—Most of the publications on modern therapy of neovascular age-related macular degeneration focus on the effect of the treatment. The purpose of this study is to determine the frequency of non-responders to anti-vascular endothelial growth factor (anti-VEGF) treatment and find possible reasons for their failure to respond.

*Methods.*—The records of patients treated until the end of 2008 the first time with either bevacizumab or ranibizumab were reviewed. Based on the availability of measurable results and according to prior publications showing the effect of the therapy, loss of three lines of distance acuity, increase of retinal thickness or lesion size were identified as indicators of non-responders. Two of these three signs had to be present.

*Results.*—334 eyes of 283 patients were included; 74.55% received bevacizumab and 25.45% received ranibizumab. Overall 14.37% of the eyes were identified as non-responders (14.06% in the bevacizumab group and 15.29% in the ranibizumab group). Baseline distance acuity and vitreoretinal adhesions were significantly correlated with non-responders. Correlations with age, gender, lesion type, other morphologic features, and the kind of anti-VEGF agent failed to be significant. 10.4% of the non-responders showed a delayed but good response to anti-VEGF treatment.

*Conclusions.*—About 15% did not sufficiently respond to anti-VEGF treatment. Vitreo-retinal adherences were the only ophthalmologic factor which could be identified to be significantly correlated with insufficient response.

▶ While most patients with neovascular age-related macular degeneration respond to anti-vascular endothelial growth factor (anti-VEGF) treatments, the incidence and reasons for poor response are not well understood. This Austrian study was a retrospective study that evaluated patients who were treated with bevacizumab or ranibizumab. Loss of 3 lines of distance visual acuity, increase of retinal thickness, or increase in lesion size were defined as the 3 criteria for nonresponders. Two of these 3 signs had to be present. The authors studied 334 eyes in which about three-quarters received bevacizumab and the remaining quarter received ranibizumab. In this cohort, about 15% were identified as nonresponders. Approximately the same amount of nonresponders were reported in the bevacizumab arm (14.06%) compared with the ranibizumab arm (15.29%). Baseline distance acuity and vitreoretinal adhesions were significantly correlated with nonresponders. Correlations with age, gender, lesion type, other morphologic features, and the kind of anti-VEGF agent failed to be significant. Of the nonresponders, 10.4% showed a delayed but good response to anti-VEGF treatment. As more treatments emerge that attack choroidal neovascular membranes from other pathophysiologic mechanisms, we hope that the rate of nonresponders will decrease.

**O. P. Gupta, MD**

**Genetic Influences on the Outcome of Anti-Vascular Endothelial Growth Factor Treatment in Neovascular Age-related Macular Degeneration**

Abedi F, Wickremasinghe S, Richardson AJ, et al (Univ of Melbourne, Victoria, Australia)

*Ophthalmology* 120:1641-1648, 2013

*Purpose.*—To determine the association of genetic variants in known age-related macular degeneration (AMD) risk-associated genes with outcome of anti-vascular endothelial growth factor (VEGF) treatment in neovascular AMD.

*Design.*—Prospective cohort study.

*Participants.*—We enrolled 224 consecutive patients with neovascular AMD at the Royal Victorian Eye and Ear Hospital, Australia.

*Methods.*—Patients were treated with 3 initial monthly ranibizumab or bevacizumab injections followed by 9 months of "as required" injections based on clinician's decision at each follow-up visit according to retreatment criteria. Seventeen single nucleotide polymorphisms (SNPs) in known AMD risk-associated genes including *CFH* (rs800292, rs3766404, rs1061170, rs2274700 and rs393955), *HTRA1* (rs11200638), *CFHR1-5* (rs10922153, rs16840639, rs6667243, and rs1853883), *LOC387715/ARMS2* (rs3793917 and rs10490924), *C3* (rs2230199 and rs1047286), *C2* (rs547154), *CFB* (rs641153) and *F13B* (rs6003) were examined. Multivariate analysis was used to determine the role of each SNP in treatment outcome.

*Main Outcome Measures.*—The influence of selected SNPs on mean change in visual acuity (VA) at 12 months.

*Results.*—Mean baseline VA was 51 ± 16.8 Early Treatment Diabetic Retinopathy Study letters. Overall, the mean change in VA from baseline was +3.2 ± 14.9 letters at 12 months. The AA (homozygote risk) genotype at rs11200638 - *HTRA1* promoter SNP ($P = 0.001$) and GG (homozygote risk) genotype at rs10490924 (*A69S*) in *LOC387715/ARMS2* ($P = 0.002$) were each significantly associated with poorer VA outcome at 12 months after multiple correction. Mean ± standard deviation change in VA from baseline in patients with AA genotype at rs11200638 was −2.9 ± 15.2 letters after 12 months compared with +5.1 ± 14.1 letters in patients with AG or GG genotypes at this SNP. Patients with either of these genotypes were also significantly more likely to lose > 15 letters after 12 months. SNPs rs11200638 and rs10490924 were in high linkage disequilibrium ($r^2 = 0.92$). None of the other examined SNPs was associated with outcome.

*Conclusions.*—The *HTRA1* promoter SNP (rs11200638) and *A69S* at *LOC387715/ARMS2* were associated with a poorer visual outcome for ranibizumab or bevacizumab treatment in neovascular AMD, suggesting strong pharmacogenetic associations with anti-VEGF treatment. This finding could aid in applying more individualized treatment regimens based on patients' genotype to achieve optimal treatment response in AMD.

▶ There is a growing body of evidence that neovascular age-related macular degeneration (AMD) consists of several genotypes and phenotypes. This became very obvious with patients experiencing a variable response to treatment despite having similar presentations. This study examined 17 single nucleotide polymorphisms (SNPs) in known AMD risk-associated genes. They used multivariate analysis to determine the role of each SNP in treatment outcome, and the influence of selected SNPs on mean change in visual acuity (VA) at 12 months was the main outcome measure. Among these 17 SNPs, 2 were found to be significantly correlated with a poor visual outcome. In particular, the HTRA1 promoter SNP (rs11200638) and A69S at LOC387715/ARMS2 were also more likely to lose more than 15 letters at 1 year. While this area of investigation is still at its infancy, it does validate clinical observations of variable response to anti–vascular endothelial growth factor agents. Initially, identifying these high-risk alleles is important. Catering treatment regimens based on genotype might then become a reality.

**O. P. Gupta, MD**

---

**Randomized Clinical Trial Evaluating Intravitreal Ranibizumab or Saline for Vitreous Hemorrhage From Proliferative Diabetic Retinopathy**

Diabetic Retinopathy Clinical Research Network (Valley Retina Inst, McAllen, TX; Southeast Retina Ctr, Augusta, GA; et al)

*JAMA Ophthalmol* 131:283-293, 2013

---

*Importance.*—Vascular endothelial growth factor plays a role in proliferative diabetic retinopathy (PDR). Intravitreal injection of saline has been shown potentially to lead to improved visual acuity compared with observation alone in eyes with vitreous hemorrhage. Therefore, it is important to determine if intravitreal anti–vascular endothelial growth factor can reduce vitrectomy rates (and risks associated with vitrectomy) compared with saline for vitreous hemorrhage from PDR that precludes placement or confirmation of complete panretinal photocoagulation.

*Objective.*—To evaluate intravitreal ranibizumab compared with intravitreal saline injections on vitrectomy rates for vitreous hemorrhage from PDR.

*Design.*—Phase 3, double-masked, randomized, multicenter clinical trial. Data reported were collected from June 2010 to March 2012 and include 16 weeks of follow-up.

*Setting.*—Community-based and academic-based ophthalmology practices specializing in retinal diseases.

*Participants.*—Two hundred sixty-one eyes of 261 study participants, who were at least 18 years of age with type 1 or type 2 diabetes mellitus. Study eyes had vitreous hemorrhage from PDR precluding panretinal photocoagulation completion.

*Intervention.*—Eyes were randomly assigned to 0.5-mg intravitreal ranibizumab (n = 125) or intravitreal saline (n = 136) at baseline and 4 and 8 weeks.

*Main Outcome Measure.*—Cumulative probability of vitrectomy within 16 weeks.

*Results.*—Cumulative probability of vitrectomy by 16 weeks was 12% with ranibizumab vs 17% with saline (difference, 4%; 95% CI, −4% to 13%) and of complete panretinal photocoagulation without vitrectomy by 16 weeks was 44% and 31%, respectively ($P = .05$). The mean (SD) visual acuity improvement from baseline to 12 weeks was 22 (23) letters and 16 (31) letters, respectively ($P = .04$). Recurrent vitreous hemorrhage occurred within 16 weeks in 6% and 17%, respectively ($P = .01$). One eye developed endophthalmitis after saline injection.

*Conclusions and Relevance.*—Overall, the 16-week vitrectomy rates were lower than expected in both groups. This study suggests little likelihood of a clinically important difference between ranibizumab and saline on the rate of vitrectomy by 16 weeks in eyes with vitreous hemorrhage from PDR. Short-term secondary outcomes including visual acuity improvement, increased panretinal photocoagulation completion rates, and reduced recurrent vitreous hemorrhage rates suggest biologic activity of ranibizumab. Long-term benefits remain unknown. Whether vitrectomy rates after saline or ranibizumab injection are different than observation alone cannot be determined from this study.

*Trial Registration.*—The study is listed on www.clinicaltrials.gov, under identifier NCT00996437 (website registration date October 14, 2009).

▶ The management of nonclearing vitreous hemorrhage in the setting of proliferative diabetic retinopathy remains controversial. The Diabetic Retinopathy Clinical Research Network compared the use of intravitreal ranibizumab vs intravitreal saline. Although there is sound clinical rationale behind the use of anti-Vascular Endothelial Growth Factor agents in diabetic retinopathy, it did not reduce the rate of vitrectomy compared with the intravitreal saline arm. An interesting subsequent study may consider investigating the cause of the persistent hemorrhage. Vitreous traction pays an important role and most likely is one common reason why intravitreal ranibizumab failed and why a surgical option was more definitive.

**O. P. Gupta, MD**

## Seven-Year Outcomes in Ranibizumab-Treated Patients in ANCHOR, MARINA, and HORIZON: A Multicenter Cohort Study (SEVEN-UP)

Rofagha S, for the SEVEN-UP Study Group (Univ of California, San Francisco; et al)

*Ophthalmology* 120:2292-2299, 2013

*Purpose.*—To assess long-term outcomes 7 to 8 years after initiation of intensive ranibizumab therapy in exudative age-related macular degeneration (AMD) patients.

*Design.*—Multicenter, noninterventional cohort study.

*Participants.*—Sixty-five AMD patients originally treated with ranibizumab in the phase 3 Anti-VEGF Antibody for the Treatment of Predominantly Classic Choroidal Neovascularization in AMD (ANCHOR) trial, Minimally Classic/Occult Trial of the Anti-VEGF Antibody Ranibizumab in the Treatment of Neovascular AMD (MARINA) trial, and Open-Label Extension Trial of Ranibizumab for Choroidal Neovascularization Secondary to Age-Related Macular Degeneration (HORIZON).

*Methods.*—Fourteen clinical trial sites recruited their original subjects for a return evaluation. Individual subject comparisons were obtained from the ANCHOR, MARINA, and HORIZON databases.

*Main Outcome Measures.*—The primary end point was percentage with best-corrected visual acuity (BCVA) of 20/70 or better; secondary outcomes included mean change in letter score compared with previous time points and anatomic results on fluorescein angiography, spectral-domain ocular coherence tomography (OCT), and fundus autofluorescence (FAF).

*Results.*—At a mean of 7.3 years (range, 6.3–8.5 years) after entry into ANCHOR or MARINA, 37% of study eyes met the primary end point of 20/70 or better BCVA, with 23% achieving a BCVA of 20/40 or better. Thirty-seven percent of study eyes had BCVA of 20/200 or worse. Forty-three percent of study eyes had a stable or improved letter score (≥0-letter gain) compared with ANCHOR or MARINA baseline measurements, whereas 34% declined by 15 letters or more, with overall a mean decline of 8.6 letters ($P < 0.005$). Since exit from the HORIZON study, study eyes had received a mean of 6.8 anti-vascular endothelial growth factor (VEGF) injections during the mean 3.4-year interval; a subgroup of patients who received 11 or more anti-VEGF injections had a significantly better mean gain in letter score since HORIZON exit ($P < 0.05$). Active exudative disease was detected by spectral-domain OCT in 68% of study eyes, and 46% were receiving ongoing ocular anti-VEGF treatments. Macular atrophy was detected by FAF in 98% of eyes, with a mean area of 9.4 $mm^2$; the area of atrophy correlated significantly with poor visual outcome ($P < 0.0001$).

*Conclusions.*—Approximately 7 years after ranibizumab therapy in the ANCHOR or MARINA trials, one-third of patients demonstrated good visual outcomes, whereas another third had poor outcomes. Compared with baseline, almost half of eyes were stable, whereas one-third declined by 15 letters or more. Even at this late stage in the therapeutic course, exudative AMD patients remain at risk for substantial visual decline.

▶ It is hard to believe that it has been almost 10 years since the start of formally using intravitreal ranibizumab for neovascular age-related macular degeneration. This cohort analysis investigated the long-term anatomic and visual outcomes in patients recruited in the Anti-VEGF Antibody for the Treatment of Predominantly Classic Choroidal Neovascularization in AMD (ANCHOR) trial, Minimally Classic/Occult Trial of the Anti-VEGF Antibody Ranibizumab in the Treatment of Neovascular AMD (MARINA) trial, and Open-Label Extension Trial of Ranibizumab for Choroidal Neovascularization Secondary to Age-Related Macular Degeneration (HORIZON) trial. Overall, 23% of patients achieved a visual acuity of 20/40 or better. However, about one-third of patients declined by 3 lines of vision at mean of 7.3 years follow-up. In addition, despite almost half the patients receiving continued injections, 98% of eyes showed macular atrophy. In addition, central fibrotic scars were noted in approximately one-third of patients. Since the start of enrollment in these trials, the treatment regimen has changed. In particular, patients are treated much more frequently than outlined in the HARBOR protocol. Consequently, these results may be different with more aggressive treatment. Nevertheless, this study documents the revolution in standard of care that has occurred with anti-VEGF agents. It also reminds us that there is still a portion of the disease process that is not being treated with anti-VEGF agents.

**O. P. Gupta, MD**

---

**Long-term Outcomes of Ranibizumab Therapy for Diabetic Macular Edema: The 36-Month Results from Two Phase III Trials: RISE and RIDE**

Brown DM, on behalf of the RIDE and RISE Research Group (The Methodist Hosp, Houston, TX; et al)

*Ophthalmology* 120:2013-2022, 2013

---

*Purpose.*—To report 36-month outcomes of RIDE (NCT00473382) and RISE (NCT00473330), trials of ranibizumab in diabetic macular edema (DME).

*Design.*—Phase III, randomized, multicenter, double-masked, 3-year trials, sham injection–controlled for 2 years.

*Participants.*—Adults with DME (n = 759), baseline best-corrected visual acuity (BCVA) 20/40 to 20/320 Snellen equivalent, and central foveal thickness (CFT) ≥275 μm on optical coherence tomography.

*Methods.*—Patients were randomized equally (1 eye per patient) to monthly 0.5 mg or 0.3 mg ranibizumab or sham injection. In the third year, sham patients, while still masked, were eligible to cross over to monthly 0.5 mg ranibizumab. Macular laser was available to all patients starting at month 3; panretinal laser was available as necessary.

*Main Outcome Measures.*—The proportion of patients gaining ≥15 Early Treatment Diabetic Retinopathy Study letters in BCVA from baseline at month 24.

*Results.*—Visual acuity (VA) outcomes seen at month 24 in ranibizumab groups were consistent through month 36; the proportions of patients who gained ≥15 letters from baseline at month 36 in the sham/0.5 mg, 0.3 mg, and 0.5 mg ranibizumab groups were 19.2%, 36.8%, and 40.2%, respectively, in RIDE and 22.0%, 51.2%, and 41.6%, respectively, in RISE. In the ranibizumab arms, reductions in CFT seen at 24 months were, on average, sustained through month 36. After crossover to 1 year of treatment with ranibizumab, average VA gains in the sham/0.5 mg group were lower compared with gains seen in the ranibizumab patients after 1 year of treatment (2.8 vs. 10.6 and 11.1 letters). Per-injection rates of endophthalmitis remained low over time (~0.06% per injection). The incidence of serious adverse events potentially related to systemic vascular endothelial growth factor inhibition was 19.7% in patients who received 0.5 mg ranibizumab compared with 16.8% in the 0.3 mg group.

*Conclusions.*—The strong VA gains and improvement in retinal anatomy achieved with ranibizumab at month 24 were sustained through month 36. Delayed treatment in patients receiving sham treatment did not seem to result in the same extent of VA improvement observed in patients originally randomized to ranibizumab. Ocular and systemic safety was generally consistent with the results seen at month 24.

► The treatment of fovea-involving diabetic macular edema (DME) has radically changed over the last several years. Focal laser photocoagulation has been the mainstay for treatment. The RISE and RIDE trials were focused on intravitreal ranibizumab for patients with vision loss from DME. Focal laser was available for all patients as a rescue therapy. This study is the 36-month results from these 2 trials. The visual and anatomic outcomes were significantly better for the treatment arms compared with the sham arm that only received focal laser. The improvements that were noted at the 24-month time point were sustained at 36 months. Interestingly, the rate of panretinal photocoagulation was lower in the treatment arm compared with the sham arm. These rates were 0% to 4% and 12% to 14%, respectively. Another interesting observation is that the rate of endophthalmitis was quite low (0.06%). This is especially important given the fact that preinjection and postinjection antibiotics were not used for any injections. This study also supports the growing body of literature that antibiotics are not necessary for intravitreal injections. Lastly, the results of the 0.3-mg and 0.5-mg treatment arms were very similar. In review of these results, the US Food and Drug Administration along with key retinal opinion leaders approved the use of 0.3 mg of ranibizumab. This is different than the dose for the treatment of neovascular age-related macular degeneration (0.5 mg). Although much advancement has been made in the treatment of DME, there are still many clinical scenarios that remain unresolved. In particular, patients with DME without visual acuity loss (excluded from this study) and the efficacy of bevacizumab are 2 topics that need to be explored.

**O. P. Gupta, MD**

**Incidence of Choroidal Neovascularization in the Fellow Eye in the Comparison of Age-related Macular Degeneration Treatments Trials**

Maguire MG, for the Comparison of Age-Related Macular Degeneration Treatments Trials (CATT Research Group) (Univ of Pennsylvania, Philadelphia; et al)

*Ophthalmology* 120:2035-2041, 2013

*Objective.*—To assess the influence of drug; dosing regimen; and traditional, nontraditional, and genetic risk factors on the incidence of choroidal neovascularization (CNV) in the fellow eye of patients treated for CNV with ranibizumab or bevacizumab.

*Design.*—Cohort study of patients enrolled in a multicenter, randomized clinical trial.

*Participants.*—Patients with no CNV in the fellow eye at the time of enrollment in the Comparison of Age-Related Macular Degeneration Treatments Trials (CATT).

*Methods.*—Eligibility criteria for the clinical trial required that study eyes have evidence on fluorescein angiography and optical coherence tomography of CNV secondary to age-related macular degeneration (AMD) and visual acuity between 20/25 and 20/320. Treatment for the study eye was assigned randomly to either ranibizumab or bevacizumab and to 3 different regimens for dosing over a 2-year period. The genotypes for 4 single nucleotide polymorphisms (SNPs) associated with risk of AMD were determined. Only patients without CNV in the fellow eye at baseline were considered at risk. The CATT ophthalmologists examined patients every 4 weeks through 2 years and recorded treatment for CNV in the fellow eye.

*Main Outcome Measures.*—Development of CNV in the fellow eye.

*Results.*—Among 1185 CATT participants, 727 (61%) had no CNV in the fellow eye at enrollment. At 2 years, CNV had developed in 75 (20.6%) of 365 patients treated with ranibizumab and in 60 (16.6%) of 362 patients treated with bevacizumab (absolute difference, 4.0%; 95% confidence interval [CI], −1.7% to 9.6%; $P = 0.17$). The risk ratio for pro re nata dosing relative to monthly dosing was 1.1 (95% CI, 0.8–1.6). Greater elevation of the retinal pigment epithelium and fluid in the foveal center of the study eye were associated with increased incidence of CNV in the fellow eye. Incidence was not associated with genotype on rs1061170 (*CFH*), rs10490924 (*ARMS2*), rs11200638 (*HTRA1*), and rs2230199 (C3; $P > 0.35$).

*Conclusions.*—Through 2 years, there was no statistically significant difference between ranibizumab and bevacizumab in incidence of CNV in the fellow eye. Genotype on 4 SNPs previously found to be associated with AMD did not affect the risk of CNV in the fellow eye among CATT patients.

▶ In the Comparison of Age-Related Macular Degeneration Treatment Trials, ophthalmologists evaluated patients every 4 weeks for 2 years. For patients being treated with ranibizumab and bevacizumab in the study eye, the study examiners noted development of choroidal neovascularization (CNV) in the fellow eye. In addition to the influence of the drug, dosing regimen and genetic risk factors were also evaluated. At the 2-year endpoint, 16% to 20% of fellow eyes developed CNV. There was no difference in the rate of conversion to neovascular age-related macular degeneration (AMD) between ranibizumab and bevacizumab. In addition, there was no difference in conversion when the treatment regimen was considered. In particular, pro re nata (PRN) and monthly dosing regimen did not affect rate of conversion to fellow eye CNV. Lastly, the investigators also evaluated 4 single nucleotide polymorphisms (SNPs) associated with AMD. The incidence of fellow eye CNV was not associated with any of these SNPs. A greater elevation of the retinal pigment epithelium and fluid in the foveal center of the study eye were the only features that were correlated with a higher incidence of CNV in the fellow eye. These types of studies are incredibly important. Once a patient presents with neovascular AMD in one eye, fellow eye conversion is a concern for the patient and provider alike. Identifying clinical features and risk stratifying patients will be incredibly useful in determining follow-up of those patients.

**O. P. Gupta, MD**

## No Face-Down Positioning and Broad Internal Limiting Membrane Peeling in the Surgical Repair of Idiopathic Macular Holes

Iezzi R, Kapoor KG (Mayo Clinic, Rochester, MN)
*Ophthalmology* 120:1998-2003, 2013

*Objective.*—To demonstrate the efficacy of broad internal limiting membrane (ILM) peeling and 20% sulfur hexafluoride ($SF_6$) endotamponade with no face-down positioning in the surgical repair of idiopathic macular holes (MHs).

*Design.*—Retrospective study.

*Participants.*—Sixty-eight idiopathic MH cases in 68 eyes of 65 patients.

*Methods.*—All idiopathic MH surgeries by 1 surgeon between March 2009 and December 2012, performed using broad ILM peeling, 20% $SF_6$, and no face-down positioning, were reviewed. No cases were excluded. Surgeon method included 23-gauge or 25-gauge pars plana vitrectomy with induction of posterior vitreous detachment (if necessary). Indocyanine green dye (0.08 mg/ml in D5W) was injected slowly, allowed to stain for 60 seconds, and then removed. The ILM was broadly peeled to the vascular arcades (approximately 8000 µm in diameter), followed by 2 fluid–air exchanges, separated by 5 minutes, and an air–20% $SF_6$

exchange. Patients maintained reading position for 3 to 5 days and were followed up at least for 1 month. Exact binomial distributions were used to establish 95% confidence intervals, and the 1-way analysis of variance was used to compare preoperative and postoperative intraocular pressures (IOPs).

*Main Outcome Measures.*—Single-procedure MH closure rate, mean postoperative best-corrected visual acuity (BCVA), incidence of cataract, and IOP.

*Results.*—Three patients (4.6%) had bilateral MH and 9 patients (13.8%) had recurrent MH (mean duration from previous surgery, 8.3 ± 5.5 years; range, 1–16 years). Twenty-one MH (30.9%) were stage 2, 27 (39.7%) were stage 3, and 20 (29.4%) were stage 4. Five MH had a basal diameter of more than 1000 μm. Mean MH basal diameter was 609.6 ± 226.2 μm. Mean preoperative BCVA was 0.68 ± 0.29 logarithm of the minimum angle of resolution (logMAR) units (Snellen equivalent, 20/95), and mean most recent postoperative BCVA was 0.28 ± 0.18 logMAR units (Snellen equivalent, 20/38). The single-procedure MH closure rate was 100% (95% confidence interval, 95%–100%), and no complications were observed.

*Conclusions.*—Macular hole surgery with broad ILM peeling, 20% $SF_6$ gas, and no face-down positioning is highly effective in the surgical treatment of idiopathic MH with efficacy comparable with methods that use longer-acting gas endotamponade, face-down positioning, or both. In our series, this method eliminated the morbidity associated with postoperative face-down positioning.

▶ It is interesting to challenge some of the basic tenets of surgical retina. Many of the tenets have some scientific merit, whereas others are carried forward from generation to generation "because we have always done it that way." Face-down positioning after macular hole surgery is one of the most dreaded features of all retinal procedures. Many reports have investigated the duration of face-down positioning, surgical technique of membrane peeling, whether to membrane peel at all, and the type of gas that is necessary. This study evaluated the success rate of macular hole repair without face-down positioning. The authors reported outcomes of 68 eyes and had a 100% closure rate. This was done with broad internal limiting membrane peeling from arcade to arcade as well as nasally to the nerve and temporally equal to the nasal peel. They also used indocyanine green (ICG) and allowed the dye to stain for 60 seconds. There is concern about ICG toxicity to the retinal pigment epithelial cells; therefore, some surgeons will not use ICG for any surgical procedure. This study not only challenges the basic tenet for the need of face-down positioning, but also supports the use of ICG in this setting. The mean visual acuity improved from 20/95 preoperatively to 20/38 postoperatively. Lastly, some surgeons consistently used C3F8 for all of their macular hole cases or at least the cases that are chronic or large macular holes. All of the eyes in this study were filled with the short-acting gas sulfur hexafluoride. There were 5 holes in the current study that were 1000 μm in size. While this is a small, uncontrolled, nonrandomized, retrospective study, the data are compelling and will certainly tempt surgeons to change their surgical technique regarding these cases.

**O. P. Gupta, MD**

---

**_CFH_ and _ARMS2_ Genetic Polymorphisms Predict Response to Antioxidants and Zinc in Patients with Age-related Macular Degeneration**

Awh CC, Lane A-M, Hawken S, et al (Tennessee Retina, Nashville; Harvard Med School, Boston, MA; Ottawa Hosp Res Inst Clinical Epidemiology Program, Canada; et al)

*Ophthalmology* 120:2317-2323, 2013

---

*Objective.*—The Age-Related Eye Disease Study (AREDS) demonstrated that antioxidant and zinc supplementation decreases progression to advanced age-related macular degeneration (AMD) in patients with moderate to severe disease. We evaluated the interaction of genetics and type of nutritional supplement on progression from moderate to advanced AMD.

*Design.*—Genetic analysis of a randomized, prospective clinical trial.

*Participants.*—White patients with AREDS category 3 AMD in 1 eye and AREDS categories 1 through 4 AMD in the fellow eye enrolled in the AREDS with available peripheral blood-derived DNA (995).

*Methods.*—Subjects were evaluated for known AMD genetic risk markers and treatment category. The progression rate to advanced AMD was analyzed by genotypes and AREDS treatment group using Cox regression.

*Main Outcome Measures.*—The effect of inherited gene polymorphisms on treatment group–specific rate of progression to advanced AMD.

*Results.*—Over an average of 10.1 years, individuals with 1 or 2 complement factor H (*CFH*) risk alleles derived maximum benefit from antioxidants alone. In these patients, the addition of zinc negated the benefits of antioxidants. Treatment with zinc and antioxidants was associated with a risk ratio (RR) of 1.83 with 2 *CFH* risk alleles ($P = 1.03E\text{-}02$), compared with outcomes for patients without *CFH* risk alleles. Patients with age-related maculopathy sensitivity 2 (*ARMS2*) risk alleles derived maximum benefit from zinc-containing regimens, with a deleterious response to antioxidants in the presence of *ARMS2* risk alleles. Treatment with antioxidants was associated with an RR of 2.58 for those with 1 *ARMS2* risk allele and 3.96 for those with 2 *ARMS2* risk alleles ($P = 1.04E\text{-}6$), compared with patients with no *ARMS2* risk alleles. Individuals homozygous for *CFH* and *ARMS2* risk alleles derived no benefit from any category of AREDS treatment.

*Conclusions.*—Individuals with moderate AMD could benefit from pharmacogenomic selection of nutritional supplements. In this analysis, patients with no *CFH* risk alleles and with 1 or 2 *ARMS2* risk alleles derived maximum benefit from zinc-only supplementation. Patients with one or two *CFH* risk alleles and no *ARMS2* risk alleles derived maximum benefit from antioxidant-only supplementation; treatment with zinc was associated with increased progression to advanced AMD. These recommendations could lead to improved outcomes through genotype-directed therapy.

▶ Genotype-directed therapy in the treatment of age-related macular degeneration (AMD) has been a major focus in recent years. This has been partially prompted by the clinical observations regarding the varied natural history and response to therapy. For example, there are some patients with dry AMD in which the maculopathy does not progress compared with others with significant progression between visits. There are other patients with neovascular AMD that respond very well to treatment compared with others that have persistent exudation despite monthly injections. In this study, the authors explored the impact of the age-related maculopathy sensitivity 2 (ARMS2) risk alleles and complement factor H (CFH) risk alleles in the setting of dry AMD. In particular, the authors show that patients with the CFH risk alleles showed the most benefit with antioxidant treatment alone. The addition of zinc resulted in faster progression of dry AMD compared with placebo. However, the rate of dry AMD progression was slowest in patients with ARMS2 risk alleles who were taking zinc supplements. The addition of antioxidants negated the benefit of zinc supplementation, and patients with the CFH risk alleles who were taking antioxidants alone progressed faster than those taking placebo. These results are compelling, but are tempered by the fact that it is a retrospective, subgroup analysis that was not sufficiently powered. Future studies will most likely be designed to explore these risk alleles further along with others. Additional studies will also investigate the genetic risk factors that result in varied clinical response to neovascular AMD therapies.

**O. P. Gupta, MD**

# 6 Oculoplastic Surgery

**Bleeding complications in both anticoagulated and nonanticoagulated surgical patients**

Kent TL, Custer PL (Washington Univ in St. Louis, MO)

*Ophthal Plast Reconstr Surg* 29:113-117, 2013

*Purpose.*—This study was performed to ascertain the incidence of anticoagulant use in oculoplastic surgical patients and the reliability of patient medication disclosure. Differences in perioperative bleeding complications among patients continuing anticoagulants, those who withheld the medications, and those not anticoagulated were investigated.

*Methods.*—Following institutional review board approval, a retrospective chart review was conducted (January 1, 2008, to June 30, 2010). Anticoagulant medications and their management during the perioperative period were reviewed. Type of surgical procedure and perioperative complications were documented.

*Results.*—Charts were reviewed for 1130 surgeries in 1015 patients. Eighteen percent of patients failed to accurately disclose their medication use. Aspirin use was not reported in 12% of patients. There were no intraoperative complications and a single postoperative orbital hematoma among 682 patients not using anticoagulants. There were 3 intraoperative complications and 1 postoperative hemorrhage in the 207 patients whose anticoagulants were withheld. In the 145 patients who continued their anticoagulation therapy throughout the surgical period, there were no intraoperative bleeding complications, and one postoperative hemorrhage. None of the study patients sustained permanent visual deficit or deformity related to hemorrhage.

*Conclusions.*—Forty percent of patients undergoing oculoplastic procedures were using anticoagulants; yet, many patients failed to disclose their medication usage. The decision to operate and whether to discontinue these medications must be individualized considering the nature of the procedure and the patient's medical condition. It may be appropriate to continue anticoagulants in certain patients at increased risk for a vascular event, ensuring adequate hemostasis throughout the procedure.

▶ This was a retrospective chart review of 1130 surgeries looking at bleeding complications in patients who stopped their anticoagulants, those who did not stop their anticoagulants, and those that were never taking anticoagulants.

There were no statistical significant differences in the intraoperative bleeding complications between those patients who were taking anticoagulants and stopped them and those who were taking anticoagulants and did not stop them. The difference in the rate of intraoperative bleeding complication for those not on anticoagulation was lower and statistically significantly lower from those who held their anticoagulants. The rate of postoperative complications was not statistically different in the 3 groups.

The study also found that 18% of patients did not accurately disclose the medications they were taking, and 12% did not disclose aspirin use preoperatively.

This study really does not give an answer as to the value of stopping anticoagulants before oculoplastic surgery. It suggests that patients on anticoagulants may have a similar risk of bleeding during and after surgery as those who stop it. The retrospective nature of the study and the fact that all anticoagulants were grouped together (Tables 1 and 2 in the original article) makes any such conclusion of questionable validity. It does suggest that surgery with patients on anticoagulants may not have a high risk of bleeding and that weighing the risk/benefit ratio of stopping these medications on an individual basis is still the best approach.

**R. B. Penne, MD**

---

**Prophylactic postoperative antibiotics for enucleation and evisceration**

Fay A, New England Oculoplastics Society Study Group (Harvard Med School, Boston, MA)

*Ophthal Plast Reconstr Surg* 29:281-285, 2013

---

*Purpose.*—To investigate the necessity and usefulness of prophylactic postoperative antibiotics in patients undergoing enucleation or ocular evisceration.

*Methods.*—A retrospective, multicenter, comparative case series was designed. After obtaining Institutional Review Board authorization, a medical records' review was conducted. Demographics, indication for surgery, surgical technique, postoperative antibiotic dosing, and postoperative course were evaluated. Records were grouped according to antibiotic protocols, and presence or absence of postoperative wound infection (orbital cellulitis) was recorded. Rates of postoperative infection were analyzed statistically.

*Results.*—Between 1996 and 2011, 666 evisceration or enucleation surgeries were conducted at 4 institutions. Six hundred forty-eight records were available for analysis, of which 4 were excluded due to insufficient follow-up data. All the remaining 644 patients received a single, perioperative, intravenous dose of antibiotics. Five hundred seventy-eight patients (90%) received an orbital implant, while 66 (10%) did not. Three hundred eighty-one patients (59%) received postoperative antibiotics, and 263 patients (41%) did not. Two cases were identified with signs suggestive of infection, but no culture-positive infections were found, and no patient was admitted to the hospital for management. Of the 2 suspicious cases, 1 was found in the group that received postoperative antibiotics (group 1) and 1 in the group that did not receive postoperative antibiotics (group

2). No statistically significant difference in postoperative infection rate was noted between the 2 groups ($p = 0.52$). While patients with infectious indications for surgery were more likely to receive postoperative antibiotics ($p < 0.001$), there was no statistically significant difference in rates of infection among patients with infectious indications for surgery based on receiving or not receiving postoperative antibiotics ($p = 0.79$), and no patients with infectious indications for surgery not receiving postoperative antibiotics developed a postoperative infection.

*Conclusions.*—This study demonstrates the clinical safety of withholding postoperative prophylactic antibiotics in orbital surgery even when implanting alloplastic material in a sterile field. Furthermore, Centers for Disease Control and Prevention guidelines mandate cessation of postoperative antibiotics within 24 hours of surgery. Surgeons are cautioned not to generalize these results to nonsterile surgery such as sinonasal or nasolacrimal surgery.

▶ The prophylactic use of antibiotics after orbital surgery is fairly common. This report addresses the use of prophylactic antibiotics after an enucleation or evisceration. The study was a retrospective chart review of 644 patients. All patients received a single dose of intravenous antibiotics perioperatively. Postoperatively, 59% of the patients received postoperative antibiotics and 41% did not. The results showed no statistically significant difference in the postoperative infection rate with both groups having a single infection.

This is a simple study and the conclusion is simple. There is no reason to use postoperative antibiotics after enucleation or evisceration as long as the patient receives an intravenous dose of antibiotics perioperatively.

**R. B. Penne, MD**

---

**Medial conjunctival resection for tearing associated with conjunctivochalasis**

Petris CK, Holds JB (Univ of Missouri, Columbia)

*Ophthal Plast Reconstr Surg* 29:304-307, 2013

---

*Purpose.*—Conjunctivochalasis is an age-dependent redundancy or laxity of the conjunctiva. It may result in epiphora (tearing) through mechanical disruption of the normal tear flow or exacerbate dry eye symptoms by disruption of an already unstable tear film. In this study, the authors performed a retrospective analysis of the benefits of a simple medial conjunctival resection for tearing associated with conjunctivochalasis.

*Methods.*—A review of medical records identified 18 patients (25 eyes) who underwent a medial conjunctivoplasty for tearing between 2000 and 2012. The degree of epiphora was graded for each patient from 0 (no tearing) to 3 (persistent tearing requiring surgical correction). All patients were given an initial preoperative score of 3. Patients were excluded from the study if more than 1 eyelid procedure that would affect the lacrimal pump function was performed at the time of conjunctivoplasty or if clinically significant entropion, ectropion, or nasolacrimal duct obstruction was present at the time of conjunctivoplasty.

*Results.*—At an average of 2.7 months post-conjunctivoplasty (range 4 weeks to 12 months), 80% of patients improved to a score of 2 or better and 60% improved to 1 or better. Six patients ultimately needed an additional surgical procedure for unresolved or recurrent tearing.

*Conclusions.*—The data suggest that conjunctivoplasty using a simple medial conjunctival resection is an effective treatment for patients with epiphora secondary to conjunctivochalasis.

▶ Conjunctivochalasis is a cause of tearing that can be frustrating to diagnose and treat. Although a potential cause of tearing, not every patient with conjunctivochalasis has tearing. Thus caution must be used when determining whether tearing is caused but conjunctivochalasis. In addition, the treatment is not always simple.

This article does offer a simple procedure that can be done in the office without sutures to treat conjunctivochalasis (Fig 2a, b in the original article). The results found that 6 of 18 patients (Table 2 in the original article) needed additional procedures to resolve their tearing. Looking at Table 2 in the original article, that large number of patients who had undergone previous eyelid procedures shows the difficulty in determining if conjunctivochalasis is really the cause of tearing. This procedure is simple, and I believe it offers a valuable tool for dealing with conjunctivochalasis.

**R. B. Penne, MD**

---

**Comparison of preferences between onabotulinumtoxinA (Botox) and incobotulinumtoxinA (Xeomin) in the treatment of benign essential blepharospasm**

Chundury RV, Couch SM, Holds JB (Saint Louis Univ, MO)

*Ophthal Plast Reconstr Surg* 29:205-207, 2013

---

*Purpose.*—To evaluate subjective outcomes and preferences in patients with benign essential blepharospasm (BEB) treated with both onabotulinumtoxinA (Botox) and incobotulinumtoxinA (Xeomin).

*Methods.*—An institutional review board approved retrospective review of 128 patients treated with onabotulinumtoxinA for BEB by 1 author (J.B.H.). Fifty of these patients were switched to incobotulinumtoxinA as an alternate drug. At scheduled follow up, patients decided to continue with incobotulinumtoxinA or switch to onabotulinumtoxinA. Patient preferences regarding treatment with onabotulinumtoxinA versus incobotulinumtoxinA were recorded. The preference groups were analyzed using unpaired Student t test, with statistical significance set at $p < 0.05$.

*Results.*—Of the 50 incobotulinumtoxinA patients, the mean age was 64.9 years; 39 (78%) were women and 11 (22%) were men. In all, 26 (52%) preferred incobotulinumtoxinA and 24 (48%) preferred onabotulinumtoxinA. Most frequently, those who preferred incobotulinumtoxinA believed that it was "more effective" (N = 10, 29%), whereas those who preferred onabotulinumtoxinA concluded that it had a "longer duration" (N = 11, 37%). The mean treatment interval was 13.0 weeks (standard deviation [SD] = 6.39) in those who preferred onabotulinumtoxinA, whereas it was 10.2 weeks (SD = 2.15) in those who preferred incobotulinumtoxinA ($p = 0.017$). There was no statistical difference when comparing mean disease duration, number of total treatments, and number of units/treatment between the 2 preference groups.

*Conclusions.*—This study demonstrates that patients who prefer incobotulinumtoxinA over onabotulinumtoxinA had a statistically significant shorter treatment interval. In addition, those who preferred incobotulinumtoxinA thought it was more effective, whereas those patients who preferred onabotulinumtoxinA thought it had a longer duration. This information can be used when counseling both newly diagnosed and long-standing BEB patients regarding their therapeutic options.

▶ There has been an intense marketing battle between onabotulinumtoxinA (Botox) and incobotulinumtoxinA (Xeomin). This report attempts to elucidate the differences between these medications and offers a guide to what to expect for the 2 agents.

The report's conclusions are that onabotulinumtoxinA has a longer duration of action and that incobotulinumtoxinA was more effective in relieving the spasm (Table 1 in the original article). These are the generally accepted differences between the 2, but I don't think this study really proves that scientifically. First, this was a retrospective study asking questions about subjective results that occurred in the past. Second, there were only 50 patients in the entire study.

This report does make some suggestions about possible differences in 2 forms of botulinum toxin, which may be used as a starting point in counseling patients on the choice between these 2 agents.

**R. B. Penne, MD**

---

### Mitomycin C in dacryocystorhinostomy: the search for the right concentration and duration—a fundamental study on human nasal mucosa fibroblasts

Ali MJ, Mariappan I, Maddileti S, et al (LV Prasad Eye Inst, Hyderabad, Andhra Pradesh, India)

*Ophthal Plast Reconstr Surg* 29:469-474, 2013

---

*Purpose.*—To establish primary cultures of human nasal mucosal fibroblasts (HNMFs) and to test the effect of varying concentrations of mitomycin C (MMC) and treatment durations on cellular proliferation and viability of the fibroblasts.

*Design.*—Laboratory investigation.

*Methods.*—Nasal mucosa harvested from patients undergoing a dacryocystorhinostomy was used to establish primary cultures by explant culture method. Cells were expanded and frozen at every passage, and passage 3 cells were used for further experiments. The cells were then treated with different concentrations of mitomycin C (0.1-0.5 mg/ml) for different time periods (3, 5, and 10 minutes). Cell viability was checked by MTT (3-[4,5-dimethylthiazol-2-yl]-2,5-diphenyltetrazolium bromide) assay. Cellular proliferation index was determined with bromodeoxyuridine immunostaining. Apoptotic index was measured using annexin A5 affinity assay, propidium iodide staining, and 4',6-diamidino-2-phenylindole counterstaining. The actin cytoskeletons of fibroblasts were studied using phalloidin staining.

*Results.*—The doubling time of cultured HNMFs is approximately 24 hours. Similarly, 0.4 mg/ml beyond 5 minutes and 0.5 mg/ml concentration at all time points were lethal and caused extensive cell death when compared with controls. A concentration of 0.2 mg/ml for 3 minutes of exposure prevented cell proliferation of HNMF cells by inducing cell cycle arrest, without causing extensive apoptosis.

*Conclusions.*—The minimum effective concentration appears to be 0.2 mg/ml for 3 minutes. This in vitro study could be the starting point for further clinical and histopathologic studies to validate its clinical usefulness.

▶ Mitomycin C (MMC) has become a common agent used during dacryocystorhinostomy (DCR) to prevent scarring. Despite the extensive use and multiple reports, there is no accepted dose to be used. This in vivo study looked at the time of exposure and concentration of MMC. Nasal mucosal cell cultures were treated with various concentrations and times of exposure and then evaluated. The goal was to prevent cell proliferation without causing cell death.

The conclusion was that an MMC concentration of 0.2 mg/mL (0.02%) for 3 minutes gave the best results. This is within the various dosage guidelines used for surgery. Although this was an *in vivo* study, I will now use this concentration and time for my surgery. I think it lends some scientific merit to the choice of time and concentration. I do not use MMC in my primary DCRs, but I do find it very effective in failed primary surgeries that require reoperation.

**R. B. Penne, MD**

---

**Targeted Therapy for Orbital and Periocular Basal Cell Carcinoma and Squamous Cell Carcinoma**

Yin VT, Pfeiffer ML, Esmaeli B (The Univ of Texas MD Anderson Cancer Ctr, Houston)

*Ophthal Plast Reconstr Surg* 29:87-92, 2013

---

*Purpose.*—To review the literature on targeted therapy for orbital and periocular basal cell carcinoma (BCC) and cutaneous squamous cell carcinoma (SCC) and provide examples of patients recently treated with such therapy.

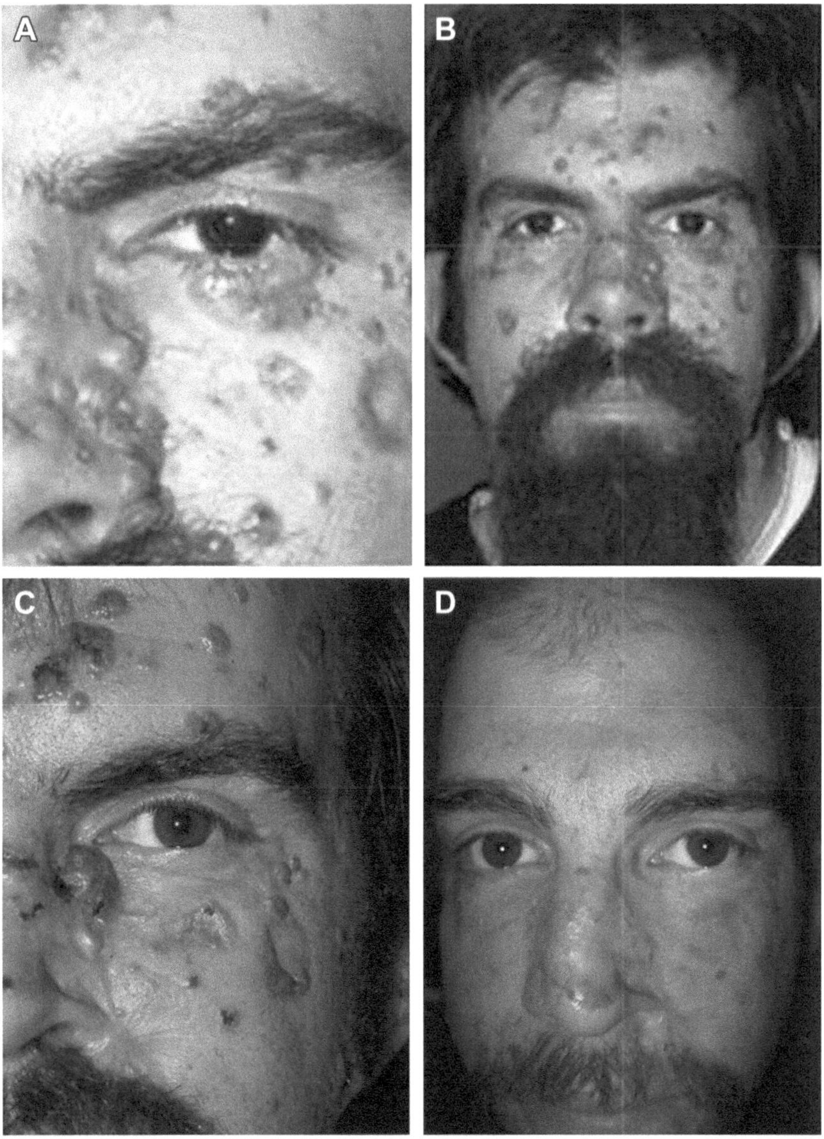


**FIGURE 1.—A, B** External photograph of a patient with basal cell nevus syndrome and multiple basal cell carcinomas (BCC) on the face including a large BCC on the left lower eyelid that was surgically removed. **C** Postoperative photo in the same patient demonstrates a nice outcome in the left lower eyelid but another large BCC has developed and is enlarging in the left medial canthus, which was subsequently excised. **D** The same patient after 16 weeks of treatment with vismodegib. He experienced significant resolution of all his facial and periorbital BCCs. (Reprinted from Yin VT, Pfeiffer ML, Esmaeli B. Targeted therapy for orbital and periocular basal cell carcinoma and squamous cell carcinoma. *Ophthal Plast Reconstr Surg.* 2013;29:87-92.)

*Methods.*—We reviewed the literature on clinical results of targeted therapy and the molecular basis for targeted therapy in orbital and periocular BCC and cutaneous SCC. We also present representative cases from our practice.

*Results.*—Mutation in the patched gene (*PTCH1*) has been implicated in BCC, and overexpression of epidermal growth factor receptor (EGFR) has been shown in SCC. Vismodegib, an inhibitor of smoothened, which is activated upon binding of hedgehog to Ptc, has been shown to significantly decrease BCC tumor size or even produce complete resolution, especially in cases of basal cell nevus syndrome. Similarly, EGFR inhibitors have been shown to significantly decrease SCC tumor size in cases of locally advanced and metastatic disease. We describe successful outcomes after vismodegib treatment in a patient with basal cell nevus syndrome with numerous bulky lesions of the eyelid and periocular region and erlotinib (EGFR inhibitor) treatment in a patient with SCC who was deemed not to be a good surgical candidate because of advanced SCC of the orbit with metastasis to the regional lymph nodes, advanced age, and multiple medical comorbidities.

*Conclusion.*—Targeted therapy using hedgehog pathway and EGFR inhibitors shows significant promise in treatment of orbital and periocular BCC and cutaneous SCC, respectively. Such targeted therapy may be appropriate for patients who are not good candidates for surgery (Fig 1).

▶ Targeted therapy is a relatively new way to treat advanced cases of orbital and periocular basal cell carcinoma (BCC) and squamous cell carcinoma (SCC). This article reviews the way that vismodegib acts to interfere with a mutation in the patched gene. This mutation has been implicated in growth of BCC. In a similar way, epidermal growth factor receptor (EGFR) overexpression has been implicated in the growth of SCC. Inhibitors of EGFR have been shown to decrease the size of SCC tumors.

The value of this article is to inform physicians about these agents and their potential use. These agents are in their early phase of use. At this point, they have potential value in advanced cases that are unresectable (Fig 1). There are side effects, and the cost of medication is high. With time this form of treatment is likely to improve and may become a mainstay of treatment of BCC and SCC.

**R. B. Penne, MD**

---

**Impact of Hospital Volume and Specialization on the Cost of Orbital Trauma Care**

Koo JJ, Wang J, Thompson CB, et al (Johns Hopkins School of Medicine, Baltimore, MD; Johns Hopkins Bloomberg School of Public Health, Baltimore, MD)

*Ophthalmology* 120:2741-2746, 2013

---

*Purpose.*—To examine the impact of hospital volume and specialization on the cost of orbital trauma care.

*Design.*—Comparative case series and database study.

*Participants.*—Four hundred ninety-nine patients who underwent orbital reconstruction at either a high-volume regional eye trauma center, its academic parent institution, or all other hospitals in Maryland between 2004 and 2009.

*Methods.*—We used a publicly available database of hospital discharge data to identify the study population's clinical and cost characteristics. Multivariate models were developed to determine the impact of care setting on hospital costs while controlling for patient demographic and clinical variables.

*Main Outcome Measures.*—Mean hospital costs accrued during hospital admission for orbital reconstruction in 3 separate care settings.

*Results.*—Almost half (n = 248) of all patients received surgical care at the regional eye trauma center and had significantly lower adjusted mean hospital costs ($6194; 95% confidence interval [CI], $5709–$6719) compared with its parent institution ($8642; 95% CI, $7850–$9514) and all other hospitals ($12 692; 95% CI, $11 467–$14 047). A subpopulation analysis selecting patients with low comorbidity scores also was performed. The eye trauma center continued to have lower adjusted costs ($4277; 95% CI, $4112–$4449) relative to its parent institution ($6595; 95% CI, $5838–$7451) and other hospitals ($7150; 95% CI, $5969–$8565).

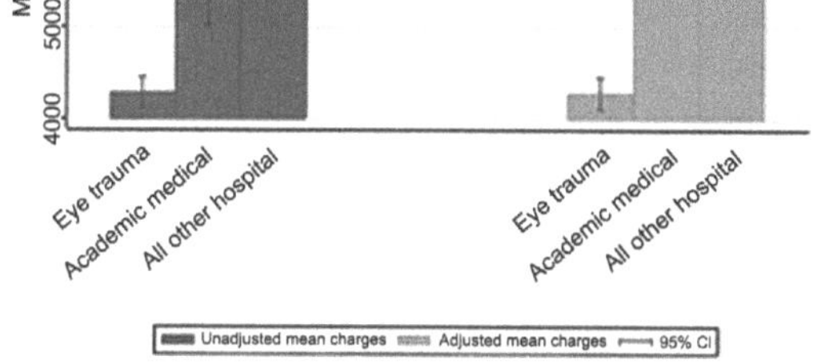


**FIGURE 2.**—Bar graph showing the subpopulation unadjusted and adjusted mean hospital charges. The subpopulation represents patients with 1-day length of stay, no intensive care unit days, and All Patient Refined Diagnosis Related Group Severity of Illness Scores of 1 or 2. Additionally, these patients were not admitted through the emergency department and were discharged to home. The eye trauma center continues to have significantly lower mean hospital charges relative to its parent institution and all other hospitals. I-bars represent 95% confidence intervals (CIs). (Reprinted from Koo JJ, Wang J, Thompson CB, et al. Impact of hospital volume and specialization on the cost of orbital trauma care. *Ophthalmology.* 2013;120:2741-2746, Copyright 2013, with permission the American Academy of Ophthalmology.)

TABLE 2.—Subpopulation Population Demographic and Clinical Characteristics by Care Setting

| | All Other Hospitals (n = 26) | Eye Trauma Center (n = 232) | Parent Institution (n = 45) | Total Group (n = 303) | *P* Value |
|---|---|---|---|---|---|
| Gender, n (%) | | | | | 0.10* |
| Female | 4 (15) | 65 (28) | 7 (16) | 76 (25) | |
| Male | 22 (85) | 167 (72) | 38 (84) | 227 (75) | |
| Race, n (%) | | | | | 0.99* |
| White | 14 (46) | 127 (55) | 25 (56) | 166 (55) | |
| Nonwhite | 12 (54) | 105 (45) | 20 (44) | 137 (45) | |
| Marital status, n (%) | | | | | 0.31* |
| Married | 7 (27) | 52 (22) | 6 (13) | 65 (21) | |
| Not married | 19 (73) | 180 (78) | 39 (87) | 238 (79) | |
| Age (yrs) | | | | | 0.76† |
| Mean (SD) | 29 (14) | 32 (17) | 31 (13) | 31 (17) | |
| Range | 4–51 | 3–90 | 9–60 | 3–90 | |
| Charlson comorbidity index | | | | | 0.66† |
| Mean (SD) | 0.12 (0.33) | 0.18 (0.59) | 0.11 (0.44) | 0.17 (0.55) | |
| Range | 0–1 | 0–6 | 0–2 | 0–6 | |
| APR DRG SOI score, n (%) | | | | | 0.77* |
| 1 | 16 (62) | 148 (64) | 31 (69) | 195 (64) | |
| 2 | 10 (38) | 84 (36) | 14 (31) | 108 (36) | |
| Readmission, n (%) | 3 (12) | 11 (5) | 3 (7) | 17 (6) | 0.26‡ |
| Fiscal year, n (%) | | | | | <0.001‡ |
| 2004 | 6 (23) | 21 (9) | 17 (38) | 44 (15) | |
| 2005 | 6 (23) | 44 (19) | 13 (29) | 63 (21) | |
| 2006 | 4 (15) | 48 (21) | 6 (13) | 58 (19) | |
| 2007 | 3 (12) | 47 (20) | 3 (7) | 53 (17) | |
| 2008 | 6 (23) | 56 (24) | 2 (4) | 64 (21) | |
| 2009 | 1 (4) | 16 (7) | 4 (9) | 21 (7) | |
| Total charge ($) | | | | | <0.001‡ |
| Mean (SD) | 7038 (3127) | 4283 (1272) | 5893 (3313) | 4759 (2112) | |
| Range | 2727–14 986 | 1224–12 551 | 1223–18 141 | 1223–18 141 | |

APR DRG SOI = All Patient Refined Diagnosis Related Groups Severity of Illness; SD = standard deviation.
*Chi-square test.
†*F* test.
‡Fisher exact test.

*Conclusions.*—Higher volume and specialization seen at a regional eye trauma center are associated with lower costs in the surgical management of orbital trauma (Fig 2, Table 2).

▶ This study looks at the cost of care for surgical repair of orbital trauma in 3 types of hospital settings: a regional eye trauma center, a large academic medical center, and all other hospitals in the state of Maryland. The study found the lowest cost was at the regional eye center followed by the academic medical center; the most expensive of the 3 locations were the other hospitals (Table 2, Fig 2). To control for the potential differences in severity of trauma, a subgroup of patients who had a 1-day length of stay, did not come through the emergency department, and had a Diagnosis-Related Group Severity of Illness score of 1 or 2 was studied. The difference in cost between these groups remained similar and was statistically significant.

This study shows that a more specialized eye care facility and one that does a high volume of surgery has the lowest cost for repair of orbital trauma. Most would agree that a high volume of any medical condition allows for more efficient care and, in most cases, high-quality care. It should be noted this study did not study quality but only cost. Studying the quality of care should be the next goal.

**R. B. Penne, MD**

## The relationship between floppy eyelid syndrome and obstructive sleep apnoea

Muniesa MJ, Huerva V, Sánchez-de-la-Torre M, et al (Hospital Universitari Arnau de Vilanova, Lleida, Spain; Institut de Recerca Biomèdica de Lleida, Spain)
*Br J Ophthalmol* 97:1387-1390, 2013

*Purpose.*—To determine the prevalence of eyelid hyperlaxity and floppy eyelid syndrome (FES) in obstructive sleep apnoea (OSA), and the presence of OSA in FES.

*Participants.*—One-hundred and fourteen patients who had been consecutively admitted for OSA evaluation and 45 patients with FES in which sleep studies were recorded.

*Methods.*—Subjects underwent eyelid laxity measurement, slit-lamp examination and polysomnography.

*Results.*—Eighty-nine patients were diagnosed of OSA. Fourteen patients with OSA had FES (16%) and 54/89 (60.67%) had eyelid hyperlaxity. Two

**TABLE 1.**—Categorisation of Patients Admitted for OSA Evaluation, Based on Reported Clinical Findings

| | OSA Patients (AHI≥10) | Non-OSA Patients Group (AHI<10) | p Value |
|---|---|---|---|
| Patients, n | 89 | 25 | |
| Age, years Mean (SD) | 55.1±9.41 | 48.6±11.15 | 0.003 |
| Gender, male | 75% | 72% | 0.79 |
| BMI (kg/m$^2$) Mean (SD) | 32.3±5.32 | 29.2±4.93 | 0.004 |
| AHI (h$^{-1}$) Mean (SD) | 43.00±23.17 | 4.43±1.88 | <0.001 |
| Epworth mean (SD) | 9.5±4.93 | 7.8±4.58 | 0.13 |
| HTA | 47% | 35% | 0.45 |
| Diabetes | 15% | 10% | 0.73 |
| Dyslipidaemia | 29% | 30% | 1 |
| Smokers | 23% | 15% | 0.80 |
| COPD | 8% | 10% | 0.67 |
| Cardiovascular diseases | 20% | 5% | 0.18 |
| FES, n (%) | 14 (16%) | 2 (8%) | 0.51 |
| Eyelid hyperlaxity, n (%) | 54 (60.67%) | 8 (32%) | 0.0474* |

AHI, apnoea–hypopnoea/h index; BMI, body mass index; COPD, chronic obstructive pulmonary disease; DM, type 2 diabetes mellitus; Epworth, Epworth Sleepiness Scale score; FES, floppy eyelid syndrome; HTA, hypertension; OSA, obstructive sleep apnoea.

*Adjusted for age and BMI.

of the 25 non-OSA patients had FES (8%) and 8 of 25 (32%) had eyelid hyperlaxity. There was a significantly higher incidence of eyelid hyperlaxity in OSA than in non-OSA patients ($p = 0.004$). Thirty-eight of the 45 patients with FES were diagnosed of OSA (85%) and 65% had severe OSA.

*Conclusions.*—OSA might be an independent risk factor for eyelid hyperlaxity and severe OSA is common in patients with FES (Table 1).

▶ The message from this report is not complicated, but is important. The incidence of floppy eyelid syndrome (FES) among patients with obstructive sleep apnea (OSA) is 16% (Table 1). However, studies have found that as high as 85% of FES patients will have OSA. It is very important that any patient with FES be evaluated for OSA. Many of the FES patients will have severe OSA, and this disease can have high morbidity and even mortality rates. The reverse, however, is not true. Most OSA patients do not have FES, although in this study 16% did.

The diagnosis of FES should indicate that the patient needs to be evaluated for OSA before any surgical therapy is considered.

**R. B. Penne, MD**

---

**Ostium Shrinkage after Endoscopic Dacryocystorhinostomy**

Chan W, Selva D (Royal Adelaide Hosp, Australia)

*Ophthalmology* 120:1693-1696, 2013

---

*Objective.*—Ostium closure after endoscopic dacryocystorhinostomy (DCR) is the commonest cause for anatomic failure. We aimed to determine the changes in size of the DCR ostium over time and investigate the correlation of ostium size and surgical outcomes.

*Design.*—A single surgeon, prospective, nonrandomized, noncomparative, interventional case series.

*Participants.*—We included a consecutive series of patients who underwent powered endonasal DCR. All patients had radiologically confirmed nasolacrimal duct or canalicular obstruction.

*Methods.*—Patients were operated on by 1 surgeon (D.S.) and follow-up was at 4 weeks and 12 months. Ostium sizes were measured at the end of surgery and at 4 weeks and 12 months after surgery.

*Main Outcome Measures.*—Intraoperative and postoperative ostium size, correlation of ostium size, and surgical outcome.

*Results.*—We included 161 patients who fulfilled the inclusion criteria. Three patients were lost to follow-up. The ostium measured 8.6 (95% confidence interval [CI], 5.0–12.2) by 13.4 (95% CI, 10.3–16.5) at the time of surgery and 5.7 (95% CI, 2.3–9.0) by 9.5 (95% CI, 6.0–13.0) at 4 weeks, and 4.8 (95% CI, 1.9–7.7) by 8.2 (95% CI, 4.5–11.9) at 12 months. There was significant ostial shrinkage from surgery to 4 weeks (mean shrinkage of 50%) and from 4 weeks to 12 months (mean shrinkage of a further 15%). The intraoperative ostium size and postoperative size were positively correlated. Ostial size was not predictive of final ostial patency and symptomatic resolution of epiphora.

*Conclusions.*—After endoscopic DCR, the final ostium size on average is 35% of the original at 12 months postoperatively. The majority of the ostium shrinkage occurs within 4 weeks postoperatively with a lesser degree of shrinkage between 1 and 12 months postoperatively. Ostium size was not predictive of overall surgical outcome.

▶ This is a prospective study that looks at the size of the surgical ostium created during endoscopic dacryocystorhinostomy (DCR) surgery in 161 patients and how the ostium changes over 1 year postoperatively. The size of the ostium was then compared with the surgical success.

This study found that the ostium size shrinks over 1 year to an average of 35% of the original size and most of this shrinkage occurs in the first 4 weeks. There was an overall 90.7% surgical success over 1 year. The ostium size did not correlate with surgical success.

The 2 take-home points from this study are that the surgical ostium will shrink, however the final size of the ostium does not correlate with surgical success. Past studies have found similar ostium shrinkage. What is different in this study is that final ostium size did not seem to correlate with surgical success.

The fact that ostium size did not correlate with surgical success may suggest to some that there is then no reason to make a larger ostium. The authors address this and I agree with their thoughts. They suggest that as large an ostium as can be made should be created. They note that in some patients, this will be larger than others because of sac size or anatomy. DCR failure is often thought to be from scarring in the area of the common internal puncta, which would go along with the thought that ostium size may not be important but should be as large as possible. The exact importance of ostium size is still not clear. For now, creating as large an ostium as possible seems to be the prudent approach.

**R. B. Penne, MD**

---

## Incidence of Canalicular Closure with Endonasal Dacryocystorhinostomy without Intubation in Primary Nasolacrimal Duct Obstruction

Cannon PS, Chan W, Selva D (Univ of Adelaide, Australia)

*Ophthalmology* 120:1688-1692, 2013

---

*Purpose.*—To describe the incidence of canalicular closure with powered endonasal dacryocystorhinostomy (DCR) without canalicular intubation in primary acquired nasolacrimal duct obstruction (PANDO).

*Design.*—A single-surgeon, prospective, nonrandomized, noncomparative, interventional case series.

*Participants.*—Consecutive patients attending a specialist clinic of an oculoplastic surgeon (DS) with radiologically confirmed diagnosis of PANDO. Cases of canalicular disease were excluded.

*Methods.*—Patients with radiologically confirmed PANDO without canalicular involvement underwent endonasal DCR without intubation. The operation was performed by 1 surgeon (DS) and follow-up was at 4 weeks and 12 months.

*Main Outcome Measures.*—Outcomes were recorded as subjective symptomatic relief at 12 months and endoscopic evidence of ostium patency and canalicular patency.

*Results.*—There were 132 cases that fulfilled the inclusion criteria. Three cases were lost to follow-up. Preoperatively, 96.3% of cases had Munk scores of >2. Of the 129 cases, 127 (98.5%) had endoscopic evidence of a patent ostium with a positive endoscopic dye test at the 12-month follow-up. All cases had a patent canalicular system as demonstrated by syringing and probing. Of the 129 cases, 117 (90.7%) had subjective improvement of epiphora at 12 months with 88.4% of cases reporting Munk scores of ≤1.

*Conclusions.*—In this prospective series of nonintubation for PANDO, there were no cases of canalicular closure or stenosis at 12 months. Anatomic and functional success was similar to reported outcomes for DCR with intubation for PANDO. We advocate that routine intubation for the purpose of maintaining canalicular patency is not necessary when performing endonasal DCR in PANDO.

*Financial Disclosure(s).*—Proprietary or commercial disclosure may be found after the references.

▶ This study looks at the need for silicone intubation as part of an endoscopic dacryocystorhinostomy (DCR). One surgeon treated 132 consecutive patients for either complete or partial nasolacrimal obstruction with an endoscopic DCR without silicone intubation. The patients were then evaluated at 12 months based on symptomatic relief of tearing and endoscopic evidence of ostium patency.

The results showed 90.4% success without lacrimal intubation, which is comparable to results using a silicone tube. One notable difference in this study from others is 40% of these patients had symptomatic tearing, but their obstruction was not complete on preoperative lacrimal irrigation. Whether this difference is significant and how it affects the final success is unknown but needs to be considered.

This study is important in that it suggests that silicone intubation of the lacrimal system may not be needed as part of an endoscopic DCR. For me, this study questions the need for silicone intubation, but because it was not randomized and because of the inclusion of so many partial obstructions, I am not ready to abandon silicone intubation yet. The study did not include patients with any canalicular scarring, and those patients do need silicone intubation of their lacrimal system.

**R. B. Penne, MD**

**Role of Oral Corticosteroids in Orbital Cellulitis**

Pushker N, Tejwani LK, Bajaj MS, et al (All India Inst of Med Sciences, Ansari Nagar, New Delhi)

*Am J Ophthalmol* 156:178-183.e1, 2013

*Purpose.*—To evaluate the role of oral corticosteroids as an anti-inflammatory adjunct in the treatment of orbital cellulitis.

*Design.*—Prospective, comparative, single-masked, interventional clinical study.

*Methods.*—*Setting*: Tertiary eye care center (All India Institute of Medical Sciences).

*Study Population*: Patients with acute onset (within 14 days) of orbital cellulitis with or without abscess.

*Intervention*: Patients were randomized into 2 groups in the ratio of 1:2. Both groups received initial intravenous antibiotics. In Group 2, oral steroids were added after an initial response to intravenous antibiotics.

*Main Outcome Measures*: Resolution of signs and symptoms, duration of intravenous antibiotics, length of hospital stay, and sequelae of disease (ptosis, proptosis, and movement restriction) were evaluated and compared between the 2 groups.

*Results.*—A total of 21 patients (age range, 11-59 years) with orbital cellulitis were studied. There were 7 patients in Group 1, who received standard intravenous antibiotics, and 14 in Group 2, who received adjuvant steroids. Patients in Group 2 showed an earlier resolution of inflammation in terms of periorbital edema ($P = .002$ at day 7), conjunctival chemosis ($P < .001$ at day 10), and pain ($P = .012$ at day 7). They also attained vision of 0.02 on logMAR earlier than Group 1 patients. Decrease in proptosis and improvement in extraocular movements were also significantly better with the use of steroids ($P = .027$ at day 10, $P = .003$ at day 14, respectively). While a significant number of patients in Group 1 had mild residual ptosis, proptosis, and movement restriction at 12 weeks, none of the patients treated with steroids had any residual changes ($P = .023$, $P = .001$, and $P = .001$, respectively). The durations of intravenous antibiotics and hospital stay were significantly less in Group 2.

*Conclusion.*—Use of oral steroids as an adjunct to intravenous antibiotic therapy for orbital cellulitis may hasten resolution of inflammation with a low risk of exacerbating infection.

▶ The benefit of corticosteroids in the treatment of orbital cellulitis has long been debated. They definitely decrease inflammation, but is there any risk of worsening the infection? This is a prospective, randomized, comparative study of the role of corticosteroids in the treatment of orbital cellulitis. The study added steroids to the treatment of patients with orbital cellulitis after 4 days of intravenous antibiotics on a randomized basis. The clinical parameters followed were pain, fever, periorbital edema, chemosis, vision, proptosis, and extraocular movements.

Patients who received steroids as part of their treatment had faster and more normalization of all parameters. The duration of antibiotics required and the length of hospital stay were also shorter. All this was statistically significant. There was no evidence that steroids worsened or prolonged the orbital infection.

Other specialties, such as ear, nose, and throat, routinely use steroids while treating an infection with good results. This study reassures me that steroid use is helpful in the treatment of orbital infections. It is important to note that the steroids were not added until the infection had responded to antibiotic (4 days in this study). Starting steroids at the same time as antibiotics has not been studied, and I would not do that until we have a study showing that it is safe.

**R. B. Penne, MD**

---

**High prevalence of IgG4-related lymphoplasmacytic infiltrative disorder in 25 patients with orbital inflammation: a retrospective case series**

Deschamps R, Deschamps L, Depaz R, et al (Fondation Ophtalmologique Adolphe de Rothschild, Paris, France; Bichat Hosp, Paris, France)

*Br J Ophthalmol* 97:999-1004, 2013

---

*Aims.*—To evaluate retrospectively the prevalence of positive IgG4-immunostaining in orbital tissue of patients with idiopathic orbital inflammation and to compare the clinical, radiographic and pathologic features among patients with and without IgG4-positive cells.

*Patients and Methods.*—25 patients with biopsy-proven idiopathic orbital in flammation examined from January 2006 through December 2011 were included. Immunohistochemistry with IgG and IgG4 immunostaining from biopsy specimens of all patients was performed. Tissue with more than 10 IgG4-positive plasma cells per high-power field and with a ratio of IgG4+/IgG+ plasma cells of more than 40% was scored as positive. Histopathologic features, demographic and clinical data, radiologic findings, treatment and follow-up information for each patient were analysed.

*Results.*—Immunohistochemical staining showed 10 cases (40%) were IgG4 positive. The symptoms and signs included eyelid or periocular swelling/mass in all, pain (3/10), extraocular muscle restriction (3/10), proptosis (5/10) and/or decreased vision (4/10). Demographic and clinical findings of these patients did not differ from those with IgG4-negative cells. The presence of positive IgG4-immunostaining in orbital tissue was significantly associated with characteristic pathological features (more background fibrosis, lymphoid hyperplasia, plasma cells and phlebitis).

*Conclusions.*—Finally, 40% of patients with biopsy-proven orbital inflammation were classified as IgG4-RD, with typical histological features, but without specific clinical or radiological findings.

▶ Immunoglobulin G4 (IgG4)-related disease is a newly recognized disease entity characterized by IgG4-positive plasma cells and T-lymphocyte infiltration into various organs. It was first described in relationship to autoimmune pancreatitis in 2001 and has since been reported in other organs, including the orbit. The question has been whether patients with idiopathic orbital inflammation (IOI) with IgG4-positive cells differ from those with non IgG4-positive cells.

This was a retrospective review of the pathology and charts of 25 patients with biopsy-proven IOI. Although 40% of the specimens were IgG4 positive, the clinical and radiologic features were no different between these 2 groups in the 25 patients studied. What was different was the pathologic features with the IgG4-positive specimens showing more fibrosis, lymphoid hyperplasia, plasma cells, and phlebitis.

This study found no significant difference in the IOI disease in the group that was IgG4-positive vs the group that was negative. There has been suggestion that patients with IgG4-positive disease may be less responsive to steroids and have more orbital fibrosis, and the disease may be more likely to involve other organs. The issue of multiorgan involvement with this inflammation was not directly studied here but was found in 3 patients who were IgG4 positive and in only one IgG4-negative patient.

The value of IgG4 staining in IOI remains unclear. The clinical course and treatment response does not seem to be different in studies so far. There is a suggestion that IgG4 staining may indicate a higher chance of involvement in other organs. Whether that is true remains to be determined, but for now it must be considered. We await further studies.

**R. B. Penne, MD**

---

**Hyaluronic Acid Gel Weight: A Nonsurgical Option for the Management of Paralytic Lagophthalmos**

Martín-Oviedo C, García I, Lowy A, et al (Gregorio Marañon Hosp, Madrid, Spain)

*Laryngoscope* 123:E91-E96, 2013

---

*Objectives/Hypothesis.*—Management of lagophthalmos should be a priority in the treatment of patients with facial palsy. The aim of the study was to evaluate the safety and efficacy of injecting hyaluronic acid gel into the upper eyelid as a nonsurgical alternative for patients with temporary facial palsy.

*Method/Study Design.*—Retrospective study of 26 patients treated with hyaluronic acid gel injected into the pretarsal region of the upper eyelid. Measurements taken before and after treatment were standardized and compared using digitized photographs. Patients were followed up for 1 year, and overall outcomes were assessed.

*Results.*—All patients initially demonstrated improvement in lagophthalmos, which decreased to 0.0 mm. After 1 month, a significant increase in lagophthalmos was observed in two patients (initial fissure of 8 and 9 mm), and a platinum weight was implanted to control keratopathy. The remaining patients (initial lagophthalmos below 6.5 mm) maintained the improvement until facial restoration. Only three patients had recurrent lagophthalmos (2 mm) due to resorption, which was resolved by injecting

**TABLE 1.**—Results and Complications

| ID | HB Score | PFAC Pre | HA Volume | PFAC 2 Months Post | PFAC 4 Months Post | HA Volume Reinjected | PFAC 6 Months Post | 1 Year Post | Complications |
|---|---|---|---|---|---|---|---|---|---|
| Patient 1 | III | 3,5 mm | 0.3 ml | 0 mm | 0 mm | NO | Recovered | Recovered | |
| Patient 22 | III | 3.5 mm | 0.3 ml | 0 mm | 0 mm | NO | Recovered | Recovered | |
| Patient 13 | III | 3.6 mm | 0.4 ml | 0 mm | 0 mm | NO | Recovered | Recovered | Transient ecchymosis |
| Patient 4 | IV | 3.8 mm | 0.4 ml | 0 mm | 0 mm | NO | 0 mm | Recovered | Transient ecchymosis |
| Patient 23 | IV | 3.8 mm | 0.4 ml | 0 mm | 0 mm | NO | Recovered | Recovered | NR blepharoptosis |
| Patient 6 | IV | 4 mm | 0.4 ml | 0 mm | 0 mm | NO | Recovered | Recovered | |
| Patient 12 | IV | 4 mm | 0.4 ml | 0 mm | 0 mm | NO | Recovered | Recovered | |
| Patient 15 | IV | 4 mm | 0.4 ml | 0 mm | 0 mm | NO | Recovered | Recovered | Transient ecchymosis |
| Patient 17 | IV | 4 mm | 0.5 ml | 0 mm | 0 mm | NO | Recovered | Recovered | |
| Patient 19 | IV | 4 mm | 0.5 ml | 0 mm | 0 mm | NO | Recovered | Recovered | |
| Patient 21 | IV | 4 mm | 0.5 ml | 0 mm | 0 mm | NO | Recovered | Recovered | |
| Patient 25 | IV | 4 mm | 0.5 ml | 0 mm | 0 mm | NO | Recovered | Recovered | |
| Patient 14 | IV | 4.2 mm | 0.5 ml | 0 mm | 0 mm | NO | Recovered | Recovered | |
| Patient 11 | IV | 4.3 mm | 0.5 ml | 0 mm | 0 mm | NO | Recovered | Recovered | |
| Patient 26 | IV | 4.3 mm | 0.6 ml | 0 mm | 0 mm | NO | 0 mm | Recovered | |
| Patient 9 | IV | 4,5 mm | 0.4 ml | 0 mm | 0 mm | NO | Recovered | Recovered | |
| Patient 10 | IV | 4,5 mm | 0.6 ml | 0 mm | 0 mm | NO | Recovered | Recovered | |
| Patient 18 | IV | 4,5 mm | 0.6 ml | 0 mm | 0 mm | NO | Recovered | Recovered | |
| Patient 24 | IV | 4,5 mm | 0.6 ml | 0 mm | 0 mm | NO | 0 mm | Recovered | |
| Patient 2 | IV | 5 mm | 0.6 ml | 0 mm | 0 mm | NO | Recovered | Recovered | |
| Patient 5 | IV | 6 mm | 0.7 ml | 0 mm | 0 mm | NO | 0 mm | Recovered | NR blepharoptosis |
| Patient 16 | V | 6 mm | 0.8 ml | 0 mm | 1 mm | 0.2 ml | 0 mm | Recovered | NR blepharoptosis |
| Patient 7 | V | 6,2 mm | 0.8 ml | 0 mm | 2 mm | 0.3 ml | 0 mm | Recovered | NR blepharoptosis |
| Patient 20 | V | 6.5 mm | 0.9 ml | 0 mm | 2 mm | 0.3 ml | 0 mm | Recovered | NR blepharoptosis |
| Patient 3 | V | 8 mm | 1 ml | 3 mm | Platinum chain | NO | Platinum chain | Recovered | |
| Patient 8 | V | 9 mm | 1 ml | 4 mm | Platinum chain | NO | Platinum chain | Recovered | |

Twenty-six patients classified according to their House-Brackman Score (HB score) and palpebral fissure with attempted closure pretreatment (PFAC pre). Hyaluronic acid gel volume injected (HA volume). Palpebral fissure with attempted closure 2, 4, 6 months posttreatment (PFAC 2, 4, 6 months post). Volume of hyaluronic acid gel reinjected (HA volume reinjected). One year of follow-up (1 year post). Complications, transient orbicular ecchymosis, and nonreabsorption blepharoptosis (NR blepharoptosis).

an additional 0.3 cc. The mean improvement in lagophthalmos was 4.6 mm (range, 3.5–6.5 mm). Complications included transient ecchymosis and minimal blepharoptosis due to nonreabsorption in five patients. These patients were successfully treated with hyaluronidase.

*Conclusions.*—Hyaluronic acid gel has proven effective in reducing paralytic lagophthalmos and controlling keratopathy in patients with temporary facial palsy, especially those with palpebral fissure with attempted closure no greater than 6.5 mm. Injection of hyaluronic acid gel is safe, quick, and easily performed. In addition, it is more cost-effective than surgery.

*Level of Evidence.*—4. (Table 1).

▶ This is another nonsurgical option to temporarily improve the closure of the eye affected by a facial palsy. Injecting hyaluronic acid gel (Restylane in these patients) in the upper lid resulted in resolution of the lagophthalmos in 24 of 26 patients. Two patients had incomplete resolution of their lagophthalmos with the injection and had implantation of a platinum chain. Three of the 24 patients required an additional injection of 0.3 mL at 4 months. The total volume of injection was on the average 0.6 mL and ranged from 0.3 to 1.0 mL. There was no guide noted in the report as to how the volume injected was determined. From Table 1 it appears that the larger the amount of lagophthalmos, the higher the volume of hyaluronic acid gel that was injected.

The results are impressive, and it is a nice way to temporarily give better eye closure in a facial palsy. The problem in the United States is that this is not reimbursable by insurance companies and is an off-label use of hyaluronic acid gel. A Botox tarsorrhaphy is a related nonsurgical tarsorrhaphy that is also not covered by insurance. Botox, however, completely closes the eye, whereas this procedure acts like an eyelid weight and gives better closure but still allowing the eye to open.

This is a technique to keep in mind, as it is very effective. At this time, the inability to get insurances to pay for the hyaluronic acid gel or the procedure will limit its clinical use in the United States.

**R. B. Penne, MD**

---

### Prevalence and Natural History of Graves' Orbitopathy in a Large Series of Patients With Newly Diagnosed Graves' Hyperthyroidism Seen at a Single Center

Tanda ML, Piantanida E, Liparulo L, et al (Univ of Insubria, Varese, Italy)
*J Clin Endocrinol Metab* 98:1443-1449, 2013

---

*Background.*—The prevalence and natural history of Graves' orbitopathy (GO) are poorly documented.

*Methods.*—A large series of 346 patients with newly diagnosed and recent onset Graves' hyperthyroidism seen at a single (nontertiary referral) center over an 8-year period were enrolled in an observational prospective study and evaluated for GO activity and severity according to the

TABLE 2.—Features of Patients at Enrollment According to the Absence or Presence (and Degree) of GO

| Feature | Absent GO | Mild and Inactive GO | Moderate-to-Severe GO | *P* Value |
|---|---|---|---|---|
| Number | 255 | 70 | 21 | |
| Age, y | 45.6 ± 13.6 | 43.9 ± 12.2 | 53.7 ± 13.6 | .01 |
| Women | 195 (76.5%) | 55 (78.6%) | 16 (76.2%) | .93 |
| Men | 60 (23.5%) | 15 (21.4%) | 5 (23.8%) | |
| Smokers | 78 (30.6%) | 34 (48.6%) | 10 (47.6%) | .01 |
| Serum FT4 (pg/mL) | 34.2 ± 15.5 | 36.5 ± 13.0 | 32.1 ± 14.9 | .38 |
| Serum FT3 (pg/mL) | 12.7 ± 8.3 | 12.8 ± 6.3 | 12.1 ± 8.1 | .93 |
| Serum TRAb (U/L) | 11.8 ± 10.8 | 15.9 ± 11.6 | 17.1 ± 13.9 | .01 |

Data are mean ± SD. Overall *P* value: F-test (ANOVA) for mean values and $\chi^2$ test for proportions. Null hypothesis: the three groups do not differ on average in the considered features.

EUGOGO (European Group on Graves' Orbitopathy) criteria. After excluding patients immediately treated for moderate-to-severe GO, patients undergoing total thyroidectomy or radioactive iodine treatment, and patients lost to follow-up, 237 patients were submitted to antithyroid drug (ATD) treatment, with ocular evaluation at 6, 12, and 18 months.

*Results.*—Among the whole cohort, at presentation 255 (73.7%) had no ocular involvement, 70 (20.2%) had mild and inactive GO, 20 (5.8%) had moderate-to-severe and active GO, and 1 (0.3%) had sight-threatening GO with dysthyroid optic neuropathy. Of the 237 patients who completed the 18-month follow-up during or after ATD treatment, 194 (81.9%) had no GO at baseline. Progression to moderate-to-severe GO occurred in 5 (2.6%) of these patients. Of the 43 (18.1%) patients with mild and inactive GO at baseline, 1 (2.4%) progressed to moderate-to-severe GO, and 25 (58.1%) experienced complete remission.

*Conclusions.*—Most patients with newly diagnosed Graves' disease have no ocular involvement. Moderate-to-severe and active GO or sight-threatening GO are rare at presentation and rarely develop during ATD treatment. Most patients (>80%) with no GO at baseline do not develop GO after an 18-month follow-up period. Remission of mild GO occurs in the majority of cases (Table 2).

▶ As an ophthalmologist, there is a tendency to see a large number of Graves' hyperthyroid patients who have Graves' orbitopathy (GO). This report looks at the prevalence of GO over time in a large group of patients that were newly diagnosed with Graves' hyperthyroidism. Patients who already had moderate-to-severe GO were excluded, as were patients who had their hyperthyroidism treated with radioactive iodine or surgical thyroidectomy (Table 2).

This study followed 237 patients for 18 months. Of the 194 that had no GO at baseline, 87.1% did not have GO, and 10.3% had mild GO. Progression to moderate-to-severe GO occurred in 5 (2.6%). Of the 43 patients who had mild GO at baseline, only 1 (2.4%) had moderate-to-severe GO, and 58% showed complete remission of eye manifestations over the 18 months.

These results are good news for GO patients. From these results, a patient newly diagnosed with GO who has mild or no ocular manifestations has a 5% chance of developing moderate-to-severe GO over time, and many who have mild signs of GO will remit in a large proportion of patients. Remember this did not include patients treated with radioactive iodine, and these patients may have a different course.

The need to stop smoking and the importance of close control of systemic thyroid levels in these patients is emphasized and may play a role in this low incidence of progression to moderate-to-severe GO.

**R. B. Penne, MD**

**Long-term Botulinum Toxin Treatment of Benign Essential Blepharospasm, Hemifacial Spasm, and Meige Syndrome**

Czyz CN, Burns JA, Petrie TP, et al (Ohio Univ/Ohio Health Doctor's Hosp, Columbus; Grant Med Ctr, Columbus, OH; et al)

*Am J Ophthalmol* 156:173-177.e2, 2013

*Purpose.*—To report the clinical success and incidence of adverse events of repetitive botulinum toxin treatment of 15 years or greater.

*Design.*—Retrospective cohort study.

*Methods.*—The study sample consisted of 37 patients from a clinical practice, 11 male and 26 female. Inclusion criteria consisted of patients treated a minimum of 15 consecutive years for facial dystonia. Seven patients had hemifacial spasm, 4 Meige syndrome, and 26 benign essential blepharospasm. Main outcome measures consisted of treatment efficacy and adverse events.

*Results.*—Mean treatment duration was 19.4 years (SD 2.2) with an average of 62 (SD 22) treatments of 70.2 (SD 20.8) neurotoxin units. Mean duration of treatment efficacy was 127 days (SD 37) with a 5% physician-reported minor adverse event rate and no major adverse events over each patient's clinical course. Patients reported no major and 20% incidence of minor adverse events over the treatment course.

*Conclusion.*—Results suggest that long-term botulinum toxin treatment produces clinical success in the alleviation of facial dystonia symptoms. Treatment produced a low incidence of major adverse events and minor adverse events. Previous studies may under-report clinical success and over-report adverse events because of study design (Table 1).

▶ This study looks at 37 patients who received botulinum toxin over 15 years or longer for hemifacial spasm, Meige syndrome, or benign essential blepharospasm. The 2 outcomes evaluated were treatment efficacy and adverse effects. Although the number of patients does not seem high when you consider keeping the same patients for 15 years or longer, it is actually a remarkable number.

The findings are fairly straightforward. There was no evidence in these patients that over time the effectiveness of treatment lessened or that the amount of botulinum toxin required to achieve a therapeutic effect increased.

TABLE 1.—Physician- and Patient-Reported Adverse Events of Botulinum Toxin Treatment for Benign Essential Blepharospasm, Hemifacial Spasm, and Meige Syndrome

| | Physician-Reported | | Patient-Reported | |
|---|---|---|---|---|
| | Major Event | Minor Event | Major Event | Minor Event |
| Treatments #1-3 | 0/111 | 6/111 (5%)<br>2.5%: diplopia (3)<br>2.5%: ptosis (3) | 0/111 | 45/111 (41%)<br>3%: diplopia (3)<br>17%: ptosis (19)<br>21%: other (23) |
| Initial treatment (treatment #4) | 0/37 | 2/37 (5%)<br>5%: diplopia (2) | 0/37 | 7/37 (19%)<br>3%: diplopia (1)<br>5%: ptosis (2)<br>11%: other (4) |
| Initial (#4) - final treatment | 0/2170 | 100/2170 (5%)<br>3%: diplopia (66)<br>2%: ptosis (34) | 0/2170 | 436/2170 (20%)<br>3%: diplopia (66)<br>7%: ptosis (156)<br>10%: other (214) |
| Final treatment | 0/37 | 0/37 | 0/37 | 7/37 (19%)<br>8%: ptosis (3)<br>11%: other (4) |

This refutes some previous studies and what may be perceived as a general belief that with long-term treatment, patients develop a resistance to botulinum toxin.

Looking at adverse effects, most importantly, there were no major adverse effects in more than 2281 treatments, so the conclusion can be made that botulinum toxin injections for these conditions are safe. From the standpoint of minor adverse effects (ie, ptosis, diplopia, and others; Table 1), these were more common during the first 3 injections. These minor adverse effects decreased 50% when comparing the incidence of minor adverse effects during visits 1 through 3 vs the incidence of minor adverse effects after the third visit. This is likely related to modification of the injection amounts and sites during these first 3 visits to maximize the treatment effectiveness and minimize any adverse effects found during the initial injections.

This is a very reassuring study for the long-term use of botulinum toxin. It not only showed safety in its long-term use but also did not find any evidence that patients develop a resistance to botulinum toxin with long-term use.

**R. B. Penne, MD**

## Recovery from deepening of the upper eyelid sulcus after switching from bimatoprost to latanoprost

Sakata R, Shirato S, Miyata K, et al (Tokyo Metropolitan Geriatric Hosp, Itabashi, Japan; Yotsuya Shirato Eye Clinic, Tokyo, Japan; Miyata Eye Hosp, Miyazaki, Japan)
*Jpn J Ophthalmol* 57:179-184, 2013

*Purpose.*—Although useful for reducing intraocular pressure (IOP), bimatoprost (BIM) can cause deepening of the upper eyelid sulcus

(DUES), one of the symptoms of prostaglandin-associated periorbitopathy (PAP). We investigated recovery from BIM-induced DUES after switching treatment to latanoprost (LAT).

*Design.*—Prospective, observer-masked, open-label study.

*Methods.*—Twenty-five Japanese patients suffering from primary open-angle glaucoma treated with LAT in both eyes for longer than 6 months and requiring further IOP reduction were prospectively enrolled in the study. During the first 6 months after the switch to BIM, 15 of the 25 patients (60 %) developed DUES. Among these patients, 13 were switched back to LAT and re-examined for DUES at 2-month intervals for an additional 6 months.

*Results.*—Two months after the switch back to LAT, for 11 of the 13 patients (85 %) the DUES symptoms had either decreased or disappeared, and this was maintained for at least 6 months. During this time, 6 of 8 patients (75 %) subjectively positive for DUES self-reported a decrease in DUES.

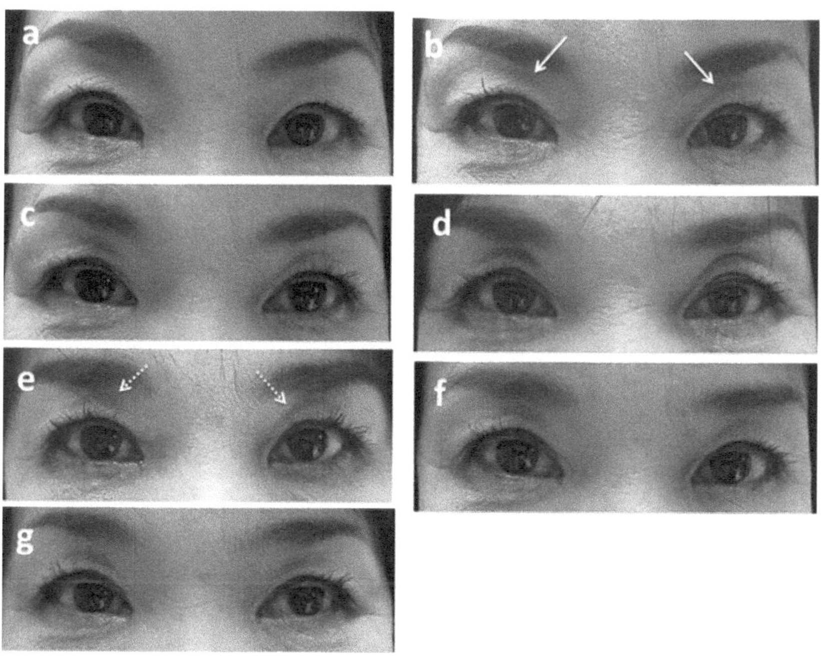


**FIGURE 1.**—A case of complete DUES recovery. For this 58-year-old woman DUES was observed 1 month after switching from LAT to BIM (**b**, *white arrow*). However, after treatment was switched back to LAT, DUES was not reported (**e**, *dotted white arrow*). Photos **a**, **b**, **c**, and **d** indicate 0, 1, 3, and 6 months, respectively, after the switch from LAT to BIM. Photos **e**, **f**, and **g** indicate 2, 4, and 6 months, respectively, after the switch back to LAT. (Reprinted from Sakata R, Shirato S, Miyata K, et al. Recovery from deepening of the upper eyelid sulcus after switching from bimatoprost to latanoprost. *Jpn J Ophthalmol.* 2013;57:179-184, with permission from Japanese Ophthalmological Society.)

*Conclusions.*—Although DUES is a frequent side effect of treatment with BIM, switching to LAT may reverse the condition for most patients (Figs 1 and 2, Tables 2 and 3).

▶ Several recent studies have found eyelid and orbital changes associated with the use of prostaglandin analogue drops for the treatment of glaucoma. The most commonly implicated drug has been bimatoprost (BIM).[1] This report looked at one aspect of the eyelid/orbital change, deepening of the upper eyelid sulcus (DUES).

The researchers identified 25 patients who were on latanoprost (LAT) for at least 6 months and needed lower intraocular pressure. These patients were switched to BIM, and within 6 months, 15 of 25 patients had developed DUES. Thirteen of the 15 were then switched back to LAT and followed up with for 6 months. Eleven of the 13 patients were noted to have a partial or full resolution of DUES (Figs 1 and 2). These results were based on photographs graded by the 4 authors. From the patients' perspectives, 8 of the 13

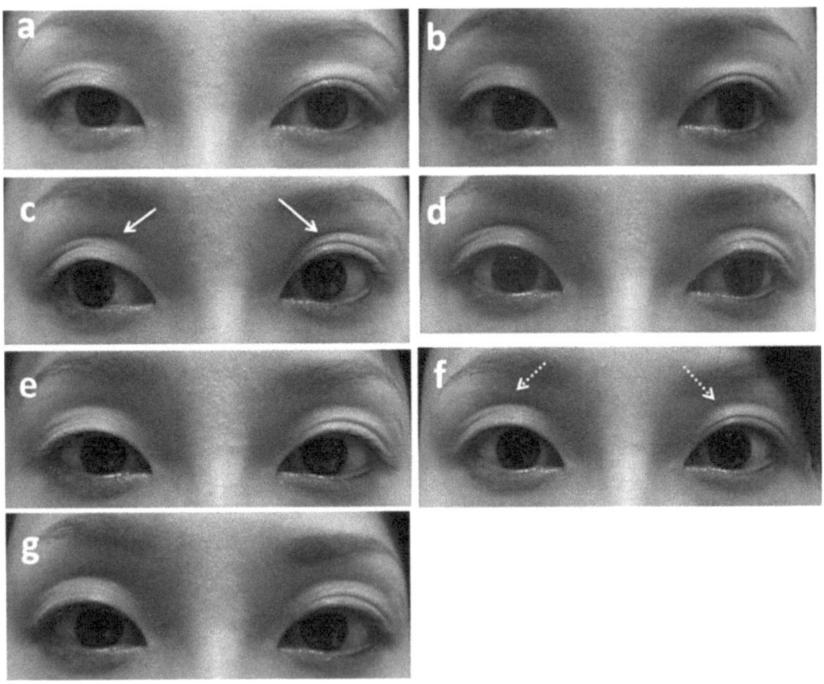


**FIGURE 2.**—A case of incomplete DUES recovery. For this 37-year-old woman DUES was observed a few months after switching from LAT to BIM (**c**, *white arrow*). After treatment was switched back to LAT, the DUES gradually decreased over a 4-month period but did not completely disappear (**f**, *dotted white arrow*). Photos **a**, **b**, **c**, and **d** indicate 0, 1, 3, and 6 months, respectively, after the switch from LAT to BIM. Photos **e**, **f**, and **g** indicate 2, 4, and 6 months, respectively, after the switch back to LAT. (Reprinted from Sakata R, Shirato S, Miyata K, et al. Recovery from deepening of the upper eyelid sulcus after switching from bimatoprost to latanoprost. *Jpn J Ophthalmol*. 2013;57:179-184, with permission from Japanese Ophthalmological Society.)

TABLE 2.—The Course of Changes in Objective DUES Measurements after the Switch Back to Latanoprost

| Objective Sign | Switch Time | 2 Months | 4 Months | 6 Months |
|---|---|---|---|---|
| DUES | | | | |
| Positive | 13/13 (100) | 2/13 (15) | 2/13 (15) | 2/13 (15) |
| Negative | 0/0 (0) | 11/13 (85) | 11/13 (85) | 11/13 (85) |

All data given represent the number of cases (%).
*DUES* deepening of the upper eyelid sulcus.

TABLE 3.—The Course of Changes in Subjectively Reported DUES after the Switch Back to Latanoprost

| Subjective Sign | Switch Time | 2 Months | 4 Months | 6 Months |
|---|---|---|---|---|
| DUES | | | | |
| Positive | 8/8 (100) | 3/8 (37) | 3/8 (37) | 2/8 (25) |
| Negative | 0/0 (0) | 5/8 (63) | 5/8 (63) | 6/8 (75) |

All data given represent the number of cases (%).
*DUES* deepening of the upper eyelid sulcus.

patients noted the DUES (Table 2) and 6 of those 8 noted a decrease in DUES (Table 3) when switched back from BIM to LAT.

This study found that early on there is a reversible component to at least some of the eyelid and orbital changes associated with prostaglandin analogues. There is still a lot we don't understand about this entity, why it happens, whom it happens to, and to what extent is it reversible. I believe it has become accepted that these eye drops do cause a change in the orbital fat, which may be much or all of the periorbital changes we see clinically. How this will modify the use of these powerful antiglaucoma drugs remains to be seen, and more studies are needed both clinically and pathologically.

**R. B. Penne, MD**

*Reference*

1. Filippopoulos T, Paula JS, Torun N, Hatton MP, Pasquale LR, Grosskreutz CL. Periorbital changes associated with topical bimatoprost. *Ophthal Plast Reconstr Surg*. 2008;24:302-307.

# 7 Pediatric Ophthalmology

## Surgical results after one-muscle recession for correction of horizontal sensory strabismus in children

Hopker LM, Weakley DR (Univ of Texas Southwestern Med Ctr, Dallas)

*J AAPOS* 17:174-176, 2013

*Purpose.*—To report the success rates in children after one-muscle recession for sensory strabismus.

*Methods.*—The medical records of consecutive patients ≤18 years of age who underwent primary unilateral horizontal surgery for sensory strabismus measuring $\leq 30^{\Delta}$ from 2004 to 2010 were retrospectively reviewed. Data collected included age at surgery, sex, length of follow-up, procedure performed, pre- and postoperative deviation, and treatment of associated vertical strabismus. Success was defined as a final deviation within $10^{\Delta}$ of orthotropia.

*Results.*—A total of 33 patients (16 males) were included. Mean age at surgery was 5.2 years (range, 6 months to 17 years) and mean follow-up was 36 months (range, 6 months-7.4 years). Age at surgery ($P = 0.37$) and follow-up ($P = 0.79$) were comparable in patients with esotropia (n = 12) and exotropia (n = 21). Mean preoperative deviation was $23.7^{\Delta}$ in the esotropia group and $24^{\Delta}$ in the exotropia group ($P = 0.875$). Successful postoperative alignment was achieved in 76% of esotropic patients and 92% of exotropic patients ($P = 0.379$). Lateral rectus recessions resulted in a mean correction of $2.8^{\Delta}$/mm of recession compared to $3.0^{\Delta}$/mm for medial rectus recessions ($P = 0.71$).

*Conclusions.*—Advantages of one-muscle recession include a high success rate, few over-corrections, relatively short duration of surgery, and an intact muscle should reoperation be indicated.

▶ Unilateral rectus muscle surgery is a safe, effective, and predictable treatment for small- to moderate-angle horizontal deviations regardless of whether the vision is significantly reduced in the involved eye. This procedure leaves other muscles untouched for repeat surgery and should be considered an excellent alternative to 2-muscle surgery for sensory strabismus of a small to moderate angle of deviation.

**L. B. Nelson, MD, MBA**

## Improved sensory status and quality-of-life measures in adult patients after strabismus surgery

Dickmann A, Aliberti S, Rebecchi MT, et al (Catholic Univ, Rome, Italy; et al)
*J AAPOS* 17:25-28, 2013

*Purpose.*—To evaluate the change in sensory status and quality-of-life measures in adults with long-standing childhood-onset constant strabismus.

*Methods.*—Consecutive patients with childhood-onset, long-term constant strabismus were enrolled. Sensory status was examined with Bagolini striated glasses test and Worth 4-dot test. Stereopsis was tested with the Lang and TNO stereopsis tests. Quality of life was studied with 2 different questionnaires (Short Form Health Survey [SF-36] and the Amblyopia and Strabismus Questionnaire [A&SQ]), which patients completed before and 3 months after strabismus surgery.

*Results.*—A total of 20 patients (age range, 18-63 years) were included, 10 of whom were esotropic and 10 of whom were exotropic. Of these, 13 obtained a satisfactory postoperative alignment and demonstrated an increase of sensory status with Bagolini striated glasses. Six patients who demonstrated suppression preoperatively achieved fusion and stereopsis postoperatively. The mean score in all domains of the A&SQ improved significantly, particularly with regard to social contact and cosmesis ($P = 0.00067$), distance estimation ($P = 0.000312$), and visual disorientation ($P = 0.004777$). Similarly, the mean score in 7 of 8 areas in the SF-36 improved significantly, particularly with regard to physical function ($P = 0.000564$), general health ($P = 0.002296$), vitality ($P = 0.002891$), social function ($P = 0.004234$), and mental health ($P = 0.000334$). The overall mean score of both questionnaires improved in all patients with a satisfactory postoperative alignment and increase of sensory status.

*Conclusions.*—Surgical treatment of strabismus in adults with long-standing childhood-onset constant strabismus can result in patients feeling that their quality of life has improved and can restore binocular sensory function.

▶ Strabismus surgery to restore ocular alignment has a significant effect on patients' self-esteem and self-confidence in patients with childhood-onset strabismus. Improving the psychosocial aspects of strabismus in adults also has a positive effect on quality of life. Even in patients with long-standing strabismus, improving alignment can increase binocularity and broaden the field of single binocular field, which also has a positive effect on these patients' quality of life.

**L. B. Nelson, MD, MBA**

**Bilateral Changes in Foveal Structure in Individuals with Amblyopia**

Bruce A, Pacey IE, Bradbury JA, et al (Univ of Bradford, UK; Bradford Teaching Hosps Foundation Trust, UK)

*Ophthalmology* 120:395-403, 2013

*Purpose.*—To examine foveal structure in amblyopia using spectral-domain optical coherence tomography (SD-OCT).

*Design.*—Prospective, cross-sectional study.

*Participants and Controls.*—Two subject groups were recruited to the study: 85 amblyopes (34 adults, 51 children) and 110 visually normal controls (44 adults, 66 children).

*Methods.*—A detailed eye examination, including an SD-OCT scan, was performed in all participants. A total of 390 eyes of 195 subjects were imaged using a 3-dimensional (3D) macula scan covering a nominal 6 × 6-mm area with a resolution of 256 × 256 (65 536 axial scans). Data from the B-scans bisecting the fovea both horizontally and vertically were fitted with a mathematical model of the fovea to determine a range of foveal parameters.

*Main Outcome Measures.*—Foveal thickness, foveal pit depth, and foveal pit slope.

*Results.*—Bilateral differences between the eyes of amblyopes compared with visually normal controls were found. The difference between foveal structure in amblyopic participants relative to structure in subjects with normal vision persisted even when variables such as age, ethnicity, axial length, and sex were taken into account. Amblyopes showed increased foveal thickness (+8.31 μm; $P = 0.006$) and a reduction in pit depth in the horizontal meridian (−10.06 μm; $P = 0.005$) but not in the vertical meridian ($P = 0.082$) when compared with subjects with normal vision. Foveal pit slopes were found to be approximately 1 degree flatter in the nasal ($P = 0.033$) and temporal ($P = 0.014$) meridians in amblyopes, but differences between amblyopes and controls in the superior ($P = 0.061$) and inferior ($P = 0.087$) meridians did not reach statistical significance. No statistically significant interocular differences were found in the foveal structure between amblyopic and fellow eyes.

*Conclusions.*—Differences were found in the foveal structure in both eyes of amblyopes compared with subjects with normal vision. These differences consisted of increased foveal thickness, reduced pit depth when measured along the horizontal meridian, and flattening of the nasal and temporal sides of the foveal pit.

► The belief that amblyopia is a deficit that is purely cortical in origin and that both eyes are structurally normal may need to be reevaluated after the finding of structural changes by optical coherence tomography in patients with amblyopia. Even if the structural changes of the fovea in amblyopes are secondary, further research is needed to determine their etiology, time course of onset, whether they are reversible with treatment, and ultimately their functional significance.

**L. B. Nelson, MD, MBA**

**Anisometropia and amblyopia in nasolacrimal duct obstruction**

Kipp MA, Kipp MA Jr, Struthers W (Wheaton Eye Clinic, IL; Univ of Notre Dame, IN; Wheaton College, IL)

*J AAPOS* 17:235-238, 2013

*Purpose.*—To investigate an association of childhood nasolacrimal duct obstruction (NLDO) with anisometropia and amblyopia.

*Methods.*—The medical records of patients from newborn to 6 years of age with a diagnosis of NLDO seen from 2000 to 2010 were retrospectively reviewed. Data collected included age at onset of NLDO, laterality of NLDO, cycloplegic refractive error, determination of clinically significant anisometropia (defined as ≥1 D), and diagnosis of amblyopia with amblyopia subtype (anisometropic vs other).

*Results.*—A total of 1,218 patients with NLDO were included. Of these, 887 cases (72.8%) were unilateral; 331 (27.2%), bilateral. Anisometropia was found in 67 (7.6%) unilateral cases and 12 (3.6 %) bilateral cases on initial examination ($\chi^2 = 5.48$, $P < 0.01$). Same-sided unilateral NLDO was significantly associated with greater hyperopia in the anisometropia patients ($\chi^2 = 33.01$, $P < 0.001$). Follow-up data were available for 482 NLDO patients and revealed an additional 26 patients with anisometropia for a total of 105 of 1218 (8.6%). Of the 482 patients, 28 (5.8%) developed amblyopia, 16 cases of which were purely attributable to anisometropia. Of 41 patients with anisometropia who were in the follow-up, 9 (22%) developed amblyopia.

*Conclusions.*—Anisometropia occurred at a greater rate in unilateral NLDO patients compared with bilateral NLDO patients and occurred at a greater rate in this NLDO cohort than expected in the general pediatric population. Several patients with anisometropia developed clinical amblyopia. Measurement of cycloplegic refraction in all NLDO patients at initial examination should be considered. Periodic follow-up is appropriate for patients with NLDO and anisometropia.

▶ It is not unusual when examining a child with a nasolacrimal duct obstruction (NLDO), especially unilateral involvement, that anisometropia is noted in the involved eye. Although the incidence of anisometropia and amblyopia for bilateral NLDOs were similar to the incidence in the general population, the incidence in unilateral NLDO was certainly significant. The etiology of the cause of increased findings of anisometropia and amblyopia in unilateral NLDO remains unknown. However, it is important that all children presenting with an NLDO, regardless of whether it is unilateral or bilateral, should have a cycloplegic refraction.

**L. B. Nelson, MD, MBA**

## Errors in Strabismus Surgery

Shen E, Porco T, Rutar T (Univ of California, San Francisco)

*JAMA Ophthalmol* 131:75-79, 2013

*Objectives.*—To determine the prevalence of and contributing factors for errors in strabismus surgery.

*Methods.*—Five hundred seventeen of 1103 strabismus surgeons (46.87%) completed a survey administered during the 2011 American Association for Pediatric Ophthalmology and Strabismus national meeting or emailed to members of the association.

*Results.*—One hundred seventy-three strabismus surgeons (33.5%) self-reported having operated on the wrong eye or muscle or performed the wrong procedure at least once. The mean error rate was 1 in 2506 (95% CI, 2128-2941) operations. Surgeons who performed fewer than the median 1500 procedures had an error rate 5.9 (95% CI, 4.1-8.2) times higher than surgeons who performed more than the median ($P < .001$). The most common factors contributing to errors were confusion between the type of deviation (esotropia/exotropia) and/or the surgical procedure (recession/resection) (34 of 114 responses [29.8%]), globe torsion (20 [17.5%]) leading primarily to inadvertent operation on the inferior rectus rather than the intended medial rectus muscle, and inattention and/or distraction (19 [16.7%]). Running more than 1 operating room ($P = .02$) and failing to mark eye muscles preoperatively ($P = .03$) were associated with an increased likelihood of error.

*Conclusions.*—Self-reported error in strabismus surgery is a complication approximately as common as periorbital cellulitis. Reducing error in strabismus surgery might entail confirming that the deviation matches the surgical plan preoperatively, more elaborate site marking, and involving an assistant in a preoperative verification of the specific eye muscles and surgical procedure.

▶ I was very surprised at how high the number of pediatric ophthalmologists (33.5%) self-reported having operated on the wrong eye or muscle or performed the wrong procedure at least once. Another surprising finding in this study was that 38.1% of surgical error cases had a timeout before performing the surgery but failed to prevent an error. To avoid errors in strabismus surgery, the authors appropriately suggested several specific modifications to the Universal Protocol. These suggestions, such as verifying the preoperative deviation matches the surgical plan, marking the eye to determine whether a resection or recession is being performed, and a more detailed timeout. Modifying the standard preoperative protocol should dramatically reduce these preventable errors in strabismus surgery.

**L. B. Nelson, MD, MBA**

## Analysis of risk factors for consecutive exotropia and review of the literature

Yurdakul NS, Ugurlu S (Izmir Atatürk Education and Res Hosp, Turkey)
*J Pediatr Ophthalmol Strabismus* 50:268-273, 2013

*Purpose.*—To evaluate the possible risk factors in patients with consecutive exotropia following esotropia surgery.

*Methods.*—Medical records of patients who had comitant esotropia surgery between June 1999 and April 2011 were reviewed. Those who developed consecutive exotropia composed the exotropia group; patients matched for age and duration of follow-up who did not develop consecutive exotropia composed the no exotropia group. The charts of the patients were reviewed and possible risk factors for development of consecutive exotropia were investigated.

*Results.*—The average ages of 47 patients in the exotropia group and 54 patients in the no exotropia group were 10.8 ± 8.7 years (range: 1 to 41 years) and 8.5 ± 6.3 years (range: 1 to 30 years), respectively ($P$ =.292). Amblyopia was detected in 31 (66%) and 12 (22.2%) patients in the exotropia and no exotropia groups, respectively ($P$ =.004). Anisometropia was observed in 20 patients (42.6%) in the exotropia group and 5 patients (9.3%) in the no exotropia group ($P$ =.003). Preoperative average esodeviation values were 42.5 ± 8.3 prism diopters (PD) (range: 25 to 60 PD) in the exotropia group and 42 ± 9.4 PD (range: 20 to 65 PD) in the no exotropia group ($P$ =.673). Postoperative deviations were 32.8 ± 23 PD exotropia (range: 10 to 90 PD exotropia) in the exotropia group and 4.4 ± 4.2 PD esotropia (range: 0 to 10 PD esotropia) in the no exotropia group ($P$ =.000). Asymmetric surgery had been performed in 61.7% of the exotropia group (n = 29) and 9.3% of the no exotropia group (n = 5) ($P$ =.000). Limitation of adduction was detected in 14 patients (29.8%) in the exotropia group; none was noted in the no exotropia group ($P$ =.000). The mean interval between the initial surgery and the onset of consecutive exotropia was 11.1 ± 15.1 months (range: 0 to 126 months).

*Conclusions.*—Anisometropia, amblyopia, asymmetric surgery, and postoperative adduction deficit were associated with the development of consecutive exotropia. Long-term follow-up should be considered because consecutive exotropia can develop after months or years.

► The authors' finding that anisometropia, amblyopia, and postoperative adduction deficit were associated with the development of consecutive exotropia is not surprising. Many of the patients with adduction deficit had undergone multiple previous surgeries. Although some patients with a hyperopia greater than +2.50 diopters were noted to develop consecutive exotropia, patients with high hyperopia and amblyopia can spontaneously develop exotropia. It is important to observe patients after surgery for exotropia long term because consecutive exotropia may develop months or years later.

**L. B. Nelson, MD, MBA**

**Strabismus among aged Medicare beneficiaries: impact of health status and region**

Repka MX, Yu F, Lum F, et al (The Johns Hopkins Univ School of Medicine, Baltimore, MD; UCLA Fielding School of Public Health; Foundation of the American Academy of Ophthalmology, San Francisco, CA; et al)
*J AAPOS* 17:391-394, 2013

*Purpose.*—To describe the effect of health status and geographic region of the United States on the prevalence of strabismus and strabismus surgery in the aged Medicare fee-for-service population.

*Methods.*—A 5% sample of Medicare claims was used to identify aged beneficiaries diagnosed with strabismus and those having strabismus surgery between 2002 and 2010. The Charlson Comorbidity Index (CCI), a measure of systemic health, was calculated. The regional analysis divided the United States into East, West, Midwest, and South. Analyses were adjusted for age, sex, race, CCI, and region.

*Results.*—The 5% sample for 2010 included 1,237,469 unique beneficiaries. Strabismus was diagnosed in 8,470 (0.68%) and strabismus surgery was performed on 197 (0.016%). Pooled data from 2002 through 2010 found the prevalence of strabismus increasing significantly with increasing comorbidity ($P < 0.0001$): 0.52% (CCI, 0), 0.65% (CCI, 1-2), 0.77% (CCI, 3-4), and 0.82% (CCI, 5 or higher). Conversely, the prevalence of strabismus surgery declined slightly with increasing comorbidity ($P = 0.088$): 0.016% (CCI, 0), 0.017% (CCI, 1-2), 0.015% (CCI, 3-4), and 0.015% (CCI, 5 or higher). The diagnosis of strabismus was made least frequently in the South ($P < 0.0001$), whereas strabismus surgery was performed more often in the West ($P = 0.006$). All significant effects remained after adjustment.

*Conclusions.*—The prevalence of strabismus increases significantly with declining health status; however, health status had little effect on the rate of strabismus surgery. Regional rates of strabismus diagnosis and surgery differ widely.

▶ It is not surprising that strabismus prevalence increases with age. With increased prevalence of central vision loss from a variety of ophthalmologic disorders, sensory strabismus will develop. Also with increasing age, medical problems such as diabetes, hypertension, and acquired neurological disorders may result in paralytic strabismus. Even though there are functional benefits of strabismus surgery in the adult population, there is a decline in strabismus surgery rate. Again, this finding is not surprising given that many of these patients may not perceive the benefit of strabismus surgery; health status may be a contraindication for surgery or the possible surgical risks of surgery.

**L. B. Nelson, MD, MBA**

## The prevalence of reoperation and related risk factors among patients with congenital esotropia

Rajavi Z, Ferdosi AA, Eslamdoust M, et al (Shahid Beheshti Univ of Med Sciences, Tehran, Iran)

*J Pediatr Ophthalmol Strabismus* 50:53-59, 2013

*Purpose.*—To determine the prevalence rate and related risk factors of reoperation among patients with congenital esotropia.

*Methods.*—One hundred fifty-seven children with congenital esotropia were divided into two groups after at least one operation: children with deviation within 10 PD (n = 89; success group) and those with deviation greater than 10 PD or history of reoperation (n = 68; failure group). The relationship of risk factors such as age at first operation and primary congenital esotropia of less than 30 or more than 50 PD and accompanying factors such as inferior oblique muscle overaction (> +1), dissociated vertical deviation, lateral rectus muscle underaction, and A-V pattern with reoperation were studied. Final sensory status of children 5 years and older was evaluated by Worth 4-dot and Titmus tests.

*Results.*—Reoperation was indicated in 32.4% of children who had residual esotropia greater than 15 PD after 3 months following their first operation. Congenital esotropia greater than 30 PD ($P = .002$) and lateral rectus muscle underaction of −1 to −2 ($P < .005$), were statistically different between the two groups. Initial operation at younger than 3 years was more likely to achieve gross stereopsis in children 5 years and older ($P = .032$).

*Conclusion.*—Congenital esotropia greater than 30 PD and lateral rectus muscle underaction were found to be risk factors of reoperation.

▶ The authors continue to mention age at the time of surgery as an important factor in success rate. However, it is not the specific age at the time of surgery that is most important but the duration in which the esotropia was present. The duration from diagnosis of esotropia to timing of surgery is the factor that most commonly determines success. The failure group had a mean preoperative deviation of approximately 72 prism diopters. However, the authors did not perform bimedial rectus recessions greater than 6 mm, which is not enough to correct these patients. Therefore, it is not surprising that this group had a higher failure rate. Finally, I was surprised at the high percentage of postoperative lateral rectus muscle under action that was found in these children by the authors. Usually after large bimedial rectus recession, children with congenital esotropia no longer cross-fixate and have normal lateral rectus function.

**L. B. Nelson, MD, MBA**

**Surgical Outcomes of Medial Rectus Recession in Esotropia with Cerebral Palsy**

Ma DJ, Yang HK, Hwang J-M (Seoul Natl Univ Bundang Hosp, Seongnam, Korea)

*Ophthalmology* 120:663-667, 2013

*Purpose.*—To determine the outcome of a reduced amount of medial rectus (MR) muscle recession in esotropes with cerebral palsy (CP) and to compare the surgical response with that of normal controls.

*Design.*—Retrospective cohort study.

*Participants.*—Thirty esotropes with CP and 60 age-matched esotropes without CP who underwent a unilateral or bilateral MR muscle recession.

*Methods.*—The surgical amount of MR muscle recession was reduced by 1 mm per muscle in patients with CP.

*Main Outcome Measures.*—Success rates, surgical response, cumulative probabilities of success, and factors affecting surgical responses evaluated by generalized linear mixed models.

*Results.*—In patients with CP, the initial success rate was higher ($P = 0.037$) and the rate of undercorrection was lower ($P = 0.037$) compared with patients without CP. At the final visit, success rates were not significantly different between both groups. However, the rate of overcorrection was higher ($P = 0.003$) compared with patients without CP. The rate of overcorrection per person-year during follow-up was 11% in patients with CP and 2% in patients without CP. Patients with CP showed a greater surgical response than did those without CP, at about 1.3 prism diopters per millimeter of MR muscle recession ($P < 0.001$).

*Conclusions.*—Even with the reduced amount of recession, esotropes with CP showed a greater surgical response to MR muscle recession than did those without CP, and the incidence of late overcorrection was significantly higher compared with that of patients without CP.

▶ There has been a concern among many in the pediatric ophthalmology community that children with cerebral palsy have a much more variable response to surgery. With that belief, many pediatric ophthalmologists are much more conservative about the amount of recessions performed on these children. As long as the examiner is able to obtain accurate measurements of a child with cerebral palsy and the indications for surgery are met, I do not believe that altering the amount of surgery is necessary. The authors actually increased their numbers and had a long-term greater overcorrection rate.

**L. B. Nelson, MD, MBA**

**Fibrin Glue for Closure of Conjunctival Incision in Strabismus Surgery: A Report by the American Academy of Ophthalmology**

Yang MB, Melia M, Lambert SR, et al (Univ of Cincinnati, OH; Jaeb Ctr for Health Res, Tampa, FL; Emory Univ, Atlanta, GA; et al)

*Ophthalmology* 120:1935-1941, 2013

*Objective.*—To evaluate the severity of postoperative inflammation, degree of patient discomfort, adequacy of wound closure, and length of operating time when using fibrin glue compared with sutures to close limbal conjunctival incisions after strabismus surgery.

*Methods.*—Literature searches of the PubMed and Cochrane Library databases were last conducted on January 24, 2013, and resulted in 24 citations, including 2 not in the English language. All citations were reviewed in full text. Five studies compared fibrin glue (68 eyes) with sutures (74 eyes) for closure of limbal conjunctival incisions in patients undergoing strabismus surgery and were included in this assessment; no studies were found that evaluated fornix incisions. A quality rating was assigned to each study using criteria specifically developed for this assessment.

*Results.*—No level I studies were found, and 5 level II studies were identified. There was significantly less postoperative inflammation and patient discomfort for 1 to 3 weeks after strabismus surgery for eyes treated with fibrin glue compared with sutures. In 3 studies that evaluated wound apposition, 2 of 50 eyes (4%) with conjunctival incisions that were initially closed using fibrin glue subsequently developed a wound gap that required suture repair. In the 2 studies that compared surgical time, fibrin glue required 1 to 5 minutes less time than suturing in 1 study and 55% less time (3.8 vs. 8.4 minutes) in a second study. These 5 studies did not evaluate the cost-effectiveness or risk of viral transmission from fibrin glue.

*Conclusions.*—Studies in the literature suggest that the off-label use of fibrin glue to close limbal conjunctival incisions in strabismus surgery resulted in less postoperative inflammation and required shorter operating time compared with sutures, but it increased the percentage of wounds requiring subsequent repair with sutures.

▶ Closure of limbal conjunctival incisions in strabismus surgery is usually performed with plain catgut suture. The suture usually dissolves within a few days. Other than a mild foreign body sensation, the suture is well tolerated by most patients. Although the fibrin glue closure is an alternative technique for closing a limbal conjunctival incision, it is more expensive. For most skilled strabismus surgeons, it does not reduce operating time, and there is a need to repair conjunctival wounds that are not adequately closed using fibrin glue.

**L. B. Nelson, MD, MBA**

**Clinical Translation of Recommendations from Randomized Clinical Trials on Patching Regimen for Amblyopia**

Jin Y-P, Chow AHY, Colpa L, et al (Univ of Toronto, Ontario, Canada; The Hosp for Sick Children, Toronto, Ontario, Canada)

*Ophthalmology* 120:657-662, 2013

*Purpose.*—To investigate whether the evidence-based recommendations by the Pediatric Eye Disease Investigator Group (PEDIG) as initial treatment of amblyopia have been implemented into clinical practice and to discuss the necessary steps in translating evidence-based knowledge to inform clinical decision making.

*Design.*—Retrospective cohort study.

*Participants.*—Children with amblyopia seen from 2007 through 2009 by academic and community ophthalmologists in a large urban center in North America that serves a population of more than 8 million. Using PEDIG criteria, moderate amblyopia was defined as visual acuity between 20/40 and 20/80 and severe amblyopia was defined as visual acuity between 20/100 and 20/400.

*Intervention.*—Patching of the sound eye.

*Main Outcome Measures.*—The number of prescribed patching hours daily and the amblyopic eye visual acuity expressed as logarithm of the minimum angle of resolution (logMAR).

*Results.*—For moderate amblyopia, the cohort ($n = 71$) was prescribed a mean of 3.2 hours of daily patching (95% confidence interval [CI]: 2.8–3.6 hours), which is significantly greater than the recommended 2 hours of daily patching for initial treatment. Only 24% (95% CI, 16%–35%) of them were prescribed the recommended initial patching hours. The amblyopic eye acuity on the 3- to 6-month visit in the cohort (0.23 logMAR) was similar to that of the 4-month visit in the PEDIG cohort (0.24 logMAR; $P = 0.74$). For severe amblyopia, the cohort ($n = 52$) was prescribed a mean of 3.9 hours of daily patching (95% CI, 3.5–4.3 hours), which is significantly lower than the recommended 6 hours of daily patching for initial treatment. Only 12% (95% CI, 5%–23%) of them were prescribed the recommended initial patching hours. The amblyopic eye acuity at the 7- to 12-month visit in the cohort (0.44 logMAR) was comparable with that of the 4-month visit in the PEDIG cohort (0.40 logMAR; $P = 0.35$).

*Conclusions.*—The evidence-based recommendations for amblyopia management have not been translated widely into changes in clinical practice in a large urban center in North America, although there is a general move from full-time to part-time patching since the PEDIG results were published. Using a well-established framework for knowledge translation, the Knowledge-to-Action Cycle, the necessary steps required to implement new knowledge into actual clinical practice are discussed.

▶ Although there continues to be a gap in implementing results from medical research in everyday clinical practice and in decision making related to health care problems, the authors were surprised that so few practices were using the results of PEDIG studies in amblyopia. Although not specifically addressed, even though the PEDIG study recommendations were obtained from multicenter studies, there are questions that many pediatric ophthalmologists have with the results. One of the main issues in studying amblyopia treatment is that the investigators are relying on information given to them from parents without necessarily having any way to verify their validity. The basic flaw in questioning why more clinical practices may not be incorporating the results of the PEDIG studies in amblyopia is whether there is a strong belief in their accuracy.

**L. B. Nelson, MD, MBA**

---

**Body Stature Growth Trajectories during Childhood and the Development of Myopia**

Northstone K, Guggenheim JA, Howe LD, et al (Univ of Bristol, UK; Cardiff Univ, UK)

*Ophthalmology* 120:1064-1073, 2013

---

*Purpose.*—Stature at a particular age can be considered the cumulative result of growth during a number of preceding growth trajectory periods. We investigated whether height and weight growth trajectories from birth to age 10 years were related to refractive error at ages 11 and 15 years, and eye size at age 15 years.

*Design.*—Prospective analysis in a birth cohort.

*Participants.*—Children participating in the Avon Longitudinal Study of Parents and Children (ALSPAC) U.K. birth cohort (minimum N = 2676).

*Methods.*—Growth trajectories between birth and 10 years were modeled from a series of height and weight measurements (N = 6815). Refractive error was assessed by noncycloplegic autorefraction at ages 11 and 15 years (minimum N = 4737). Axial length (AXL) and radius of corneal curvature were measured with an IOLMaster (Carl Zeiss Meditec, Welwyn Garden City, U.K.) at age 15 years (minimum N = 2676). Growth trajectories and an allelic score for 180 genetic variants associated with adult height were tested for association with refractive error and eye size.

*Main Outcome Measures.*—Noncycloplegic autorefraction at ages 11 and 15 years and AXL and corneal curvature at age 15 years.

*Results.*—Height growth trajectory during the linear phase between 2.5 and 10 years was negatively associated with refractive error at 11 and 15 years ($P < 0.001$) but explained <0.5% of intersubject variation. Height and weight growth trajectories, especially shortly after birth, were positively associated with AXL and corneal curvature ($P < 0.001$), predicting 1% to 5% of trait variation. Height growth after 2.5 years was not associated with corneal curvature, whereas the association with AXL continued up to 10 years. The height allelic score was associated with corneal curvature ($P = 0.03$) but not with refractive error or AXL.

*Conclusions.*—Up to the age of 10 years, shared growth mechanisms contribute to scaling of eye and body size but minimally to the development of myopia.

▶ The growth of the eye with increasing myopia when body stature is also changing suggests that a shared mechanism may be present. Although the authors found that up to age 10 years, there was a connection between increasing body stature and myopia, the relationship was not a strong one. Many children have increases in either height or myopia, and therefore, the subtle association of these conditions may be explained by other unidentified courses that future studies may uncover.

**L. B. Nelson, MD, MBA**

**Three Horizontal Muscle Surgery for Large-Angle Infantile or Presumed Infantile Esotropia: Long-term Motor Outcomes**

Chatzistefanou KI, Ladas ID, Droutsas KD, et al (Univ of Athens Med School, Greece)

*JAMA Ophthalmol* 131:1041-1048, 2013

*Importance.*—Bilateral medial rectus muscle recession and one lateral rectus muscle resection surgery for the correction of large-angle infantile esotropia may be associated with a favorable long-term motor outcome. A consecutive exotropic drift was encountered more commonly than a recurrent esotropic drift in the long run, especially in the smaller (50-69 prism diopters [Δ]) range of preoperative esodeviation.

*Objective.*—To outline the short- and long-term motor outcomes of graded bilateral medial rectus muscle recession and one lateral rectus muscle resection for the correction of large-angle esotropia (≥50Δ).

*Design.*—Retrospective analysis.

*Setting.*—Strabismus service, tertiary care university referral center.

*Participants.*—A total of 194 consecutive patients with infantile or presumed infantile esotropia.

*Exposure.*—All patients underwent bilateral medial rectus recession and a lateral rectus resection in the nondominant eye by the same surgeon.

*Main Outcomes and Measures.*—Short-term (8 weeks) and long-term rates of postoperative successful alignment (±10Δ), undercorrection, and overcorrection.

*Results.*—The median age of patients at surgery was 2.7 years (range, 20 months–36 years). The median follow-up time was 4.5 years (range, 6 weeks–25 years). The mean preoperative deviation was 68.2Δ. Of the 194 patients, 121 (62.4%) were successfully aligned at the last follow-up visit or prior to reoperation, and 154 (79.4%) were successfully aligned at the 8-week postoperative evaluation. A comparison of early vs late outcomes revealed a higher rate of late overcorrections (5.15% vs 24.1%, respectively; $P = .001$) but the same rate of undercorrections (15.4% vs

15.1%; *P* =.85). The outcome of surgery was not associated with the presence of amblyopia, high hyperopia, or the total amount of millimeters of surgery but was adversely influenced by the presence of inferior oblique overaction and the magnitude of the preoperative esodeviation. Delayed consecutive exotropia was more prevalent in the 50Δ to 69Δ range of preoperative esodeviation.

*Conclusions and Relevance.*—Three horizontal muscle surgery for the correction of large-angle esotropia is associated with a high success rate. Long-term follow-up indicated that an exotropic drift may be expected 3 times more often than an esotropic drift.

▶ I commend the authors being able to obtain long-term follow-up on patients with congenital esotropia. However, the 3-muscle surgery for congenital esotropia does not appear to be a better procedure then performing large bimedial recessions. I believe that, as the authors pointed out, factors other than surgical planning or a particular surgical procedure may influence the alignment outcome beyond 6 months after surgery. If a child with congenital esotropia is orthophoric 6 months postoperatively and 5 years later develops a recurrent esotropia, other factors may be involved beyond which surgical procedure was initially performed. Therefore, performing a large bimedial recession is easier, requires lens anesthesia time, and leaves the lateral recti untouched in case further surgery is necessary.

**L. B. Nelson, MD, MBA**

**Prismatic Correction of Consecutive Esotropia in Children after a Unilateral Recession and Resection Procedure**

Lee EK, Hwang J-M (Seoul Natl Univ Bundang Hosp, Seongnam, Korea)
*Ophthalmology* 120:504-511, 2013

*Purpose.*—To determine the long-term efficacy of prismatic correction in consecutive esotropia after a unilateral recession and resection (RR) procedure for primary exotropia.

*Design.*—Retrospective cohort study.

*Participants.*—A total of 110 patients with esodeviation of 5 prism diopters (PD) or more at 4 weeks after the unilateral RR procedure for primary exotropia who were fitted with prism glasses and were followed up for a minimum of 2 years after primary surgery.

*Methods.*—Patients were divided into 2 groups based on whether they were weaned off the prism glasses within 1 year: (1) the prism-weaned group whose esotropia decreased enough for them to be weaned off the prism within 1 year; (2) the prism-wearing group who wore prism glasses for more than 1 year. Clinical characteristics and changes in deviation angle were compared between groups.

*Main Outcome Measures.*—The period of prism wearing, the rate of decline in deviation angle after prismatic correction, and preoperative and postoperative motor and sensory outcomes.

*Results.*—The average age of patients was 4.7 years. Overall, the average period of prism wearing was 20.9 months, and the rate of decrease in the deviation angle was 2.9 PD per 6 months. Thirty-four patients (32%) were weaned off the prism glasses within 1 year. The prism-weaned group showed more preoperative constant deviation and anisometropia compared with the prism-wearing group. Overall, successful motor outcome was achieved in 71% of patients. The rate of recurrence during follow-up was higher in the prism-weaned group, and the rate of overcorrection was higher in the prism-wearing group ($P = 0.003$). No patients demonstrated new onset amblyopia, and 1 of the 105 patients (0.95%) demonstrated loss of stereoacuity as a result of overcorrection. At the final visit, stereoacuity was improved or was maintained in 92% of patients compared with preoperative values.

*Conclusions.*—Prismatic correction can lead to good motor outcomes while maintaining favorable sensory status in most patients with consecutive esotropia. Patients showed different clinical manifestations and outcome according to the period of prismatic correction. Patients in the prism-weaned group showed a faster change in esodeviation after prismatic correction and more exotropic drift after prism weaning, resulting in a higher rate of recurrence of exotropia.

▶ Although temporary prismatic correction of consecutive esotropia in children may be successful, there were several problems with this study. It is unclear to me why the authors only included overcorrections from patients who underwent a resect/recess surgery. The authors stated it was because the preoperative characteristics between these 2 procedures differ greatly. However, a greater deviation and performing either procedure should not affect the postoperative management. Also, the overcorrection rate for the resect/recess patients was 54.5%, which is much greater than expected.

**L. B. Nelson, MD, MBA**

# 8 Neuro-ophthalmology

## Visual Loss in Early-Stage Chronic Lymphocytic Leukemia

Gonsalves WI, Zent CS, Pulido JS, et al (Mayo Clinic, Rochester, MN)
*J Clin Oncol* 31:e280-e282, 2013

*Background.*—Chronic lymphocytic leukemia (CLL) is a common lymphoproliferative disorder in North America, but involvement of the optic nerve rarely occurs. A patient with CLL suffered progressive visual loss caused by optic neuritis.

*Case Report.*—Man, 75, was found to have lymphocytosis as an incidental finding on a preoperative complete blood count (CBC). Hypercellular results on a bone marrow biopsy with nodular interstitial infiltrate of CLL cells and trisomy 12 detected on conventional cytogenetic tests and interphase fluorescent in situ hybridization identified him as at intermediate risk for CLL. With no palpable lymphadenopathy or hepatosplenomegaly, he was observed for 1 year, when he complained of pain in the right eye plus blurry vision, floaters, and bright halos. Funduscopic evaluation showed bilateral disc edema worse on the right, magnetic resonance imaging (MRI) showed normal orbits, and cerebrospinal fluid (CSF) analysis found lymphocytosis. The clinical diagnosis was optic neuritis, for which the patient was given prednisone 1 mg/kg for 14 days. He experienced marked improvement in vision within a week of beginning treatment. A subsequent evaluation found his white blood cell (WBC) count was $48.5 \times 10^9$/L and an absolute lymphocyte count of $34.9 \times 10^9$/L. CSF analysis showed 29 total nucleated cells per $\mu$L, with 96% lymphocytes. Fifty percent of the lymphocytes were clonal. The probability of multiple sclerosis was lowered because of the absence of oligoclonal bands and normal CSF immunoglobulin G index. The right eye disc had persistent edema, blurring, and peripapillary hemorrhages. A corticosteroid dose taper was initiated, but visual symptoms recurred. There was marked visual field loss in the right eye plus progressive chronic changes of papilledema and disc blurriness indicative of perioptic nerve infiltration or chronic papilledema. CSF revealed 20 total nucleated cells per $\mu$L, with 87% lymphocytes (35% clonal). Infection was ruled out through serum and CSF testing, and MRI T1-weighted images demonstrated abnormally enhanced right optic nerve. Optic nerve infiltration by CLL was diagnosed by exclusion, with treatment using fludarabine 20 mg/m$^2$ per day on days 2, 3, and 4 and rituximab 375 mg/m$^2$ on day 1. Visual symptoms improved progressively, with full resolution by the end of the second cycle of treatment. Both eyes had a marked decrease in optic disc edema, with resolution of the optic neuritis confirmed by orbital MRI.

*Conclusions.*—Optic nerve infiltration by CLL cells causing neuritis and impaired vision is rare but can lead to permanent blindness if not treated. It can be challenging to identify the problem before permanent vision loss because MRI and clinical findings are nonspecific and a nerve biopsy, which is quite destructive, is required to confirm CLL nerve infiltration. Therefore the condition is diagnosed by exclusion. One test used to exclude other conditions is CSF analysis by flow cytometry. Treatment for CLL optic neuritis includes orbital or whole-brain radiation, intrathecal therapy with methotrexate, and systemic chemotherapy with chlorambucil and fludarabine. In this case fludarabine plus rituximab proved effective.

▶ Visual loss in any patient with a recent or remote history of cancer must trigger an investigation for cancer as the cause of the visual loss. In fact, any neuro-ophthalmic development including double vision, nystagmus, proptosis, and migraine-like symptoms must also trigger the same approach.

Careful and complete examination must be followed by neuroimaging directed at the base of the skull and orbits with and without gadolinium (Figs 1 and 2 in the original article). Magnetic resonance imaging scans of the brain do not examine the critical anatomic regions of the cranial nerves controlling the afferent and efferent visual systems.

This case report is an instructive reminder of how to think about this condition and how to establish a diagnosis.

**R. C. Sergott, MD**

---

**Tournay's description of anisocoria on lateral gaze: Reaction, myth, or phenomenon?**

Robert MP, Plant GT (Hôpital Universitaire Necker-Enfants Malades, Paris; Natl Hosp for Neurology and Neurosurgery, Queen Square, London)

*Neurology* 82:452-456, 2014

---

The year 1917 witnessed the opening of a great debate in neuro-ophthalmology, with Tournay's description of a phenomenon thought to be universal: anisocoria in lateral gaze, due to mydriasis of the abducting pupil and a minor miosis of the fellow one. Through many publications, this phenomenon was soon assessed and confirmed to be physiologic, while the cause of the pupil reaction in lateral gaze was extensively discussed. Cases of abolition and reversal of the phenomenon were also reported in specific clinical situations, such as neurosyphilis, and its study became part of the neuro-ophthalmologic examination. Publications on the phenomenon declined after 1934, with only one publication appearing between 1934 and 1974 (1957). In 1974, the demise of the Tournay phenomenon was secured after 2 pupillographic studies showed it to be rare and marginal. This story is reviewed. Hypotheses are proposed in order to help unfold the controversy; anisocoria in lateral gaze should not be regarded as a myth, nor does it—or only rarely—correspond to a pupil reaction, or noumenon: it can usually be accounted for by a specific optical distortion (apparent without real anisocoria) and hence fits the Kantian definition of a phenomenon. An understanding of Tournay phenomenon is therefore of current relevance to the examination of the pupils to avoid misinterpretation of observed changes in the pupil.

▶ This is a wonderful report providing exquisite historical detail and perspective about Tournay's phenomenon, anisocoria on lateral gaze. The current consensus is that this phenomenon does occur on occasion but does not have pathologic significance.

It is important for clinicians to be aware of these episodic phenomena so that pathologic importance is not attached to it. Unfortunately, I can cynically imagine a scenario in which this phenomenon is noticed after some sort of mishap and medical legal damages are sought.

**R. C. Sergott, MD**

---

**Sport-Related Concussion and Sensory Function in Young Adults**

Moore RD, Broglio SP, Hillman CH (Univ of Illinois, Urbana-Champaign; Univ of Michigan, Ann Arbor)

*J Athl Train* 49:36-41, 2014

---

*Context.*—The long-term implications of concussive injuries for brain and cognitive health represent a growing concern in the public consciousness. As such, identifying measures sensitive to the subtle yet persistent effects of concussive injuries is warranted.

*Objective.*—To investigate how concussion sustained early in life influences visual processing in young adults. We predicted that young adults with a history of concussion would show decreased sensory processing, as noted by a reduction in P1 event-related potential component amplitude.

*Design.*—Cross-sectional study.

*Setting.*—Research laboratory.

*Patients or Other Participants.*—Thirty-six adults (18 with a history of concussion, 18 controls) between the ages of 20 and 28 years completed a pattern-reversal visual evoked potential task while event-related potentials were recorded.

*Main Outcome Measure(s).*—The groups did not differ in any demographic variables (all $P$ values <.05), yet those with a concussive history exhibited reduced P1 amplitude compared with the control participants ($P$ =.05).

*Conclusions.*—These results suggest that concussion history has a negative effect on visual processing in young adults. Further, upper-level neurocognitive deficits associated with concussion may, in part, result from less efficient downstream sensory capture.

▶ Concussions and concussion centers are now proliferating throughout America at a rate usually reserved for nonmedical enterprises. Although there is no doubt that traumatic brain injury and concussions are an ever-increasing problem, we recommend that these centers undergo some sort of certification process backed by validated ophthalmic clinical and basic research so that patients and their families are not victimized by pseudoscience, and health care dollars are not wasted on investigations that are costly but not necessarily valuable for the care of the patient.

This article reports some interesting findings, but readers must be cautious of any data reported in cross-sectional studies. Without baseline studies performed in and around the episode of trauma, the data from an isolated event during the patient's clinical course are difficult to interpret.

We hope that concussion centers do not become a vehicle to recommend a variety of visual training exercises, for which credible research from Europe and the United States lacks validation when studied in a rigorous manner.

**R. C. Sergott, MD**

---

**Temporal reorganization to overcome monocular demyelination**

Raz N, Chokron S, Ben-Hur T, et al (Hadassah Hebrew-Univ Med Ctr, Jerusalem, Israel; Fondation Ophtalmologique Rothschild, Paris, France)

*Neurology* 81:702-709, 2013

---

*Objective.*—To identify the source of delayed visual evoked potential (VEP) latencies in the fellow eyes of patients with optic neuritis (ON) and determine whether these latencies stem from clinically silent demyelination or reflect an adaptive process for synchronization with the affected eyes.

*Methods.*—The study sample comprised 17 patients whom we followed for 12 to 26 months after unilateral first-ever ON diagnosis and 17 age-matched controls. To avoid confounding effects of axonal loss, only intact fellow eyes (except for VEPs) were included. Subjects underwent standard visual evaluation, motion perception, as well as static and time-constrained stereo tasks. Assessments included VEP, optical coherence tomography, high-resolution MRI, and diffusion tensor imaging.

*Results.*—We observed delayed VEP peaks (P100) in both affected and fellow eyes. However, while these were derived from prolonged time-to-start in the affected eyes, supporting the existence of demyelination, time-to-start in the fellow eyes was intact. VEP latencies in the fellow eyes could not be explained by demyelinative lesions along postchiasmal pathways (assessed by diffusion tensor imaging). Delayed peaks in fellow eyes resulted from a wider waveform, which evolved over time and occurred with a concomitant decrease in the gap in time between VEP peaks of both eyes. These changes offered a functional advantage; synchronization of inputs highly correlated with improved time-constrained binocular perception.

*Conclusion.*—Delayed latencies in the fellow eyes may reflect adaptive mechanisms at the cortical level that improve binocular integration over time to adjust for the damage incurred. These data provide a unique demonstration of temporal reorganization that compensates for delayed transmittal of visual information to the cortex.

▶ This is a very intriguing report that challenges the traditional explanation for abnormal visual evoked potential in eyes unaffected by optic neuritis after the contralateral eye has had an attack. Although the information from this report will not be used in your offices tomorrow, clinicians should be aware of this hypothesis as we begin to try to understand how the visual system, brain, and spinal cord adapt to demyelinating events. Increased understanding of these adaptive strategies will need to be considered in clinical trials with multiple sclerosis and the visual system. This is a very elegant study providing a new perspective about an issue that we thought we understood perfectly.

**R. C. Sergott, MD**

---

**Trans-Synaptic Axonal Degeneration in the Visual Pathway in Multiple Sclerosis**

Gabilondo I, Martínez-Lapiscina EH, Martínez-Heras E, et al (Hosp Clinic of Barcelona, Spain)

*Ann Neurol* 75:98-107, 2014

---

*Objective.*—To evaluate the association between the damage to the anterior and posterior visual pathway as evidence of the presence of retrograde and anterograde trans-synaptic degeneration in multiple sclerosis (MS).

*Methods.*—We performed a longitudinal evaluation on a cohort of 100 patients with MS, acquiring retinal optical coherence tomography to measure anterior visual pathway damage (peripapillary retinal nerve fiber layer [RNFL] thickness and macular volume) and 3T brain magnetic resonance imaging (MRI) for posterior visual pathway damage (volumetry and spectroscopy of visual cortex, lesion volume within optic radiations) at inclusion and after 1 year. Freesurfer and SPM8 software was used for MRI analysis. We evaluated the relationships between the damage in the anterior and posterior visual pathway by voxel-based morphometry (VBM), multiple linear regressions, and general linear models.

*Results.*—VBM analysis showed that RNFL thinning was specifically associated with atrophy of the visual cortex and with lesions in optic radiations at study inclusion ($p < 0.05$). Visual cortex volume ($\beta = +0.601$,

95% confidence interval [CI] = +0.04 to +1.16), N-acetyl aspartate in visual cortex ($\beta = +1.075$, 95% CI = +0.190 to +1.961), and lesion volume within optic radiations ($\beta = -2.551$, 95% CI = −3.910 to −1.192) significantly influenced average RNFL thinning at study inclusion independently of other confounders, especially optic neuritis (ON). The model indicates that a decrease of $1cm^3$ in visual cortex volume predicts a reduction of 0.6μm in RNFL thickness. This association was also observed after 1 year of follow-up. Patients with severe prior ON (adjusted difference = −3.01, 95% CI = −5.08 to −0.95) and mild prior ON (adjusted difference = −1.03, 95% CI = −3.02 to +0.95) had a lower adjusted mean visual cortex volume than patients without ON.

*Interpretation.*—Our results suggest the presence of trans-synaptic degeneration as a contributor to chronic axon damage in MS (Figs 1 and 2).

▶ For decades, trans-synaptic degeneration was considered heresy in neuro-ophthalmology, discussion of which could lead to excommunication from the

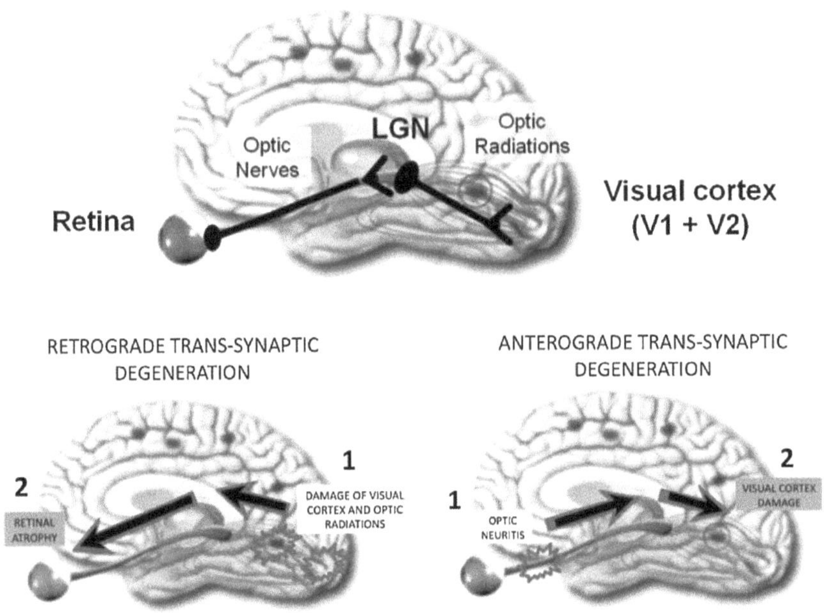


FIGURE 1.—The visual pathway as a model to study trans-synaptic neuronal degeneration in multiple sclerosis. The afferent visual pathway has a distinct anatomy that can be simplified into 2 neuronal pathways: the anterior pathway, composed of the retina, optic nerves, chiasm, and optic tracts; and the posterior pathway, composed of the optic radiations and visual cortex. Both pathways are connected by a single synaptic relay, the lateral geniculate nuclei (LGN). At the bottom left, the model for retrograde trans-synaptic degeneration is represented as the effect of the damage to the posterior visual pathway (visual cortex [V1 + V2] atrophy and lesions within the optic radiations) on retinal atrophy. At the bottom right, the model for anterograde trans-synaptic degeneration is represented as the effect of optic neuritis on the posterior visual pathway (visual cortex [V1 + V2] atrophy). (Reprinted from Gabilondo I, Martínez-Lapiscina EH, Martínez-Heras E, et al. Trans-synaptic axonal degeneration in the visual pathway in multiple sclerosis. *Ann Neurol.* 2014;75:98-107, with permission from Annals of Neurology and John Wiley and Sons, www.interscience.wiley.com.)

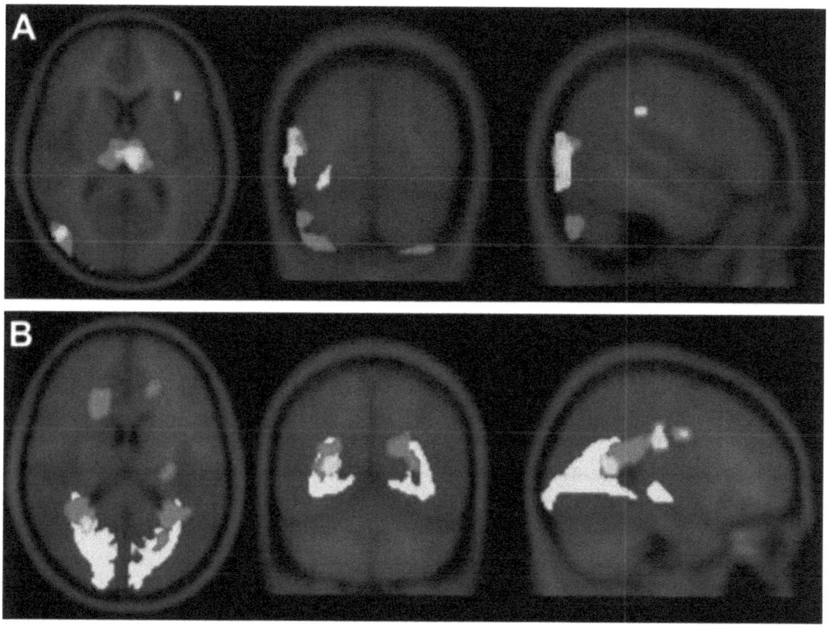


FIGURE 2.—Topography of regional gray matter (GM) atrophy and white matter (WM) lesion distribution in the brain associated with retinal nerve fiber layer (RNFL) thinning. (A) Correlation analysis between GM volume and retina thickness by voxel-based morphometry (VBM). GM voxels correlated with average RNFL thickness in the overall cohort (dark blue) and for the patients without prior optic neuritis (ON; light blue). No significant clusters where found in cases with ON history. WM total lesion load was used as an additional covariate in this model. (B) Correlation analysis between WM lesion distribution and retina thickness by VBM. WM lesions correlated with average RNFL thickness in the overall cohort (dark blue) and in patients without prior ON (light blue). The Jülich probabilistic mask for Optic Radiations (OR, represented in yellow) was used to evaluate the volume of lesion clusters within OR. Results of VBM analysis were analyzed at the cluster level with familywise error correction ($p < 0.05$, uncorrected threshold at voxel level of $p < 0.001$). Resulting clusters are represented in axial, coronal, and sagittal planes of 1mm per the Montreal Neurological Institute template. For Interpretation of the references to color in this figure legend, the reader is referred to web version of this article. (Reprinted from Gabilondo I, Martínez-Lapiscina EH, Martínez-Heras E, et al. Trans-synaptic axonal degeneration in the visual pathway in multiple sclerosis. *Ann Neurol.* 2014;75:98-107, with permission from Annals of Neurology and John Wiley and Sons, www.interscience.wiley.com.)

academic establishment of the subspecialty community. Enter new medical technology, specifically, spectral domain optical coherence tomography and volumetric magnetic resonance imaging scanning.

The results from this very well-done study show that the concept of trans-synaptic degeneration was indeed correct. We just had to wait for technologic advances to prove the concept. Prior therapies for multiple sclerosis (MS) have been directed at the inflammatory component of this disease. This study, and others, now forces us to think about potential therapeutic pathways aimed at the axon and synapses. Now we must ask if similar mechanisms exist for glaucoma and other ophthalmic diseases that do not have obvious neurologic connections such as MS.

**R. C. Sergott, MD**

## Morning Glory Disc Anomaly: Characteristic MR Imaging Findings

Ellika S, Robson CD, Heidary G, et al (Children's Hosp Boston and Harvard Med School, MA)
*AJNR Am J Neuroradiol* 34:2010-2014, 2013

Establishing the diagnosis of morning glory disc anomaly is crucial to appropriate patient treatment. Although typically made clinically, the diagnosis is not always straightforward, especially in circumstances where physical examination is limited. The goal of this study was to define the spectrum and frequency of orbital findings in a series of patients with funduscopically-confirmed morning glory disc anomaly by using MR imaging. MR imaging demonstrated 3 findings in all patients: 1) funnel-shaped morphologic pattern of the posterior optic disc with elevation of the adjacent retinal surface; 2) abnormal tissue associated with the distal intraorbital segment of the ipsilateral optic nerve, with effacement of the regional subarachnoid spaces; and 3) discontinuity of the uveoscleral coat. These findings were not observed in any of the unaffected globes of the study patients. In summary, these consistent and characteristic findings of morning glory disc anomaly should allow for accurate differentiation from other ocular anomalies and have the potential to guide appropriate management of this patient population.

▶ The morning glory syndrome has been characterized by a triad of funduscopic findings: (1) an enlarged, funnel-shaped excavation in the optic disc with an annulus of chorioretinal pigmentary changes that surrounds the optic disc excavation; (2) a central glial tuft overlying the optic disc; and (3) a radial orientation of unusually straight and narrow retinal blood vessels emerging from the periphery of the abnormal disc.

This report adds a triad of neuroradiologic diagnostic findings to this rare but important syndrome because of its association with intracranial pathology: (1) funnel-shaped morphologic pattern of the posterior optic disc with elevation of the adjacent retinal surface; (2) abnormal tissue associated with the distal intraorbital segment of the ipsilateral optic nerve, with effacement of the regional subarachnoid spaces; and (3) discontinuity of the uveoscleral coat (Figs 1-3 in the original article).

Morning glory must be distinguished from optic disc colobomas. The morning glory syndrome is a sporadic condition, whereas colobomas are often familial and associated with multisystem malformations.

Patients with morning glory syndrome require neuroradiologic evaluation for possibly associated central nervous system vascular abnormalities that can range from a focal defect in the Circle of Willis to Moyamoya disease with a progressive vasculopathy. Skull base abnormalities such as encephaloceles have also been reported.

**R. C. Sergott, MD**

### Sweep visually evoked potentials and visual findings in children with West syndrome

de Freitas Dotto P, Cavascan NN, Berezovsky A, et al (Universidade Federal de São Paulo – UNIFESP, Brazil)
*Eur J Paediatr Neurol* 18:201-210, 2014

*Background.*—West syndrome (WS) is a type of early childhood epilepsy characterized by progressive neurological development deterioration that includes vision.

*Aim.*—To demonstrate the clinical importance of grating visual acuity thresholds (GVA) measurement by sweep visually evoked potentials technique (sweep-VEP) as a reliable tool for evaluation of the visual cortex status in WS children.

*Methods.*—This is a retrospective study of the best-corrected binocular GVA and ophthalmological features of WS children referred for the Laboratory of Clinical Electrophysiology of Vision of UNIFESP from 1998 to 2012 (Committee on Ethics in Research of UNIFESP n° 0349/08). The GVA deficit was calculated by subtracting binocular GVA score (logMAR units) of each patient from the median values of age norms from our own lab and classified as mild (0.1–0.39 logMAR), moderate (0.40–0.80 logMAR) or severe (>0.81 logMAR). Associated ophthalmological features were also described.

*Results.*—Data from 30 WS children (age from 6 to 108 months, median = 14.5 months, mean ± SD = 22.0 ± 22.1 months; 19 male) were analyzed. The majority presented severe GVA deficit (0.15–1.44 logMAR; mean ± SD = 0.82 ± 0.32 logMAR; median = 0.82 logMAR), poor visual behavior, high prevalence of strabismus and great variability in ocular positioning. The GVA deficit did not vary according to gender ($P$ =.8022), WS type ($P$ =.908), birth age ($P$ =.2881), perinatal oxygenation ($P$ =.7692), visual behavior ($P$ =.8789), ocular motility ($P$ =.1821), nystagmus ($P$ =.2868), risk of drug-induced retinopathy ($P$ =.4632) and participation in early visual stimulation therapy ($P$ =.9010).

*Conclusions.*—The sweep-VEP technique is a reliable tool to classify visual system impairment in WS children, in agreement with the poor visual behavior exhibited by them.

▶ West syndrome or, as it is also called, *infantile spasms (IS)*, is a tragic cause of epilepsy and neurologic impairment in the pediatric age group. Control of the spasms and chaotic electroencephalogram pattern of hypsarrhythmia is mandatory to try to limit long-term neurologic and cognitive impairment. Because of the young age of these patients, evaluation of the visual system has been difficult.

The treatment of this condition is limited to adrenocorticotropic hormone and vigabatrin. The treatment paradigm becomes more complicated, as vigabatrin has been blamed for concentric visual field constriction and retinal toxicity.

This retrospective study is valuable because it provides data about the visual system of patients with IS and also demonstrates that no statistical association exists between these deficits and the vigabatrin therapy.

The development of IS is a pediatric neurology emergency requiring aggressive therapy to control the spasms. These data, and other information developing from longitudinal studies in epilepsy patients, indicate that abnormalities of the afferent visual system may be a comorbidity of the underlying neurologic condition of epilepsy and not invariably linked to therapy with anti-epileptic medications.

**R. C. Sergott, MD**

## The long-term outcomes of ocular tics in a pediatric neuro-ophthalmology practice

Bisker ER, McClelland CM, Brown LW, et al (Univ of Pennsylvania, Philadelphia; Washington Univ, St Louis, MO; Children's Hosp of Philadelphia, PA)
*J AAPOS* 18:31-35, 2014

*Purpose.*—To describe the outcome and comorbidities of ocular tics in children evaluated by a pediatric neuro-ophthalmologist.

*Methods.*—The medical records of all consecutive patients in a pediatric neuro-ophthalmology practice diagnosed with ocular tics (eye rolling, blinking, and widening) were retrospectively reviewed. Children with known secondary causes for tics were excluded. Patients, parents, and/or guardians were contacted by telephone to obtain follow-up information.

*Results.*—A total of 43 patients were included in the retrospective cohort, with a mean age of 7.8 ± 4.8 years at diagnosis. Thirty-two patients participated in the follow-up survey, with an average follow-up of 6.1 ± 3.9 years. None of the 43 children carried a diagnosis of Tourette syndrome or obsessive-compulsive disorder (OCD) at presentation; 1 child had attention deficit hyperactivity disorder (ADHD). At follow-up, 14 of the 32 children (44%) had persistent ocular tics, 3 (9%) reported new nonocular motor tics, 5 (16%) reported new vocal tics, and 4 (13%) developed both nonocular motor and vocal tics. One patient (3%) was formally diagnosed with Tourette syndrome during the follow-up interval, and 3 (9%) were diagnosed with ADHD.

*Conclusions.*—Almost half of the children with ocular tics at presentation had persistent ocular tics on follow-up. New nonocular motor and vocal tics occurred in several patients.

▶ This is a valuable retrospective study about a somewhat rare but always troubling condition to patients, parents, and clinicians. The results from this study fill a gap about the long-term prognosis of these patients.

Fourteen of 32 patients still had a persistent ocular tic at the end of the study period, and some of these patients also had nonocular motor and vocal tics. One patient had Tourette syndrome and 3 had attention deficit hyperactivity disorder, which is a surprisingly low number, but a longer-term study of this cohort will be of value.

**R. C. Sergott, MD**

**Microcystic Macular Edema: Retrograde Maculopathy Caused by Optic Neuropathy**

Abegg M, Dysli M, Wolf S, et al (Univ of Bern, Switzerland)

*Ophthalmology* 121:142-149, 2014

*Purpose.*—To investigate retrograde axonal degeneration for its potential to cause microcystic macular edema (MME), a maculopathy that has been previously described in patients with demyelinating disease. To identify risk factors for MME and to expand the anatomic knowledge on MME.

*Design.*—Retrospective case series.

*Participants.*—We included 117 consecutive patients and 180 eyes with confirmed optic neuropathy of variable etiology. Patients with glaucoma were excluded.

*Methods.*—We determined age, sex, visual acuity, etiology of optic neuropathy, and the temporal and spatial characteristics of MME. Eyes with MME were compared with eyes with optic neuropathy alone and to healthy fellow eyes. With retinal layer segmentation we quantitatively measured the intraretinal anatomy.

*Main Outcome Measures.*—Demographic data, distribution of MME in the retina, and thickness of retinal layers were analyzed.

*Results.*—We found MME in 16 eyes (8.8%) from 9 patients, none of whom had multiple sclerosis or neuromyelitis optica. The MME was restricted to the inner nuclear layer (INL) and had a characteristic perifoveal circular distribution. Compared with healthy controls, MME was associated with significant thinning of the ganglion cell layer and nerve fiber layer, as well as a thickening of the INL and the deeper retinal layers. Youth is a significant risk factor for MME.

*Conclusions.*—Microcystic macular edema is not specific for demyelinating disease. It is a sign of optic neuropathy irrespective of its etiology. The distinctive intraretinal anatomy suggests that MME is caused by retrograde degeneration of the inner retinal layers, resulting in impaired fluid resorption in the macula (Fig 2).

▶ This is an important article that confirms observations made anecdotally by others that microcystic macular edema is not specific for multiple sclerosis as had been originally reported. Be cautious of any article coming from a subspecialty clinic because, by virtue of seeing almost all one disease entity, every new finding is usually attributed to the disease for which the subspecialty clinic has been named.

This report is important in not only defining the occurrence of this finding in other entities but also in defining a typical parafoveal circular distribution. The retinal nerve fiber layer and ganglion cell layers were thinned, but the inner nuclear area was thickened. Younger patients may be more at risk for this change.

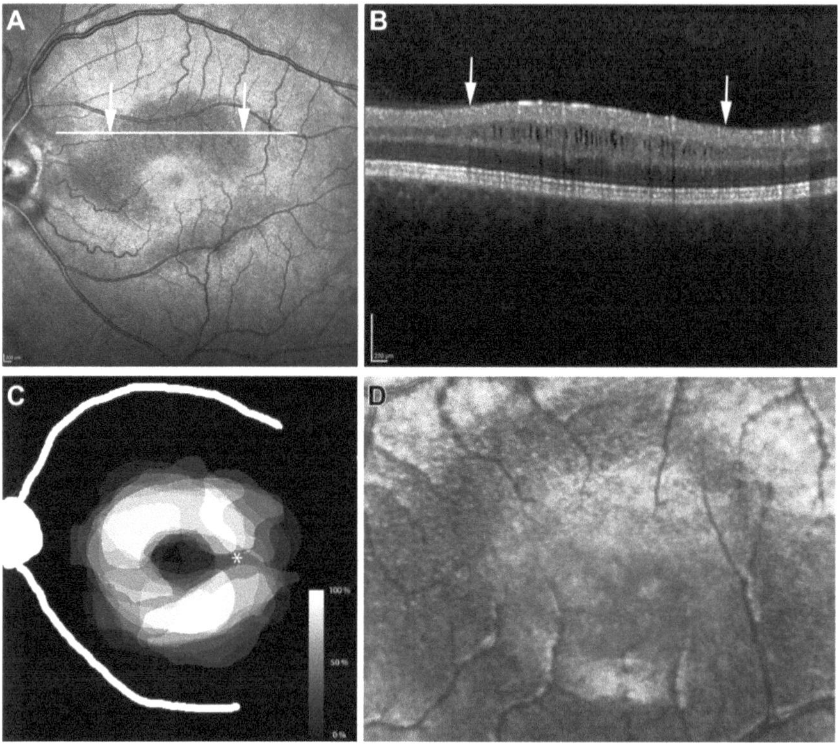


FIGURE 2.—Anatomic characteristics of microcystic macular edema (MME). **A**, A 30° infrared image of the left eye of a patient with MME. The microcysts cause a diffraction of the infrared reflex originating from layers below the edema, thereby leading to a dark appearance of the MME in infrared images. The location of the optical coherence tomography (OCT) section is indicated with a white horizontal line and arrows. **B**, The OCT section shows that microcystic inclusions are located in the inner nuclear layer (INL) but not in the other layers. The presence of microcysts corresponds well with the dark area in the infrared image (white vertical arrows). **C**, Cumulative probability of MME location (16 eyes). The scale bar indicates the percentage of patients with MME in a given area. White areas indicate that all patients had MME in that area; black indicates that MME was present in none of the patients in the MME group. The MME shows a characteristic perifoveal distribution in all patients. Asterisk indicates location of the temporal raphe. **D**, Magnified and contrast-enhanced infrared example of MME. The speckled area shows that microcysts can be detected in the infrared image, illustrating the use of infrared imaging for detecting MME. (Reprinted from Abegg M, Dysli M, Wolf S, et al. Microcystic macular edema: retrograde maculopathy caused by optic neuropathy. *Ophthalmology*. 2014;121:142-149, Copyright 2014, with permission from American Academy of Ophthalmology.)

This finding was actually reported histopathologically in *Investigative Ophthalmology and Visual Science* in an article by Gills et al in a patient with a compressive optic neuropathy from a pituitary tumor.

**R. C. Sergott, MD**

**A randomised double-blind, cross-over trial of 4-aminopyridine for downbeat nystagmus—effects on slowphase eye velocity, postural stability, locomotion and symptoms**

Claassen J, Spiegel R, Kalla R, et al (Univ Hosp Munich, Bavaria, Germany; et al)

*J Neurol Neurosurg Psychiatry* 84:1392-1399, 2013

*Objective.*—The effects of 4-aminopyridine (4-AP) on downbeat nystagmus (DBN) were analysed in terms of slow-phase velocity (SPV), stance, locomotion, visual acuity (VA), patient satisfaction and side effects using standardised questionnaires.

*Methods.*—Twenty-seven patients with DBN received 5 mg 4-AP four times a day or placebo for 3 days and 10 mg 4-AP four times a day or placebo for 4 days. Recordings were done before the first, 60 min after the first and 60 min after the last drug administration.

*Results.*—SPV decreased from 2.42 deg/s at baseline to 1.38 deg/s with 5 mg 4-AP and to 2.03 deg/s with 10 mg 4-AP ($p < 0.05$; post hoc: 5 mg 4-AP: $p = 0.04$). The rate of responders was 57%. Increasing age correlated with a 4-AP-related decrease in SPV ($p < 0.05$). Patients improved in the 'get-up-and-go test' with 4-AP ($p < 0.001$; post hoc: 5 mg: $p = 0.025$; 10 mg: $p < 0.001$). Tandem-walk time (both $p < 0.01$) and tandem-walk error (4-AP: $p = 0.054$; placebo: $p = 0.059$) improved under 4-AP and placebo. Posturography showed that some patients improved with the 5 mg 4-AP dose, particularly older patients. Near VA increased from 0.59 at baseline to 0.66 with 5 mg 4-AP ($p < 0.05$). Patients with idiopathic DBN had the greatest benefit from 4-AP. There were no differences between 4-AP and placebo regarding patient satisfaction and side effects.

*Conclusions.*—4-AP reduced SPV of DBN, improved near VA and some locomotor parameters. 4-AP is a useful medication for DBN syndrome, older patients in particular benefit from the effects of 5 mg 4-AP on nystagmus and postural stability.

▶ Nystagmus is one of the most difficult and frustrating conditions for both patients and clinicians. The involuntary dancing movements of the eyes produce not only visual symptoms such as decreased vision, oscillopsia, and double vision but also neurologic symptoms including imbalance, vertigo, and gait disturbances. Any new therapeutic approach as offered by this excellent clinical trial is most welcome.

For several years, anecdotal reports of the beneficial effect of 4-aminopyridine for downbeat nystagmus have been published. This provides the best evidence of a therapeutic benefit using a double-blind, crossover trial design.

Clinicians now have excellent data to justify the use of this medication for patients with downbeat nystagmus. Now, the challenge will be obtaining approval from insurance carriers to pay for this medication.

**R. C. Sergott, MD**

**Long-term outcomes of pars plana vitrectomy without internal limiting membrane peeling for optic disc pit maculopathy**

Avci R, Yilmaz S, Inan UU, et al (Retina Eye Hosp, Bursa, Turkey; Kocatepe Univ Med School Dept of Ophthalmology, Afyonkarahisar, Turkey; et al)

*Eye* 27:1359-1367, 2013

*Purpose.*—To evaluate the results of surgical treatment of maculopathy secondary to congenital optic pit anomaly with pars plana vitrectomy (PPV), endolaser to the temporal edge of the optic disc and C3F8 tamponade without internal limiting membrane (ILM) peeling.

*Patients and Methods.*—Thirteen eyes of 12 patients with serous macular detachment and/or macular retinoschisis secondary to congenital optic disc pit (ODP) were included in the study. All eyes underwent PPV, posterior hyaloid removal, endolaser photocoagulation on the temporal margin of the optic disc and 12% C3F8 gas tamponade. Anatomic success and functional outcome determined retrospectively by optical coherence tomography and measurement of best corrected visual acuity (BCVA), respectively were the main outcome parameters.

*Results.*—Two lines or more improvement in BCVA was obtained in 11 eyes and 6 of these eyes had 20/40 or better BCVA at the final visit. Subretinal or intraretinal fluid was completely resorbed postoperatively in 12 eyes but a little intraretinal fluid persisted in one eye at the 16-month follow-up. Better visual improvement was observed in patients treated by earlier surgical intervention.

*Conclusion.*—PPV, C3F8 gas tamponade and endolaser to the optic disc margin without ILM peeling may yield favourable results in the treatment of ODP maculopathy (Fig 2).

▶ Spectral domain optical coherence tomography is revealing more and more interaction of the optic nerve and retina in many syndromes that were previously classified as either an optic neuropathy or maculopathy. Now, with spectral domain optical coherence tomography (OCT), essentially a high-resolution qualitative and quantitative ophthalmoscope, we can see these 2 structures interacting with several pathologic processes.

This report shows this connection with optic pits and a serous detachment of the macula or macular schisis. Although this syndrome has been recognized for many years, it is only with OCT that we can visualize and quantitate the degree of involvement, facts that will guide us in the timing of therapeutic intervention.

This group of patients benefitted from the outlined surgical approach, and we would advocate intervention when significant disruption of the ellipsoid zone of the photoreceptors develops.

Once again, better technology results in earlier, more accurate diagnosis and the opportunity to treat disease processes earlier in their course, yielding better long-term results.

Because of the frequent interaction and overlap of optic nerve and macular conditions, we recommend that the first OCT for any patient with cryptic visual

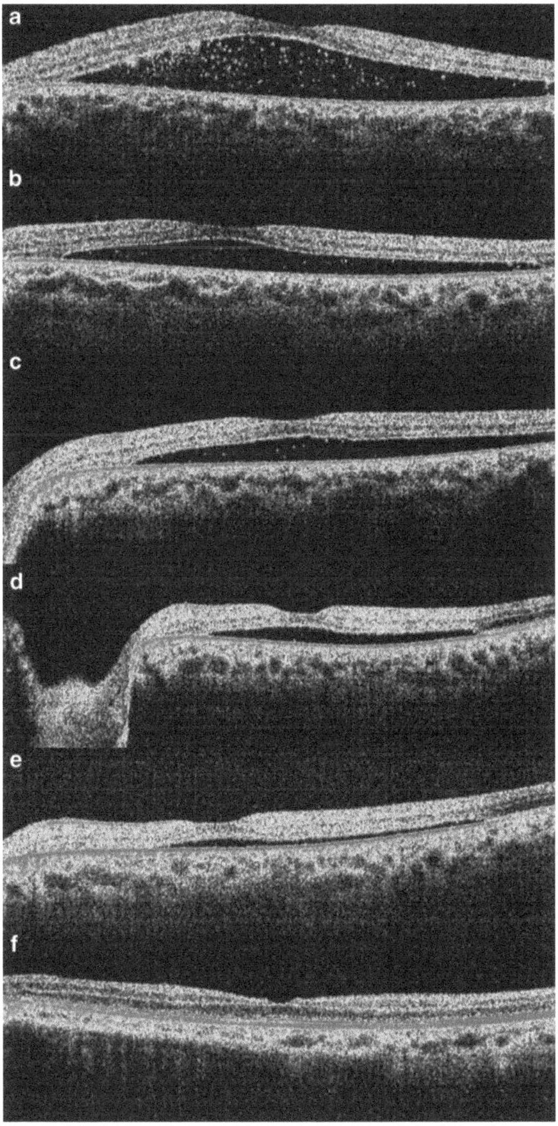


FIGURE 2.—Preoperative serous macular detachment in patient 9 (preoperative VA was 20/100 (a), gradual resolving of subretinal fluid at month 1 (20/80) (b), month 3 (20/63) (c), month 6 (20/40) (d), month 9 (20/40) (e) and month 14 (20/32) (f). (Reprinted from Avci R, Yilmaz S, Inan UU, et al. Long-term outcomes of pars plana vitrectomy without internal limiting membrane peeling for optic disc pit maculopathy. *Eye*. 2013;27:1359-1367, with permission from Macmillan Publishers Limited.)

loss or with clinically apparent optic disc or macular edema include both the optic nerves and maculas.

**R. C. Sergott, MD**

**Analysis of spectral domain optical coherence tomography measurements in optic neuritis: Differences in neuromyelitis optica, multiple sclerosis, isolated optic neuritis and normal healthy controls**

Park K-A, Kim J, Oh SY (Sungkyunkwan Univ School of Medicine, Seoul, Korea)

*Acta Ophthalmol* 92:e57-e65, 2014

*Purpose.*—To compare the retinal layer thickness of eyes with optic neuritis (ON) and that of control eyes and ON eyes with and without neuromyelitis optica (NMO) or multiple sclerosis (MS).

*Methods.*—Horizontal and vertical SD-OCT scans of the fovea were undertaken for 56 patients with ON with and without NMO or MS and for 24 healthy controls. Patients with ON were divided into three groups: NMO, MS and isolated ON without NMO or MS. The thickness of each retinal layer was compared between ON and healthy control eyes, and between ON eyes with and without NMO or MS.

*Results.*—Compared with healthy control eyes, ON eyes showed significant thinning of the ganglion cell layer plus the inner plexiform layer (GCL + IPL) at all eight inner and outer macular locations. Significant differences in thickness were observed for the retinal layers of NMO, MS and isolated ON without NMO or MS at several retinal locations.

*Conclusions.*—Our SD-OCT data revealed a notable difference in the GCL + IPL thickness between ON and healthy control eyes. It also showed differences in the thickness of several retinal layers for ON subgroups including NMO, MS and isolated ON. This may be helpful for distinguishing the aetiology of ON.

▶ This study addresses the clinically important problem of differentiating the inflammatory optic neuropathy associated with multiple sclerosis (MS) compared with neuromyelitis optic (NMO) or the clinically isolated syndrome (CIS) of optic neuritis without clinical or neuroradiologic evidence of MS.

The authors investigated a relatively large cohort of 56 patients who were relatively well balanced demographically and in terms of patient numbers.

Using spectral-domain optical coherence tomography (SD-OCT) with excellent resolution and reproducibility, the authors found that the ganglion cell layer and inner plexiform layers were thinnest in the NMO group compared with the MS and CIS patients. The authors suggest that this increased thinning correlates with the histopathology of NMO that produces necrosis and cavitation of the optic nerves and spinal cord. There was a suggestion that different macular areas may be affected differently in NMO versus MS.

Although these observations are interesting, this observational cross-sectional study does not provide enough data to use SD-OCT to differentiate NMO from optic neuritis associated with MS or CIS. To achieve that goal, we still need a longitudinal study from the time of onset of visual loss with serial observations for at least 6 months. We now test all patients who have acute optic neuritis for NMO with serial testing as the treatment approaches for these 2 disorders is currently quite different. There is sufficient overlap in the clinical findings of NMO and MS to make serial testing essential.

**R. C. Sergott, MD**

**Effect of chlorzoxazone in patients with downbeat nystagmus: A pilot trial**

Feil K, Claaßen J, Bardins S, et al (Univ Hosp Munich, Germany)

*Neurology* 81:1152-1158, 2013

*Objective.*—Downbeat nystagmus (DBN) is the most frequent form of acquired persisting fixation nystagmus with different symptoms such as unsteadiness of gait, postural instability, and blurred vision with reduced visual acuity (VA) and oscillopsia. However, different symptomatic therapeutic principles are required, such as 3,4-diaminopyridine and 4-aminopyridine, that effectively suppress DBN. Chlorzoxazone (CHZ) is a nonselective activator of small conductance calcium-activated potassium (SK) channels that modifies the activity of cerebellar Purkinje cells. We evaluated the effects of this agent on DBN in an observational proof-of-concept pilot study.

*Methods.*—Ten patients received CHZ 500 mg 3 times a day for 1 or 2 weeks. Slow-phase velocity of DBN, VA, postural sway, and the drug's side effects were evaluated. Recordings were conducted at baseline, 90 minutes after first administration, and after 1 or 2 weeks.

*Results.*—Mean slow-phase velocity significantly decreased from a baseline of 2.74°/s ± 2.00 to 2.29°/s ± 2.12 (mean ± SD) 90 minutes after first administration and to 2.04°/s ± 2.24 ($p < 0.001$; post hoc both $p = 0.024$) after long-term treatment. VA significantly increased and postural sway in posturography showed a tendency to decrease on medication. Fifty percent of patients did not report any side effects. The most common reported side effect was abdominal discomfort and dizziness.

*Conclusions.*—The treatment with the SK-channel activator CHZ is a potentially new therapeutic agent for the symptomatic treatment of DBN.

*Classification of Evidence.*—This study provides Class IV evidence that CHZ 500 mg 3 times a day may improve eye movements and visual fixation in patients with DBN.

▶ For several years, we have had no real new therapeutic information concerning downbeat nystagmus. Now, this year, we have 2 excellent studies from the center in Munich, Germany.

This study explores the possible beneficial effect of chlorzoxazone, a nonselective activator of small conductance calcium-activated potassium channels with a modifying effect on cerebellar Purkinje cells.

This proof-of-concept study examined the response of 10 patients receiving 500 mg 3 times a day for 1 or 2 weeks. The slow-phase velocity of the nystagmus decreased compared with baseline both after the first dose and after longer-term treatment. Visual acuity and postural stability also improved. The most common adverse events were abdominal pain and dizziness.

Although limited conclusions can be drawn from such a small study, the data are nonetheless promising, and the pharmacologic rationale to target selectively Purkinje cells is intriguing. Because of the major disability that can be produced by downbeat nystagmus, we welcome any new therapeutic advance.

**R. C. Sergott, MD**

# 9 Imaging

**High prevalence of IgG4-related lymphoplasmacytic infiltrative disorder in 25 patients with orbital inflammation: a retrospective case series**

Deschamps R, Deschamps L, Depaz R, et al (Adolphe de Rothschild, Paris, France; Bichat Hosp, Paris, France; et al)

*Br J Ophthalmol* 97:999-1004, 2013

*Aims.*—To evaluate retrospectively the prevalence of positive IgG4-immunostaining in orbital tissue of patients with idiopathic orbital inflammation and to compare the clinical, radiographic and pathologic features among patients with and without IgG4-positive cells.

*Patients and Methods.*—25 patients with biopsy-proven idiopathic orbital inflammation examined from January 2006 through December 2011 were included. Immunohistochemistry with IgG and IgG4 immunostaining from biopsy specimens of all patients was performed. Tissue with more than 10 IgG4-positive plasma cells per high-power field and with a ratio of IgG4+/IgG+ plasma cells of more than 40% was scored as positive. Histopathologic features, demographic and clinical data, radiologic findings, treatment and follow-up information for each patient were analysed.

*Results.*—Immunohistochemical staining showed 10 cases (40%) were IgG4 positive. The symptoms and signs included eyelid or periocular swelling/mass in all, pain (3/10), extraocular muscle restriction (3/10), proptosis (5/10) and/or decreased vision (4/10). Demographic and clinical findings of these patients did not differ from those with IgG4-negative cells. The presence of positive IgG4-immunostaining in orbital tissue was significantly associated with characteristic pathological features (more background fibrosis, lymphoid hyperplasia, plasma cells and phlebitis).

*Conclusions.*—Finally, 40% of patients with biopsy-proven orbital inflammation were classified as IgG4-RD, with typical histological features but without specific clinical or radiological findings.

► In this retrospective study, Deschamps et al retrospectively evaluated the prevalence of positive immunoglobulin IgG4 immunostaining in the orbital tissue of patients with idiopathic orbital inflammation and compared the clinical, radiographic, and pathologic features among patients with and without IgG4-positive cells. Forty percent of their patients with idiopathic orbital inflammation had IgG4-related disease. They report similar imaging findings on magnetic resonance imaging (MRI) for IgG4-related disease as before (hypointensity on T2-weighted MRI and homogeneous enhancement pattern). Notably, they found no significant differences between IgG4-related disease and IgG4-negative idiopathic orbital inflammations on imaging; however, the IgG4-positive and IgG4-negative groups were distinctly different pathologically in their study. Therefore, pathology likely represents the primary diagnostic tool for this disease process.

**K. Talekar, MD**

**Ocular adnexal IgG4-related disease: CT and MRI findings**

Song YS, Choung H-K, Park S-W, et al (Seoul Natl Univ College of Medicine, Korea; Boramae Med Ctr, Seoul, Korea)

*Br J Ophthalmol* 97:412-418, 2013

*Background/Aims.*—To evaluate CT and MRI findings of histopathologically proven ocular adnexa IgG4-related disease.

*Methods.*—Study subjects included 18 patients with histopathologically proven ocular adnexal IgG4-related disease. CT (n = 16) and MR (n = 3) images were retrospectively evaluated for location, laterality, shape, margin, attenuation on precontrast CT images, T1 and T2 signal intensity on precontrast MRI , internal architecture, ocular adnexal lesion enhancement patterns, sialadenitis of major salivary glands, cervical lymph node enlargement and perilesional bony change.

*Results.*—Lacrimal gland enlargement was observed in 16 cases. Extraglandular lesions were observed in the medial canthus (n = 2) and extraconal space (n = 2). Bilateral supraorbital and infraorbital nerves, pterygopalatine fossa and cavernous sinus involvement were observed in one case. All ocular adnexal lesions showed well defined margins, isoattenuation on precontrast CT images, isointensity on T1- and hypointensity on T2-weighted images, homogenous internal arcithecture and enhancement patterns and bone remodelling without destruction.

*Conclusions.*—Ocular adnexal IgG4-related disease can involve the lacrimal gland, medial canthus, extraconal space, supraorbital and infraorbital nerves, pterygopalatine fossa and cavernous sinus. A diagnosis of ocular adnexal IgG4-related disease should be considered in lesions with the typical imaging features described herein.

▶ Immunoglobulin G4-related disease is a recently described syndrome consisting of diseases that share specific pathologic findings of tumorlike swelling of involved organs, a lymphoplasmacytic infiltrate with abundant IgG4-positive plasma cells, and fibrosis. More than 50% of these patients have elevated serum concentrations of IgG4. It is a multiorgan disease that is found to involve the ocular adnexa with various manifestations including dacroadenitis and orbital inflammation including myosin. It mimics lymphoma and other inflammatory orbital diseases clinically and on imaging. Diagnosis of this disease entity has therapeutic implications as it is steroid responsive; therefore, more aggressive forms of treatment can be avoided. There is a dearth of imaging literature on this newly described disease entity. Radiologic features that have been reported for IgG4-related disease in the head and neck include soft tissue attenuation on computed tomography, hypointensity on T2-weighted magnetic resonance imaging and a homogeneous and gradual enhancement pattern.[1,2] These 2 retrospective studies have reported fairly similar imaging findings of this disease process. Song et al report that differentiating IgG4-related disease from lymphoma (and other orbital inflammatory processes) is difficult. Especially, many of the imaging features of lymphoma overlap with those of IgG4-related diseases; however, they suggest that certain features such as lobulation of the margin and the lesional T2 signal intensity may be helpful in differentiating ocular adnexal IgG4-related diseases from orbital lymphomas because ocular adnexal IgG4-related diseases tend to show hypointensity on T2-weighted images and well-defined margin without lobulation. Ginat et al[3] suggest that routine imaging findings are unreliable in differentiating IgG4-related disease from lymphoma. Given the lack of specificity of the imaging finding, pathologic diagnosis should be sought to make this differentiation. Both these articles are somewhat limited because of the retrospective nature of these studies and small patient populations.

**K. Talekar, MD**

*References*


1. Toyoda K, Oba H, Kutomi K, et al. MR Imaging of IgG4-related disease in the head and neck and brain. *AJNR Am J Neuroradiol.* 2012;33:2136-2139.
2. Katsura M, Mori H, Kunimatsu A, et al. Radiological features of IgG4-related disease in the head, neck, and brain. *Neuroradiology.* 2012;54:873-882.
3. Ginat DT, Freitag SK, Kieff D, et al. Radiographic Patterns of Orbital Involvement in IgG4-Related Disease. *Ophthal Plast Reconstr Surg.* 2013;29:261-266.


---

**Radiographic Patterns of Orbital Involvement in IgG4-Related Disease**

Ginat DT, Freitag SK, Kieff D, et al (Massachusetts General Hosp, Boston; Massachusetts Eye and Ear Infirmary, Boston)

*Ophthal Plast Reconstr Surg* 29:261-266, 2013

---

*Purpose.*—Immunoglobin G4 (IgG4)-related disease is a systemic condition characterized by lymphoplasmacytic infiltrates that can involve the orbit. The purpose of this study was to identify the various patterns of orbital IgG4-related disease on imaging.

*Methods.*—Retrospective review of radiologic examinations including CT, MRI, and positron emission tomography was performed in patients with proven cases of IgG4-related disease.

*Results.*—A total of 9 patients with orbital IgG4-related disease were identified, including 9 with CT, 4 with MRI, and 4 with 18-fluorodeoxyglucose positron emission tomography. Patterns of involvement included lacrimal gland enlargement, lacrimal sac involvement, extraocular muscle thickening, preseptal involvement, orbital fat involvement, and cranial nerve involvement, many of which occurred simultaneously. Associated demineralization of the orbital wall was evident on CT in 2 cases. On T2-weighted MRI, the lesions appeared as hypointense in 2 cases, heterogeneously hypointense to isointense in 1 case, and hyperintense in 1 case. Diffuse enhancement was present in all 3 cases in which postcontrast T1-weighted sequences were available. The lesions were hypermetabolic on positron emission tomography in 3 of 4 cases. There was definite extra-orbital involvement by IgG4-related disease in 3 of the 9 patients and suspected involvement in another 3 of the 9 patients.

*Conclusions.*—IgG4-related disease displays a wide variety of imaging manifestations in the orbit. Extraorbital disease is often present and can help suggest the diagnosis.

▶ Immunoglobulin (Ig)G4-related disease is a recently described syndrome consisting of diseases that share specific pathologic findings of tumorlike swelling of involved organs, a lymphoplasmacytic infiltrate with abundant IgG4-positive plasma cells, and fibrosis. More than 50% of patients with this syndrome have elevated serum concentrations of IgG4. It is a multiorgan disease that has been shown to involve the ocular adnexa with various manifestations including dacryoadenitis and orbital inflammation including myosin. It mimics lymphoma and other inflammatory orbital diseases clinically and on imaging. Diagnosis of this disease entity has therapeutic implications because it is responsive to steroids, and therefore, more aggressive forms of treatment can be avoided. There is a dearth of imaging literature on this newly described disease entity. Radiologic features that have been reported for IgG4-related disease in the head and neck include soft tissue attenuation on computed tomography, hypointensity on T2-weighted magnetic resonance imaging, and a homogeneous and gradual enhancement pattern.[1,2] These 2 retrospective studies cited here have reported fairly similar imaging findings of this disease process. Song et al[3] reported that differentiating IgG4-related disease from lymphoma (and other orbital inflammatory processes) is difficult. In particular, many of the imaging features of lymphoma overlap with those of IgG4-related diseases. However, they suggest that certain features such as lobulation of the margin and the lesional T2 signal intensity may be helpful in differentiating ocular adnexal IgG4-related diseases from orbital lymphomas because ocular adnexal IgG4-related diseases tend to show hypointensity on T2-weighted images and a well-defined margin without lobulation. Ginat et al suggest that routine imaging findings are unreliable in differentiating IgG4-related disease from lymphoma. Given the lack of specificity of the imaging finding, pathologic diagnosis should be sought to make this differentiation. Both these articles are somewhat limited because of the retrospective nature of these studies and small patient populations.

**K. Talekar, MD**

*References*


1. Toyoda K, Oba H, Kutomi K, et al. MR Imaging of IgG4-Related Disease in the Head and Neck and Brain. *AJNR Am J Neuroradiol.* 2012;33:2136-2139.
2. Katsura M, Mori H, Kunimatsu A, et al. Radiological features of IgG4-related disease in the head, neck, and brain. *Neuroradiology.* 2012;54:873-882.
3. Song YS, Choung H-K, Park S-W, et al. Ocular adnexal IgG4-related disease: CT and MRI findings. *Br J Ophthalmol.* 2013;97:412-418.

# 10 Ocular Oncology

**Reactive Retinal Astrocytic Tumors (So-called Vasoproliferative Tumors): Histopathologic, Immunohistochemical, and Genetic Studies of Four Cases**

Poole Perry LJ, Jakobiec FA, Zakka FR, et al (Harvard Med School, Boston, MA; et al)

*Am J Ophthalmol* 155:593-608, 2013

*Purpose.*—To evaluate the cellular nature of and diagnostic terminology used in connection with acquired retinal "vasoproliferative tumors."

*Design.*—Retrospective clinicopathologic study.

*Methods.*—Clinical records and microscopic slides of 4 enucleated globes were reviewed. Special stains and immunohistochemical probes for CD31, CD34, p53, glial fibrillary acidic protein (GFAP), CD163, and Ki67 (cell replication) were employed; ultrastructural and fluorescence in situ hybridization (FISH) analyses were performed.

*Results.*—Tumors were located inferotemporally in middle-aged patients. They were uniformly composed of compacted elongated, GFAP-positive spindle cells (due to intermediate filaments identified ultrastructurally) with a Ki67 index of less than 1%. Rosenthal fibers and eosinophilic granular bodies were observed. Hyalinized periodic acid-Schiff-positive vessels were widely separated. CD31 and CD34 revealed a sparse microvasculature. Tumor-associated exudate spread predominantly subretinally. The retinal pigment epithelium had undergone extensive placoid fibrous metaplasia with focal ossification. P53 upregulation, *BRAF-KIAA* gene rearrangement, and *IDH1 R132H* mutation typically associated with low-grade astrocytic neoplasms were absent.

*Conclusions.*—Retinal "vasoproliferative" tumors have been mischaracterized, because they actually display a paucity of microvessels. Proliferating fibrous astrocytes with a very low proliferation index predominate, without immunohistochemical or genetic evidence favoring a neoplasm. Subretinal exudate appeared capable of provoking widespread fibrous metaplasia of the pigment epithelium that was mainly responsible for secondary retinal damage. The term "reactive retinal astrocytic tumor" is proposed as more appropriate for this entity. In carefully selected progressive lesions, consideration should be given to earlier surgical intervention before extensive subretinal exudate accumulates and pigment epithelial proliferation with fibrous metaplasia ensues.

▶ Retinal vasoproliferative tumors (VPT) were first described in 1983[1] as a vascular mass believed to be an acquired nonfamilial retinal hemangioma. This mass was distinguished from the retinal hemangioblastoma of von Hippel Lindau (VHL) disease by its onset in older patients without features of markedly dilated retinal vessels. The lack of VHL was confirmed in these cases by genetic testing. Since then, there have been numerous names for this tumor, including the most common term of *retinal vasoproliferative tumor*[2] and other less common terms of *acquired retinal angioma, angioma-like mass, retinal angiomatous mass, retinal angiomas in the aged, angioma-like lesion, glioangiosis, presumed acquired retinal hemangioma, hemangioma-like masses of the retina,* and a few others. Despite the numerous names, this reactive tumor appears to behave in a benign fashion but with progressive leakage of subretinal fluid and exudation. Most cases are managed with cryotherapy, laser photocoagulation, or plaque radiotherapy, with little need for enucleation.

In a more current study of 334 patients with VPT, Shields et al[3] identified primary VPTs as those that are idiopathic without evident cause and secondary VPT as those caused by underlying disease, including pars planitis, retinitis pigmentosa, Coats' disease, and others. A comparison of primary vs secondary types of tumor found that secondary VPT was more often bilateral, multiple, and larger than primary VPT. Additionally, secondary VPT occurred at an earlier age and was associated with poorer visual acuity than primary VPT.

In this report, Poole Perry et al provided histopathologic evaluation of 4 eyes that came to enucleation after therapy for retinal VPT. They noted that these tumors had a prominent finding of compacted bipolar cells, with slender, elongated bland nuclei and long cytoplasmic processes, similar to pilocytic astrocytes. The vascular component was "remarkably inconspicuous" in their 4 cases. They speculate that the precise cell of origin of VPT could be fibrous astrocytes or the Müller cell. They propose renaming this tumor as reactive retinal astrocytic tumor because of the predominant astrocytic component.

**C. L. Shields, MD**

*References*

1. Shields JA, Decker WL, Sanborn GE, Augsburger JJ, Goldberg RE. Presumed acquired retinal hemangiomas. *Ophthalmology.* 1983;90:1292-1300.
2. Shields CL, Shields JA, Barrett J, De Potter P. Vasoproliferative tumors of the ocular fundus. Classification and clinical manifestations in 103 patients. *Arch Ophthalmol.* 1995;113:615-623.
3. Shields CL, Kaliki S, Al-Dahmash S, et al. Retinal vasoproliferative tumors: comparative clinical features of primary vs secondary tumors in 334 cases. *JAMA Ophthalmol.* 2013;131:328-334.

## Radiation-Related Cancer Risk Associated With Surveillance Imaging for Metastasis From Choroidal Melanoma

Wen JC, Sai V, Straatsma BR, et al (Univ of California, Los Angeles; Univ of California, San Francisco)

*JAMA Ophthalmol* 131:56-61, 2013

*Objective.*—To estimate the lifetime attributable risk of cancer associated with whole-body positron emission tomography (PET)/computed tomography (CT) and with CT of the chest, abdomen, and pelvis if performed at various frequencies and for different durations for surveillance of patients with primary choroidal or ciliary body melanoma for distant metastasis.

*Methods.*—Effective radiation doses for whole-body CT and for CT of the chest, abdomen, and pelvis were calculated using Monte Carlo simulation studies. The effective dose of the PET scan was estimated by multiplying fludeoxyglucose F18 radioactivity with dose coefficients. Lifetime attributable risks of cancer were calculated using the approach described in the Biological Effects of Ionizing Radiation VII report.

*Results.*—For a 50-year-old patient, an annual CT of the chest, abdomen, and pelvis for 10 years carries an estimated lifetime attributable risk of cancer of 0.9% for male patients and 1.3% for female patients, whereas an annual PET/CT each year for 10 years carries an estimated lifetime attributable risk of cancer of 1.6% for male patients and 1.9% for female patients. Lifetime risk was found to be higher in younger, female patients. The lifetime attributable risk of cancer was estimated to be as high as 7.9% for a 20-year-old female patient receiving a PET/CT scan every 6 months for 10 years.

*Conclusions.*—Aggressive surveillance protocols incorporating CT scanning or PET/CT scanning for detection of metastasis from primary choroidal or ciliary body melanoma appear to confer a significant substantial risk of a secondary malignant tumor in patients who do not succumb to metastatic melanoma within the first few posttreatment years.

▶ Choroidal melanoma shows a 10-year cumulative rate of metastasis at approximately 25% to 34%, primarily based on tumor size and genetic structure.[1-3] The most common sites for metastatic disease are the liver, lung, and skin. There is interest in identifying those patients at risk and providing screening for metastatic disease at an early point to minimize morbidity and mortality. Methods of monitoring include chest radiograph; liver function tests; liver imaging with computed tomography (CT), magnetic resonance imaging (MRI), or ultrasonography; and whole-body imaging with CT, MRI, or positron emission testing (PET) coupled with CT.

PET CT is a common way to monitor and stage cutaneous melanoma with relatively high sensitivity and specificity. PET CT exposes the body to a substantial dose of radiation. Radiation exposure is generally measured in milliSieverts. The risk for cancer induction increases with increasing exposure. The lifetime attributable risk (LAR) for cancer associated with radiation dosages is a method widely used to estimate risks after studies like mammogram, CT, and PET CT.

Wen et al calculated that the LAR for second cancer at 10 years for men with uveal melanoma who were imaged with PET CT every 6 months was 2% for a 70-year-old, 4% for 50-year-old, and 5% for a 20-year-old. Similarly, the rates were highest in the youngest population of women, as PET CT-induced LAR for second cancer was 2% for a 70-year-old, 5% for a 50-year-old, and 8% for a 20-year-old woman.

Wen et al pleaded that clinicians consider the patient age, sex, and disease prognosis when providing an opinion on imaging for metastatic disease. For a young patient with small melanoma and excellent prognosis, such testing may not be beneficial for the patient.

**C. L. Shields, MD**

*References*


1. Shields JA, Shields CL. *Intraocular Tumors. An Atlas and Textbook*. 2nd edition. Philadelphia, PA: Lippincott Williams and Wilkins; 2008.
2. Diener-West M, Reynolds SM, Agugliaro DJ, et al. Collaborative Ocular Melanoma Study Group. Development of metastatic disease after enrollment in the COMS trials for treatment of choroidal melanoma: Collaborative Ocular Melanoma Study Group Report No. 26. *Arch Ophthalmol.* 2005;123:1639-1643.
3. Shields CL, Furuta M, Thangappan A, et al. Metastasis of uveal melanoma millimeter-by-millimeter in 8033 consecutive eyes. *Arch Ophthalmol.* 2009;127: 989-998.


**Vitreoretinal Lymphoma. A 20-Year Review of Incidence, Clinical and Cytologic Features, Treatment, and Outcomes**

Levasseur SD, Wittenberg LA, White VA (Univ of British Columbia, Vancouver, Canada)

*JAMA Ophthalmol* 131:50-55, 2013

*Objectives.*—To determine the incidence and clinical and cytologic diagnostic accuracy of vitreoretinal lymphoma (VRL) and to evaluate its clinical features, management, and outcomes in a cohort of patients who underwent diagnostic vitrectomy.

*Methods.*—Retrospective medical record review of 463 diagnostic vitrectomy specimens from 430 patients collected from October 1, 1990, through December 31, 2010, from Vancouver General Hospital and the British Columbia Cancer Agency.

*Results.*—A total of 22 patients were diagnosed as having VRL with a preoperative clinical diagnostic sensitivity of 77%, specificity of 73%, positive predictive value of 13%, and negative predictive value of 98%. The cytologic diagnostic sensitivity was 87% (27 of 31 specimens). The incidence of VRL in British Columbia doubled from 1990 to 2010, with a final incidence of 0.047 cases per 100 000 people per year. The mean age at diagnosis was 66 years. Seventeen patients (77%) were women. The initial diagnosis of lymphoma was VRL in 19 patients (86%), of whom 7 (37%) had concurrent central nervous system lymphoma. Recurrent disease was found in 11 patients. Large B-cell lymphoma was diagnosed in 20 patients (91%). The median progression-free survival was 11 months, and the median survival was 33 months from the initial diagnosis.

*Conclusions.*—Vitreoretinal lymphoma remains a clinical diagnostic challenge. Early clinical suspicion with subsequent diagnostic vitrectomy for cytologic analysis and collaboration with the oncology department is critical to appropriate and prompt staging and treatment. More interdisciplinary studies are required to further characterize VRL and maximize the therapeutic options, thus improving the morbidity and mortality associated with the disease.

▶ Vitreoretinal lymphoma (VRL), also know as *vitreous large cell lymphoma, vitreous reticulum cell sarcoma*, and *primary intraocular lymphoma*, is a rare disease with extremely poor prognosis. This is a form of high-grade lymphoma that affects both the brain and eye in elderly or immunosuppressed patients, leading to death at a mean of 2 to 3 years after diagnosis. The difficulty stems from the similarity of VRL with uveitis, and often there is a long delay from symptoms to establishment of the true diagnosis.

VRL was first described in 1951 and represents less than 1% of all non-Hodgkin lymphoma. There is a 3-fold increase in this disease since 1980 because of increasing numbers of immunocompromised and immunosuppressed patients, but this condition can occur also in immunocompetent patients. VRL can manifest as a bilateral or unilateral condition with vitreous cells and decreased visual acuity. At presentation of the ocular findings, approximately 33% to 50% of patients have brain involvement.[1,2]

Levasseur et al reviewed the 463 diagnostic vitrectomy specimens in an ophthalmic pathology laboratory in Vancouver, British Columbia, Canada. They found only a small number of 22 cases of VRL in this large sample. They identified that VRL was becoming more common in their population, as the incidence in 1990 to 1995 was 0.023 per 100 000 population and in 2005 to 2010 was 0.048 per 100 000. By Kaplan Meier analysis, survival rate was 80% at 2 years, 50% at 5 years, and 10% at 10 years.

They conclude that VRL continues to have poor prognosis with no strict treatment guidelines or remotely successful therapy. They advise brain and systemic screening by an oncologist after the eye diagnosis is established. Screening should continue for life.

**C. L. Shields, MD**

*References*

1. Whitcup SM, de Smet MD, Rubin BI, et al. Intraocular lymphoma: clinical and histopathologic diagnosis. *Ophthalmology.* 1993;100:1399-1406.
2. Fardeau C, Lee CPL, Merle-Béral H, et al. Retinal fluorescein, indocyanine green angiography, and optic coherence tomography in non-Hodgkin primary intraocular lymphoma. *Am J Ophthlamol.* 2009;147:886-894.

## Molecular pathology of uveal melanoma

Coupland SE, Lake SL, Zeschnigk M, et al (Univ of Liverpool, UK; Universitätsklinikum Essen, Germany)
*Eye (Lond)* 27:230-242, 2013

Like other cancers, uveal melanomas (UM) are characterised by an uncontrolled, clonal, cellular proliferation, occurring as a result of numerous genetic, and epigenetic aberrations. Signalling pathways known to be disrupted in UM include: (1) the retinoblastoma pathway, probably as a result of cyclin D1 overexpression; p53 signalling, possibly as a consequence of MDM2 overexpression; and the P13K/AKT and mitogen-activated protein kinase/extracellular signal-related kinase pathway pathways that are disturbed as a result of PTEN and GNAQ/11 mutations, respectively. Characteristic chromosomal abnormalities are common and include 6p gain, associated with a good prognosis, as well as 1p loss, 3 loss, and 8q gain, which correlate with high mortality. These are identified by techniques such as fluorescence *in situ* hybridisation, comparative genomic hybridisation, microsatellite analysis, multiplex ligation-dependent probe amplification, and single-nucleotide polymorphisms. UM can also be categorised by their gene expression profiles as class 1 or class 2, the latter correlating with poor survival, as do *BRCA1-associated* protein-1 (BAP1) inactivating mutations. Genetic testing of UM has enhanced prognostication, especially when results are integrated with histological and clinical data. The identification of abnormal signalling pathways, genes and proteins in UM opens the way for target-based therapies, improving prospects for conserving vision and prolonging life.

▶ There is intense interest in the understanding of the molecular genetic abnormalities that lead to the development of uveal melanoma. This interest is fueled by the development of medications that inhibit signaling pathways in melanoma evolution. This could lead to targeted therapy for prevention of metastatic disease, once melanoma is diagnosed and evaluated by molecular genetics.

The most common aberrations in uveal melanoma involve chromosome 1p loss, 1q gain, 3 loss, 6p gain, 6q loss, 8p loss, and 8q gain. Of these, only 6p gain is favorable, associated with good prognosis. The rest are associated with poor prognosis, particularly 3 loss and 8q gain. In all cases, this testing requires the clinician to obtain tissue by gross specimen or fine-needle biopsy. In our clinic, we have had extensive experience with fine-needle aspiration biopsy of uveal melanoma in more than 2000 cases for samples for genetic analysis. In an analysis of 500 consecutive cases, we found chromosome 3 loss in approximately 23% of small melanoma, 30% of medium melanoma, and 50% of large melanoma.[1] Factors related to chromosome 3 loss include larger melanoma size and peripheral tumor location.

Coupland et al emphasize that investigation of the signaling pathways for uveal melanoma development could shed light on potential targeted therapies for inhibition of metastases. Some of these agents include inhibitors of MAPK/MEK signaling pathway, P13K/AKT pathway at the level of AKT, mTOR, mTOR blockade combined with an insulinlike growth factor—1R antibody, tyrosine kinases, c-Met pathway, CXCR4, and histone deacetylase.

**C. L. Shields, MD**

*Reference*

1. Shields CL, Ganguly A, Bianciotto CG, Turaka K, Tavallali A, Shields JA. Prognosis of uveal melanoma in 500 cases using genetic testing of fine-needle aspiration biopsy specimens. *Ophthalmology*. 2011;118:396-401.

**SD-OCT and autofluorescence characteristics of autoimmune retinopathy**

Pepple KL, Cusick M, Jaffe GJ, et al (Duke Univ Eye Ctr, Durham, NC; Eye Consultants of Pennsylvania, Wyomissing)

*Br J Ophthalmol* 97:139-144, 2013

*Aims.*—To report abnormal fundus hyperautofluorescence (hyper-AF) and loss of outer retinal layers by spectral domain optical coherence tomography in patients with autoimmune retinopathy (AIR).

*Methods.*—Retrospective, observational case series of 14 eyes of 7 patients diagnosed with an AIR for whom colour fundus photographs, fundus AF images and spectral domain optical coherence tomograms (SD-OCT) were obtained at presentation.

*Results.*—Seven patients were identified ranging in age from 24 to 73 years. Six had a history of cancer and were diagnosed with cancer associated retinopathy or melanoma associated retinopathy. Among the seven patients, six (86%) had abnormalities by AF or SD-OCT including loss of outer retinal layers in association with hyper-AF. One patient with melanoma associated retinopathy did not have any imaging abnormalities. In one patient with cancer associated retinopathy followed over 8 months, progressive loss of retinal architecture was associated with the formation of a hyper-AF ring.

*Conclusions.*—Patients with AIR can present with structural abnormalities that are detectable by fundus AF and SD-OCT. The areas of hyper-AF correspond to loss of outer-retinal structures such as the inner segment/outer segment junction, the external limiting membrane and outer nuclear layer. These imaging modalities may be useful in establishing the diagnosis of this rare disease, monitoring disease progression and evaluating response to therapy.

► Autoimmune retinopathy (AIR) includes a set of rare, immune-mediated retinal degenerations that can lead to impaired visual field and reduced visual acuity. These conditions are also known as *paraneoplastic retinopathies* and include cancer-associated retinopathy (CAR), melanoma-associated retinopathy (MAR), lymphoma-associated retinopathy (LAR), and simple autoimmune retinopathy without underlying cancer. In this set of conditions, the symptoms are often vague with acute or chronic vision loss, night blindness, and photopsia. Fundus evaluation is usually normal in appearance but can show retinal pigment epithelial (RPE) mottling, vascular attenuation, waxy optic disc pallor, and rare vitreous cell. The diagnosis is suspected based on electroretinogram abnormalities with rod or cone reduced responses and visual field ring scotoma with constriction. However, the diagnosis is established with documentation of retinal or optic disc autoantibodies in the patient serum.

One of the problems with AIR is that some patients with normal visual function manifest circulating autoantibodies to retina. Therefore, there is no single test to confirm this disease spectrum.

In this report, Pepple et al describe 2 new methods of imaging patients with AIR, including autofluorescence and spectral domain optical coherence tomography

(SD OCT). They studied 7 patients with CAR or MAR and found hyperautofluorescence in 5 and SD OCT loss of outer retinal structures in 6. The autofluorescence findings typically represented RPE abnormalities and correlated with the SD OCT findings. Most commonly, there was a central parafoveal ring of hyperautofluorescence surrounding the normofluorescent fovea. This correlated with loss of the outer retinal layers including photoreceptor tips, ellipsoid layer, external limiting membrane, and outer nuclear layer. The foveal anatomy was preserved, and this correlates to the classic ring scotoma.

This information adds to our understanding of AIR, The combination of accurate history, ocular findings, and diagnostic testing contributes to the diagnosis of this often elusive disease.

**C. L. Shields, MD**

## Lesions Simulating Retinoblastoma (Pseudoretinoblastoma) in 604 Cases: Results Based on Age at Presentation

Shields CL, Schoenberg E, Kocher K, et al (Thomas Jefferson Univ, Philadelphia, PA)

*Ophthalmology* 120:311-316, 2013

*Purpose.*—To determine the types and frequency of ocular conditions that simulate retinoblastoma (pseudoretinoblastoma) based on age at presentation.

*Design.*—Retrospective case series.

*Participants.*—Two thousand seven hundred seventy-five patients.

*Methods.*—Chart review.

*Main Outcome Measures.*—Conditions simulating retinoblastoma.

*Results.*—Of 2775 patients referred for management of retinoblastoma, 2171 patients (78%) had confirmed retinoblastoma and 604 patients (22%) had simulating lesions (pseudoretinoblastomas). In the pseudoretinoblastoma cohort, the mean patient age at presentation was 4 years (median, 2 years). There were 27 different pseudoretinoblastoma conditions, and the 10 most common included Coats' disease (n = 244; 40%), persistent fetal vasculature (PFV; n = 158; 28%), vitreous hemorrhage (n = 27; 5%), ocular toxocariasis (n = 22; 4%), familial exudative vitreoretinopathy (FEVR; n = 18; 3%), rhegmatogenous retinal detachment (n = 18; 3%), coloboma (n = 17; 3%), astrocytic hamartoma (n = 15; 2%), combined hamartoma of retina and retinal pigment epithelium (n = 15; 2%), and endogenous endophthalmitis (n = 10; 2%). Simulating lesions differed based on age at presentation, and children younger than 1 year were most likely to have PFV (49%), Coats' disease (20%), or vitreous hemorrhage (7%); those 2 to 5 years of age were most likely to have Coats' disease (61%), toxocariasis (8%), or PFV (7%); and those older than 5 years were most likely to have Coats' disease (57%), toxocariasis (8%), or FEVR (6%).

*Conclusions.*—The most common pseudoretinoblastomas include Coats' disease, PFV, and vitreous hemorrhage, but the spectrum varies depending on patient age.

▶ The diagnosis of retinoblastoma is based on characteristic clinical findings on examination and with diagnostic imaging.[1] This management of this malignancy is different from most other tumors that require biopsy to establish the diagnosis. In retinoblastoma management, it is imperative that the tumor not be biopsied because entry into the globe for needle biopsy or open biopsy could seed this highly aggressive malignancy into surrounding tissues, leading to risk for metastasis and death.[2] With this in mind, the clinician must be skilled and confident of diagnosis without histopathology confirmation before embarking on conservative therapies.

In this report, Shields et al examined the referring diagnosis of 2775 patients (mostly children) referred with possible diagnosis of retinoblastoma and found 78% of cases with retinoblastoma and 22% with simulating lesions. They further explored the simulators and found that they differed based on age. For the youngest group (< 1 year), persistent fetal vasculature was the leading simulator; for the 2- to 5-year age group Coats disease was the leading simulator; and for the oldest group (> 5 years), Coats disease also prevailed.

Despite the 22% misdiagnosis at referral, this is an improvement of a report previously published by our group in 1991 in which there was a 46% misdiagnosis rate.[3] Careful examination with clear understanding of the clinical features and imaging findings of retinoblastoma can improve diagnostic accuracy. The authors advised that any child with possible retinoblastoma consult with a retinoblastoma specialist, especially before enucleation or exposing the child to chemotherapy.

**C. L. Shields, MD**

*References*


1. Bianciotto C, Shields CL. Clinical features. In: Ramasubramanian A, Shields CL, eds. *Retinoblastoma.* New Delhi, India: Jaypee Brothers Medical Publishers; 2012: 37-45.
2. Kaliki S, Shields CL, Shah SU, Eagle RC Jr, Shields JA, Leahey A. Postenucleation adjuvant chemotherapy with vincristine, etoposide, and carboplatin for the treatment of high-risk retinoblastoma. *Arch Ophthalmol.* 2011;129:1422-1427.
3. Shields JA, Parsons HM, Shields CL, Shah P. Lesions simulating retinoblastoma. *J Pediatr Ophthalmol Strabismus.* 1991;28:338-340.


**Progression of Ocular Melanoma Metastasis to the Liver. The 2012 Zimmerman Lecture**

Grossniklaus HE (Univ School of Medicine, Atlanta, GA)
*JAMA Ophthalmol* 131:462-469, 2013

*Importance.*—To the best of my knowledge, this study demonstrates for the first time small, apparently dormant micrometastasis in the liver of patients with uveal melanoma.

*Objective.*—To evaluate the histological and immunohistochemical findings in metastatic uveal melanoma to the liver.

*Design.*—Samples of liver were obtained at autopsy from patients who died of metastatic uveal melanoma to the liver.

*Setting.*—L. F. Montgomery Laboratory, Emory Eye Center, Atlanta, Georgia.

*Participants.*—A total of 10 patients who died of metastatic uveal melanoma to the liver.

*Intervention.*—Sections of the liver were examined with hematoxylin-eosin, periodic acid-Schiff, Masson trichrome, or reticulin stains.

*Main Outcome Measures.*—The tumors' morphology, growth pattern, mean vascular density, and mitotic index were determined with the aid of immunohistochemical stains for S100, HMB45, CD31, and Ki67.

*Results.*—Stage 1 metastases (defined as tumor clusters ≤50 μm in diameter) were identified in the sinusoidal spaces of 9 of 10 patients (90%). Stage 1 metastases were avascular and lacked mitotic activity. Stage 2 metastases (defined as tumors measuring 51-500 μm in diameter) and stage 3 metastases (defined as tumors measuring >500 μm in diameter) were found in all patients. Immunohistochemical stains were positive for S100 or HMB45 in all tumors. Overall, stage 1 metastases outnumbered stage 2 metastases (which outnumbered stage 3 metastases). The mean vascular density and mitotic index increased from stage 2 to stage 3 metastases ($P < .05$). The architecture of stage 2 metastases mimicked the surrounding hepatic parenchyma, whereas stage 3 metastases exhibited either lobular or portal growth patterns.

*Conclusions.*—Uveal melanoma that spreads to the liver can be categorized as stage 1 (≤50 μm in diameter), stage 2 (51-500 μm in diameter), or stage 3 (>500 μm in diameter) metastases. The later stage exhibits a lobular or portal pattern of growth. During this progression, tumors become vascularized and mitotically active.

▶ Uveal melanoma is a deadly tumor, carrying an overall 40% risk for liver metastasis within 10 years. Zimmerman et al believed that enucleation of an eye with melanoma could spread melanoma cells into the system, and, in the 1970s, this theory became known as the *Zimmerman hypothesis*.[1] They speculated that the 2-year postenucleation spike in death rate was related to the enucleation surgery. Later, others calculated tumor doubling time and, working backwards mathematically, estimated that undetectable melanoma metastasis (micrometastasis) existed in the liver years before the date of intraocular tumor detection.[2,3]

In this report, Grossniklaus investigated autopsy liver metastatic disease and found that metastasis can be small (stage 1, < 50 μm), medium (stage 2, 51–500 μm), or large (stage 3, > 500 μm). Small metastases were more common than medium, which were more common than large metastatic foci. Vascular growth and mitotic activity increased with increasing stage. The author claims, based on these findings, that stage 1 metastases are subclinical and exhibit more dormant features with less mitotic activity compared with greater stages. These features suggest that the liver controls tumor progression with innate immunity, macrophage activity, and other factors. Grossniklaus further believes that the 2-year postenucleation peak in metastatic disease is a stochastic phenomenon of tumor burden in the end organ with loss of suppression.

This publication is a histopathologic confirmatory report on liver metastatic disease after treatment of uveal melanoma and is inspiring to clinicians to consider adjuvant therapy for prevention of growth of micrometastatic foci in patients at high risk.

**C. L. Shields, MD**

*References*

1. Zimmerman LE, McLean IW, Foster WD. Does enucleation of the eye containing a malignant melanoma prevent or accelerate the dissemination of tumour cells. *Br J Ophthalmol.* 1978;62:420-425.
2. Eskelin S, Pyrhönen S, Summanen P, Hahka-Kemppinen M, Kivelä T. Tumor doubling times in metastatic malignant melanoma of the uvea: tumor progression before and after treatment. *Ophthalmology.* 2000;107:1443-1449.
3. Singh AD. Uveal melanoma: implications of tumor doubling time. *Ophthalmology.* 2001;108:829-831.

**The Cytologic Composition of Dacryops: An Immunohistochemical Investigation of 15 Lesions Compared to the Normal Lacrimal Gland**

Jakobiec FA, Zakka FR, Perry LP (Harvard Med School, Boston, MA)

*Am J Ophthalmol* 155:380-396.e1, 2013

*Purpose.*—To define the cytologic composition of the double-layered epithelial lining of dacryops (lacrimal duct cyst), improve histopathologic diagnosis, and better understand pathogenesis.

*Design.*—Clinicopathologic retrospective study with immunohistochemical studies of 15 lesions compared with normal lacrimal gland.

*Methods.*—Clinical data from 14 patients were reviewed and microscopy was performed with routine stains and immunohistochemical probes for epithelial membrane antigen (EMA), gross cystic disease fluid protein-15 (GCDFP-15), cytokeratin 7 (CK7), and smooth muscle actin (SMA).

*Results.*—The major lacrimal gland was involved in 13 lesions; 2 lesions arose in an accessory gland of Krause. One case was bilateral; the average age of the patients was 50.7 years. Neither visual acuity nor motility was disturbed. No lesion was discovered to have recurred after excision. Microscopically, in all dacryops specimens goblet cells and luminal pseudoapocrine apical cytoplasmic projections were identified. Lacrimal acinar cells immunoreacted with GCDFP-15 and CK7, whereas the normal ducts and the epithelium of the dacryops lesions reacted diffusely only with CK7. SMA-positive myoepithelial cells were found in the acini but not in the normal ducts or dacryops epithelium.

*Conclusions.*—Negative GCDFP-15 staining ruled out apocrine metaplasia in dacryops. Normal ducts and dacryops showed no immunohistochemical evidence for the presence of myoepithelial cells. Pathogenetic theories of dacryops that implicate a failure of ductular "neuromuscular" contractility must therefore be revised. A dysfunction of the rich neural plexus around the ductules may play a role in the development of dacryops in conjunction with periductular inflammation and induced scarring.

▶ *Dacryops* is a Greek word for *dacryo* (tear of lacrimal gland or sac) and *ops* (eye). This cyst originates from the ducts that drain the lacrimal gland. The biologic properties of the dacryops lining have not yet been definitively elucidated until this report.

In this report, Jakobiec et al describe the histopathology of 15 cases of dacryops in 14 patients. The authors sought to define the cause of obstruction and dilation of the lacrimal duct and clarify the tissues involved.

In their analysis, they found that ectasia can occur with any lacrimal tissue in the orbit or palpebrum, in the tarsal region (Wolfring),[1] in the fornices (Krause),[2] and in the caruncle (Popoff).[3] They indicated in this small series that there was no symptom of visual loss in any case. Histopathologically, the cyst was comprised of a nonkeratinizing wall with double layer of cells surround by a fibrous wall and surrounding lacrimal gland lobules. They identified that the conjunctival forniceal cyst can closely resemble dacryops, but the absence of lacrimal tissue in the former helps to define the diagnosis.

These authors commented that dacryops can be differentiated from simulating conditions. Dacryops does not contain iron or lipofuscin within the epithelium, as is encountered with hidrocystoma. Dacryops does not have ciliated respiratory epithelium like mucocele. Dacryops does not have pilosebaceous units in the wall as do dermoid cysts. Dacryops does not have myoepithelial outer wall layer like apocrine cysts. Moreover, dacryops does have goblet cells in the wall which is absent in eccrine and apocrine cysts.

This report is a valuable clinical and histopathologic analysis of an entity that is often confused with similar conditions.

**C. L. Shields, MD**

*References*


1. Weatherhead RG. Wolfring dacryops. *Ophthalmology.* 1992;99(10):1575-1581.
2. Jastrzebski A, Brownstein S, Jordan DR, deNanassy J. Dacryops of Krause gland in the inferior fornix in a child. *Arch Ophthalmol.* 2012;130(2):252-254.
3. Stern K, Jakobiec FA, Harrison WG. Caruncular dacryops with extruded secretory globoid bodies. *Ophthalmology.* 1983;90(12):1447-1451.


## Normative Reference Ranges for the Retinal Nerve Fiber Layer, Macula, and Retinal Layer Thicknesses in Children

Yanni SE, Wang J, Cheng CS, et al (Retina Foundation of the Southwest, Dallas, TX)
*Am J Ophthalmol* 155:354-360.e1, 2013

*Purpose.*—To establish a normative database of peripapillary retinal nerve fiber layer (RNFL) thickness, macular thickness, and retinal layer thickness in healthy North American children, using spectral-domain optical coherence tomography (SD OCT).

*Design.*—Prospective cross-sectional study.

*Methods.*—This institutional study enrolled 83 healthy children (aged 5-15 years) as volunteer research subjects at the Retina Foundation of the Southwest (Dallas, Texas); all had normal visual acuity. Imaging was accomplished with the Spectralis SD OCT. Peripapillary RNFL thickness and macular thickness were assessed for 1 eye of each child using the Heidelberg Spectralis SD OCT software. Thicknesses of individual retinal layers and layer combinations were assessed using custom software to segment the line scans obtained with the Spectralis SD OCT.

*Results.*—Average global peripapillary RNFL thickness was 107.6 ± 1.2 µm and average central subfield macular thickness was 271.2 ± 2.0 µm. Peripapillary RNFL thickness was thicker than has been reported in adults, particularly the superior and inferior sectors, and central subfield macular thickness was significantly correlated with age. While the thickness of most retinal layers was comparable with those of adults, the outer segment layer was 36% thinner in children than in adults.

*Conclusions.*—SD OCT can be used to assess peripapillary RNFL thickness, macular thickness, and retinal layer thickness in children as young as 5 years. Pediatric means and normative reference ranges are provided for each measurement. The values presented herein can be used as a standard with which to compare those of children suspected of having retinal or optic nerve abnormalities.

▶ Optical coherence tomography (OCT) is a noncontact imaging method for cross-sectional delineation of the retina and choroid. Most analyses have been performed in adult patients of 18 years or older. This technology is difficult to perform in children because of cooperation and technical limitations of patient movement. In this report, the authors assess children ages 5 to 15 years who underwent imaging with spectral domain OCT (SD OCT) to compile normative data.

In their results, they found normal thickness of macula (mean 271 µm) with no difference in sex or ethnicity. However, as age increased from 5 to 15 years, central foveal thickness increased. Compared with adults, the foveal thickness was similar. The peripapillary nerve fiber layer thickness (mean 108 µm) was significantly higher than data for adult patients. The thicknesses of other macular layers were measured manually and appeared thinner than in adults.

These investigators have provided useful information in normal eyes of children that can now be used for comparison with disease states. The next step would be to investigate younger children from birth to 5 years of age, but that might necessitate examination under anesthesia

**C. L. Shields, MD**

## Three-Dimensional Tomographic Features of Dome-Shaped Macula by Swept-Source Optical Coherence Tomography

Ellabban AA, Tsujikawa A, Matsumoto A, et al (Kyoto Univ Graduate School of Medicine, Japan; et al)

*Am J Ophthalmol* 155:320-328.e2, 2013

*Purpose.*—To study the tomographic and pathomorphologic features of dome-shaped maculas with swept-source optical coherence tomography (OCT).

*Design.*—Prospective, cross-sectional study.

*Methods.*—The macular area of 51 highly myopic eyes (35 patients) with dome-shaped maculas was studied with swept-source OCT at 1050 nm. Three-dimensional (3-D) data sets were obtained with raster scanning covering a $12 \times 8\text{-mm}^2$ area; 3-D images of the posterior pole were constructed by autosegmentation of the retinal pigment epithelium (RPE).

*Results.*—In all reconstructed 3-D images of the RPE, 2 outward concavities were seen within the posterior staphyloma and a horizontal ridge was formed between these 2 concavities. In 42 of these eyes, this horizontal ridge was band shaped. The vertical OCT section through the fovea showed a convex configuration of RPE, but the horizontal section showed an almost flat RPE line. In 9 eyes, 3-D images showed a typical dome-shaped convexity within the staphyloma. OCT scans showed no outward protrusions in the external scleral surface, but marked scleral thinning was seen consistent with the 2 outward concavities of the RPE. The sclera of the fovea (518.6 ± 97.6 μm) was significantly thicker than that in all 4 quadrants of the parafoveal area (range, 277.2 to 360.3 μm; $P < .001$).

*Conclusions.*—In highly myopic eyes with a dome-shaped macula, a horizontal ridge is formed within the posterior staphyloma by uneven thinning of the sclera.

▶ Optical coherence tomography (OCT) is being investigated in numerous diseases to assist in defining the classic features. High myopia is one of the most common causes of visual disturbance in the world, particularly in Asia. Refraction and spectacle correction can improve the symptoms related to this disturbance. However, there are persisting and perplexing problems with high myopia. The topography of the eye is altered in high myopia with elongation of the axial length, posterior staphyloma, and related complications of choroidal neovascularization, macular hole, choroid and retinal atrophy, and visual field defects.

Recently, OCT has depicted a peculiar dome-shaped macula in patients with high myopia that tends to bow forward in the region of staphyloma. This bowing was attributed to changes in scleral configuration with increased thickness in the subfoveal region, leading to anterior bowing. In this report, the authors use a longer wavelength swept-source OCT, a technique that allows deeper tissue penetration into the choroid and sclera, to study eyes with high myopia.

In this analysis of 51 highly myopic eyes, every eye showed apparent biconvex thickening of the subfoveal scleral tissue with a midpoint horizontal topographic ridge. The subfoveal scleral thickness was significantly greater than extrafoveal scleral tissue. The reason and mechanism for this adaptation in highly myopic eyes is not certain. It is known that posterior staphyloma develops in highly myopic eyes over time and is not commonly seen in children. The staphyloma can slowly change over time and can be asymmetric. The authors postulate that this finding relates to regional differences in the biochemical structure of the sclera or the mechanical strength of the collagen bundles.

**C. L. Shields, MD**

# 11 Pathology

## Human Corneal Anatomy Redefined: A Novel Pre-Descemet's Layer (Dua's Layer)

Dua HS, Faraj LA, Said DG, et al (Univ of Nottingham, UK)
*Ophthalmology* 120:1778-1785, 2013

*Purpose.*—To define and characterize a novel pre-Descemet's layer in the human cornea.

*Design.*—Clinical and experimental study.

*Participants.*—We included 31 human donor sclerocorneal discs, including 6 controls (mean age, 77.7 years).

*Methods.*—Air was injected into the stroma of donor whole globes (n = 4) and sclerocorneal discs (n = 21) as in the clinical deep anterior lamellar keratoplasty procedure with the big bubble (BB) technique. The following experiments were performed: (1) creation of BB followed by peeling of the Descemet's membrane (DM); (2) peeling off of the DM followed by creation of the BB, and (3) creation of the BB and continued inflation until the bubble popped to measure the popping pressure. Tissue obtained from these experiments was subjected to histologic examination.

*Main Outcome Measures.*—Demonstration of a novel pre-Descemet's layer (Dua's layer) in the human cornea.

*Results.*—Three types of BB were obtained. Type-1, is a well-circumscribed, central dome–shaped elevation up to 8.5 mm in diameter (n = 14). Type-2, is a thin-walled, large BB of maximum 10.5 mm diameter, which always started at the periphery, enlarging centrally to form a large BB (n = 5), and a mixed type (n = 3). With type-1 BB, unlike type-2 BB, it was possible to peel off DM completely without deflating the BB, indicating the presence of an additional layer of tissue. A type-1 BB could be created after first peeling off the DM (n = 5), confirming that DM was not essential to create a type-1 BB. The popping pressure was 1.45 bar and 0.6 bar for type-1 BB and type-2 BB, respectively. Histology confirmed that the cleavage occurred beyond the last row of keratocytes. This layer was acellular, measured 10.15 ± 3.6 microns composed of 5 to 8 lamellae of predominantly type-1 collagen bundles arranged in transverse, longitudinal, and oblique directions.

*Conclusions.*—There exists a novel, well-defined, acellular, strong layer in the pre-Descemet's cornea. This separates along the last row of keratocytes in most cases performed with the BB technique. Its recognition will have considerable impact on posterior corneal surgery and the understanding

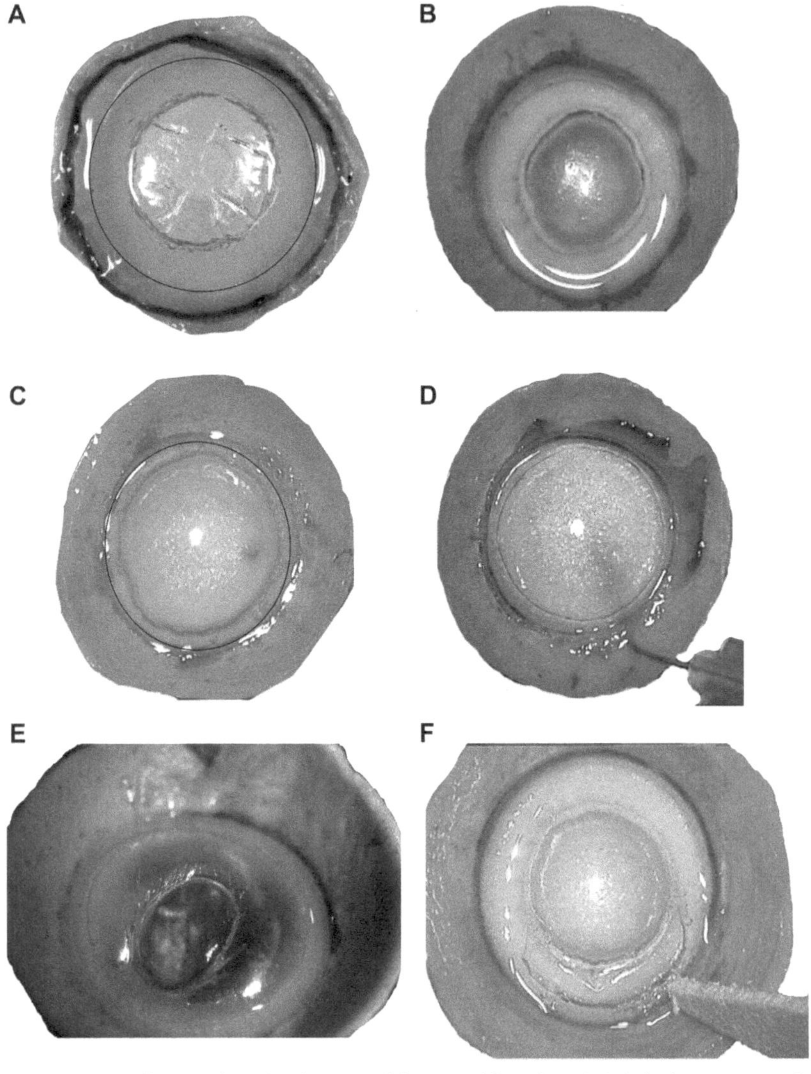


FIGURE 1.—All images show the sclerocorneal disc viewed from the endothelial side. **A**, **B**, Type-1 big bubbles (BBs). The bubble occupies the center of the sclerocorneal disc and are well circumscribed and circular. **A**, A black circle is drawn to delineate the periphery of the cornea, beyond which is a frill of sclera. **C**, **D**, Type-2 BBs. The bubbles extend almost to the periphery of the cornea, represented by the black circle drawn in C. The needle is visible in the stroma. Vision blue dye was applied to the endothelium. **E**, Mixed-type BB. A horse shoe—shaped type-2 BB is seen along 10 clock-hours (from 8 to 6 o'clock) of the sclerocorneal disc. The peripheral margin of this horse shoe—shaped bubble extends very close to the margin of the cornea. The posterior wall of the horse shoe bubble is elevated above the posterior wall of the central type-1 BB, which is seen in the hollow of the horse shoe. **F**, Another mixed-type BB where the central type-1 BB is associated with a crescent-shaped, narrower type-2 BB inferiorly. The tip of a swab points to the type-2 BB. (Reprinted from Dua HS, Faraj LA, Said DG, et al. Human corneal anatomy redefined: a novel pre-Descemet's layer (Dua's layer). *Ophthalmology.* 2013;120:1778-1785, Copyright 2013, with permission from the American Academy of Ophthalmology.)

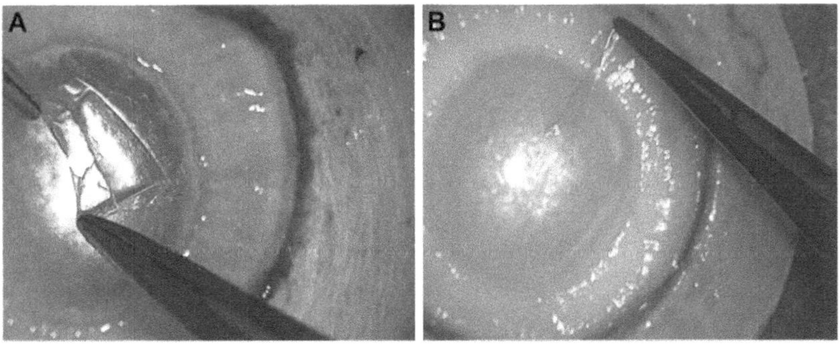


FIGURE 2.—A, The Descemet's membrane (DM) is being peeled off the surface of a type-1 big bubble (BB). The fold of the DM is clearly visible, exposing the Dua's layer underneath. The bubble has not deflated. B, A narrow strip of the DM is being peeled off another type-1 BB, which has not deflated. (Reprinted from Dua HS, Faraj LA, Said DG, et al. Human corneal anatomy redefined: a novel pre-Descemet's layer (Dua's layer). *Ophthalmology.* 2013;120:1778-1785, Copyright 2013, with permission from the American Academy of Ophthalmology.)

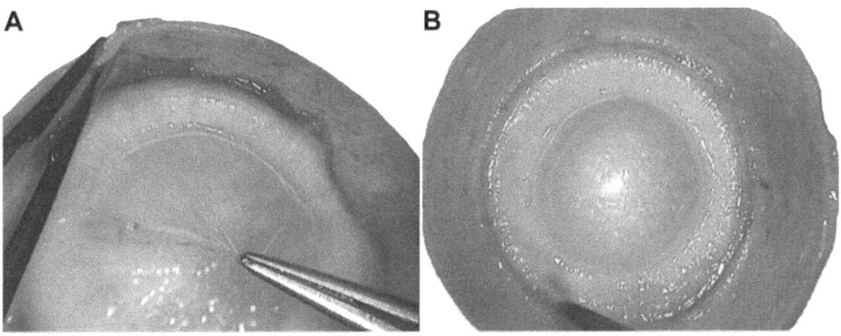


FIGURE 3.—A, Striae induced by tugging, in the Dua's layer (from which the Descemet's membrane [DM] had been removed) extending beyond the edge of the big bubble (BB) on to the adjacent uncleaved surface. B, A fully inflated type-1 BB from which the DM has been removed. Fine radial striae are seen from the edge of the BB toward the periphery of the cornea all along the circumference. (Reprinted from Dua HS, Faraj LA, Said DG, et al. Human corneal anatomy redefined: a novel pre-Descemet's layer (Dua's layer). *Ophthalmology.* 2013;120:1778-1785, Copyright 2013, with permission from the American Academy of Ophthalmology.)

of corneal biomechanics and posterior corneal pathology such as acute hydrops, Descematocele and pre-Descemet's dystrophies (Figs 1-5 and, 7).

► Dua et al have recently described a region of posterior corneal stroma characterized as a "well-defined, acellular, strong layer in the pre-Descemet's cornea" that Dua has named after himself. The findings are described in the context of lamellar keratoplasty, which is surgical removal of diseased tissues of the cornea while leaving healthy components intact. The portion removed is replaced by healthy tissue from a donor cornea. Lamellar keratoplasty is contrasted with penetrating keratoplasty in which all layers (diseased and healthy)

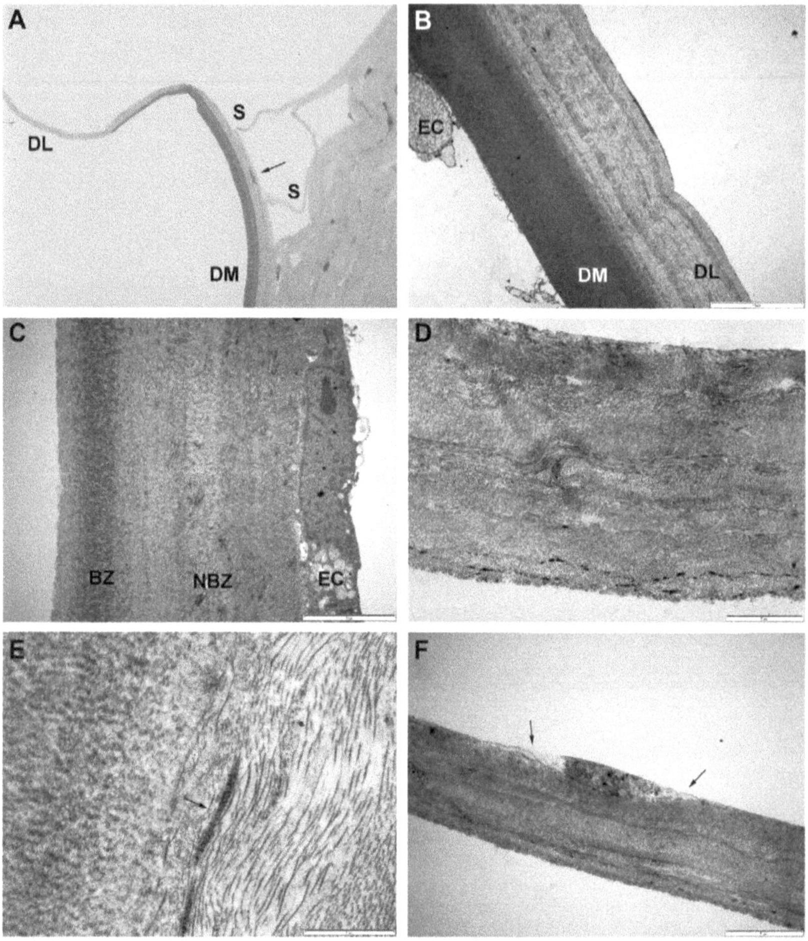


FIGURE 4.—A, Light photomicrograph of resin section stained with toluidine blue showing a type-1 big bubble (BB) from which the Descemet's membrane (DM) has been peeled off centrally to reveal the Dua's layer (DL). At the periphery of the cleavage, the DM can be seen on the posterior surface of the DL. Strands of collagen bundles (S) are seen bridging the stromal bed and posterior surface of the DL. A keratocyte (arrow) is seen in the anterior surface of the DL (objective ×40). B–F, Transmission electron micrographs. B, The posterior wall of a type-1 BB showing the DL closely applied to the DM. The DL is seen to be made of multiple thin lamellae. Part of an endothelial cell (EC) is visible on the posterior surface of the DM. Bar = 10 microns. C, The posterior wall of a type-2 BB showing that it is made up of DM and attached EC only. The banded (BZ) and nonbanded (NBZ) zones of the DM are clearly visible. This was exactly the same with the DM peeled off a type-1 BB. No split in the BZ and NBZ was seen in either instance. Bar = 5 microns. D, The DL from a type-1 BB showing multiple lamellae with collagen bundles running in longitudinal, transverse, and oblique directions. The lamellae are compactly arranged. Bar = 5 microns. E, The DL of a type-1 BB from which the DM has not been peeled off. The banded zone of the DM is seen adjacent to the DL with long-spaced collagen (arrow). Bar = 1 micron. This is also evident in (D), where it appears as dark material in the posterior lamellae of the DL. F, The DL from a type-1 BB showing a coiled end of a broken strand on its anterior surface (between the 2 arrows). Some keratocyte cellular debris is also present. (Reprinted from Dua HS, Faraj LA, Said DG, et al. Human corneal anatomy redefined: a novel pre-Descemet's layer (Dua's layer). *Ophthalmology.* 2013;120:1778-1785, Copyright 2013, with permission from the American Academy of Ophthalmology.)

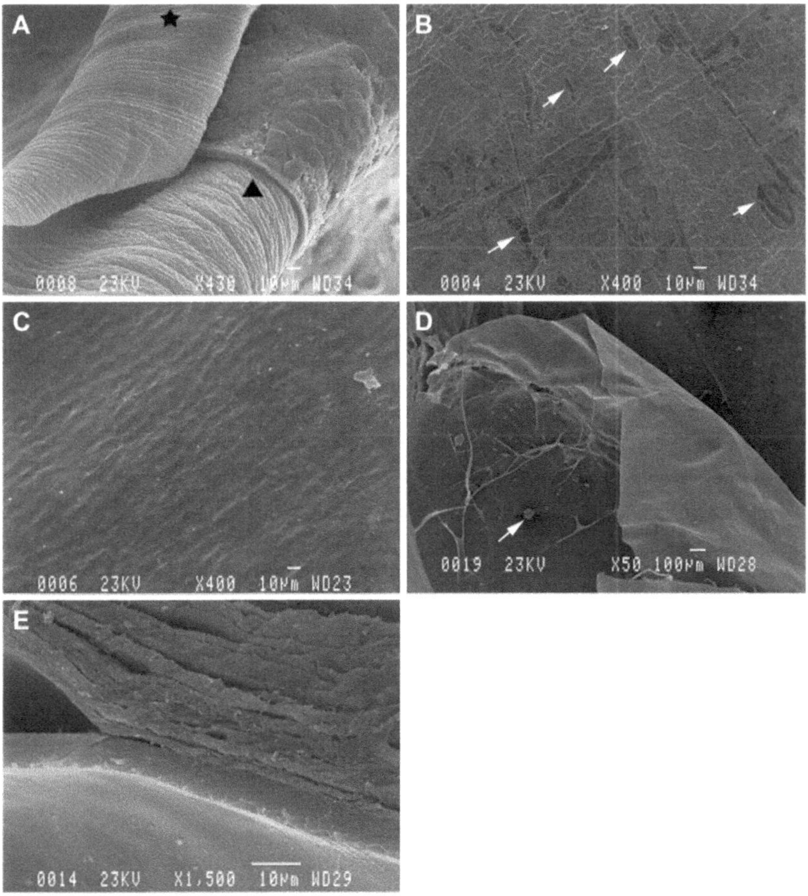


**FIGURE 5.**—Scanning electron micrographs. **A**, The anterior surface (star) of the Dua's layer (DL) showing parallel and regularly arranged collagen bundles. The posterior surface of the DL (triangle) shows a smooth pleated pattern. The edge of the Descemet's membrane (DM) is also seen. **B**, The stromal bed of a type-1 big bubble showing a crisscross pattern with gaps related to passage of air (arrows). This contrasts with the appearance of the anterior surface of the DL seen in (**A**). **C**, The anterior surface of the DM. This was the smoothest of all surfaces examined. **D**, Strands of tissue are seen bridging the stromal bed and the anterior surface of the DL. Ends of broken strands are visible as small round dots (arrow). **E**, The end of the cleavage created by the air bubble between the DL and posterior stroma is visible. The DL is seen as a distinct and compact layer. (Reprinted from Dua HS, Faraj LA, Said DG, et al. Human corneal anatomy redefined: a novel pre-Descemet's layer (Dua's layer). *Ophthalmology.* 2013;120:1778-1785, Copyright 2013, with permission from the American Academy of Ophthalmology.)

of the host cornea are surgically removed and replaced by full-thickness donor tissue.

The several types of lamellar keratoplasty are defined by the plane of separation between diseased and healthy host tissue. Epikeratoplasty, a procedure that is no longer used, actually added a lamellar lenticule to change the optical characteristics of the cornea. Deep anterior lamellar keratoplasty (DALK), the relatively new procedure referred to by Dua, removes abnormal anterior corneal

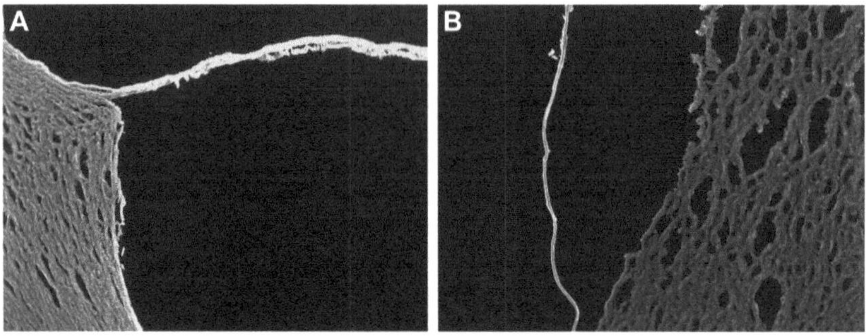


FIGURE 7.—Immunostaining for collagen and proteoglycans. A, Collagen 1. The intensity of staining of the corneal stroma and the Dua's layer (DL), seen as a thin line, is the same (Alexa Fluor 555). The nuclei appear as blue dots (4′,6-diamidino-2-phenylindole is a fluorescent stain for nuclear DNA [DAPI] at ×4). B, Collagen VI. The staining intensity is greater in the DL compared with the posterior corneal stroma (Alexa Fluor 555 and DAPI at ×4). There are no nuclei visible in the DL in either image. For Interpretation of the references to color in this figure legend, the reader is referred to web version of this article. (Reprinted from Dua HS, Faraj LA, Said DG, et al. Human corneal anatomy redefined: a novel pre-Descemet's layer (Dua's layer). *Ophthalmology.* 2013;120:1778-1785, Copyright 2013, with permission from the American Academy of Ophthalmology.)

stroma (eg, keratoconus) leaving Descemet's membrane and corneal endothelium intact (Figs 1 and 2). Descemet's membrane endothelial keratoplasty (DMEK) removes Descemet's membrane and abnormal endothelium (e.g. Fuchs' endothelial dystrophy) while leaving the host anterior cornea intact.[1]

Jester et al[2] and Maurice,[3] among many others, have described the complex functional and structural characteristics of the cornea and its adaptive ability that in most people maintain perfect optical stability throughout the life. The architecture of the cornea is able to respond and adjust to constantly changing influences such as pressures associated with the presence of the upper eyelid, the intermittent forces of the 4 rectus muscles, and the effect of hydration and dehydration from the fluid environment of its anterior and posterior surfaces as well as numerous other dynamic factors. These characteristics vary from the center to the periphery of the cornea and from the anterior to posterior cornea. Thus, each of many lamellar planes of the cornea will have different structures and functions. Each of these lamellae is logically separated into tissue planes that most likely have unique characteristics, such as relative resistance to cleavage.

In the case of DALK, the desired area of separation is in the deep posterior corneal stroma. After initial dissection of the anterior stroma to a subjectively determined depth, energy is transferred by nonquantifiable agents such as air (compressible), saline (noncompressible), or viscoelastic (noncompressible) to create and extend a cleavage plane parallel to the orientation of stromal lamella. Thus, the level dissected is likely to vary considerably from surgeon to surgeon and novice to expert. All of the agents forcefully applied to the posterior surgical field alter the homogeneity of the stromal architecture and make the deep tissue opaque and visible to the ophthalmic surgeon. The surgery then proceeds, as would any other lamellar keratectomy procedure, with the implantation of donor lamellar tissue.

The deep opaque layer was not "unknown" as alleged by Dua and associates. The region of the posterior cornea has existed for some time, but the tissue had no surgical significance until DALK was introduced. This is not the first time when a region of the eye had no pathologic or surgical significance until a new surgical technique was introduced. A good example is the irido-ciliary sulcus. This is the attachment of the iris to the anterior-internal ciliary body, which forms a circumferential concave surface in the posterior chamber. This is the natural resting place for intraocular lens loops that come to lie outside of the lens capsule. Before posterior chamber intraocular lenses, this tissue interface with the aqueous of the posterior chamber had no surgical or pathological significance. Now after 4 decades, this structure remains identified by its descriptive term but has gained neither additional surgical nor pathophysiologic significance.

This discovery of anatomy identified solely by technical surgical significance also applies to the host tissue left behind by the DALK procedure, the posterior stromal lamella (Figs 3-5, and 7). Its significance will probably be limited to this type of manual surgery that could easily be supplanted by more precise digitally guided laser procedures that consistently define a tissue depth based on measurement instead of arbitrary depth based on subjective and immeasurable force vector variables. It is likely that the addition of this nomenclature in the form of a self-designated eponym will do little to advance the understanding of the pathophysiology of "acute hydrops, Descemetocele or pre-Descemet's dystrophies."

It is not clear that Dua and associates have provided ophthalmic surgeons with a useful term because of limited precision and because of little prospect of enduring value for making intraoperative decisions.

**J. Douglas Cameron, MD, MBA**

*References*

1. Schlötzer-Schrehardt U, Bachmann BO, Tourtas T, et al. Reproducibility of graft preparations in Descemet's membrane endothelial keratoplasty. *Ophthalmology.* 2013;120:1769-1777.
2. Jester JV, Murphy CJ, Winkler M, et al. Lessons in corneal structure and mechanics to guide the corneal surgeon. *Ophthalmology.* 2013;120:1715-1717.
3. Maurice DM. Some puzzles in the microscopic structure of the stroma. *J Refract Surg.* 1999;15:692-694.

## Vitreoretinal Presentation of Secondary Large B-Cell Lymphoma in Patients With Systemic Lymphoma

Salomão DR, Pulido JS, Johnston PB, et al (Mayo Clinic, Rochester, MN)
*JAMA Ophthalmol* 131:1151-1158, 2013

*Importance.*—Intraocular lymphomas represent a diverse group of hematologic malignant neoplasms involving different tissues within the eye. Predominant involvement of the retina and vitreous without uveal infiltration in systemic lymphoma, mimicking a primary vitreoretinal lymphoma, is extremely rare. Our study emphasizes the importance of systemic evaluation in addition to central nervous system evaluation in all patients with newly diagnosed vitreoretinal lymphoma.

*Objective.*—To determine the incidence of secondary intraocular lymphoma presenting as vitreoretinal infiltrates without central nervous system involvement, mimicking primary vitreoretinal lymphoma in patients with systemic lymphoma.

*Design.*—Retrospective review of all vitreous aspiration biopsy samples acquired because malignant neoplasm was suspected clinically that were obtained at our institution from January 1, 2000, through December 31, 2010. Review included patient clinical history, radiographic study findings, cytologic and/or histologic preparations, immunophenotypic study findings, treatment, and outcomes.

*Setting.*—Mayo Clinic pathology database.

*Participants.*—Fifty-five patients with vitreous specimens available for review.

*Exposures.*—Vitreous aspiration biopsy.

*Main Outcome and Measure.*—Confirmation of the diagnosis of diffuse large B-cell lymphoma (DLBCL).

*Results.*—Of the 55 patients with vitreous specimens available for review, 3 (5%) had a DLBCL infiltration in the vitreous without any central nervous system involvement as a manifestation of systemic lymphoma. All 3 patients were men, aged 54, 66, and 73 years, and had blurred vision and floaters for several weeks before undergoing diagnostic vitrectomy. Ophthalmic examinations revealed clumps of vitreous cells but no choroidal involvement. One patient had no history of lymphoma; the diagnosis of vitreoretinal lymphoma was followed by DLBCL after a lymph node biopsy. The other 2 patients had low-grade B-cell lymphoma and chronic lymphocytic leukemia for 29 and 7 months before large-cell transformation in the eye. Patients were treated with systemic chemotherapy plus intraocular injections of rituximab or methotrexate sodium.

*Conclusions and Relevance.*—Vitreoretinal symptoms of DLBCL in patients with systemic lymphoma may be more frequent than previously thought (5% in our study). Not all lymphomas with vitreoretinal involvement represent primary intraocular lymphomas; thorough ophthalmologic evaluation in patients with visual symptoms and complete staging in patients with documented ocular lymphoma are of utmost importance (Table 2).

► Unlike the primary intraocular/vitreoretinal/central nervous system (CNS) lymphoma, which classically involves the retina and vitreous, systemic/visceral lymphoma typically involves the uveal tract of the eye. Predominant involvement of the retina and vitreous without uveal infiltration in a patient with systemic lymphoma, mimicking a primary vitreoretinal lymphoma, is extremely rare.

In this retrospective clinical-pathologic case series, Salomão et al examined their institutional experience with this phenomenon by reviewing the records of patients undergoing diagnostic vitrectomy for suspected malignant neoplasm during an 11-year period. Of 55 identified patients, 13 (24%) had evidence of lymphoma. Seven of 13 patients (54%) had primary vitreoretinal/CNS lymphoma, whereas the remaining 6 patients (46%) had vitreoretinal involvement

TABLE 2.—Results of 57 Vitreous Aspiration Biopsy Specimens From 55 Patients

| Diagnosis | No. of Patients | Sex | Age, Mean (Range), y | No. of Specimens |
|---|---|---|---|---|
| Negative for malignant neoplasm | 34 | 20 Female | 63.0 (36-91) | 21 |
| | | 4 Male | 53.9 (23-92) | 15 |
| Positive for malignant neoplasm | | | | |
| Lymphoma[a] | 13 | 6 Female | 68.8 (63-74) | 6 |
| | | 7 Male | 66.8 (54-80) | 7 |
| Other[b] | 4 | 3 Female | 63.3 (56-69) | 3 |
| | | 1 Male | 64.0 | 1 |
| Suspected lymphoma[a] | 3 | 2 Female | 62.5 (59-66) | 2 |
| | | 1 Male | 69.0 | 1 |
| Nondiagnostic | 1 | 1 Male | 85.0 | 1 |
| All | 55 | | | 57 |

[a]Patients are described in Table 3.
[b]Includes 3 uveal melanomas and 1metastatic small cell lung carcinoma.

by systemic lymphoma (Fig 1 in the original article, Table 2). In this latter group, 3 patients had concomitant CNS, ocular, and systemic involvement. The remaining 3 patients had primary vitreoretinal involvement by the diffuse large B-cell lymphoma (DLBCL), and no CNS involvement was found at the time of vitrectomy. In 1 of these 3 patients, the ocular symptoms and subsequent diagnostic vitrectomy led to the diagnosis of systemic DLBCL. This patient had persistent ocular lymphoma with no CNS involvement at 40 months of follow-up (Fig 1 in the original article). In the other 2 patients, the vitreous cavity was the primary site of large-cell transformation of low-grade B-cell malignant neoplasms and was followed subsequently by CNS involvement and, ultimately, death (Fig 3 in the original article).

Salomão's study highlights the high frequency of systemic lymphoma in patients with lymphoma involving the vitreous and retina (half of the patients). It also emphasizes the strength of association between the ocular involvement and concomitant or eventual CNS disease (12 or 13 patients, 92%). These findings indicate the importance of ophthalmologic studies in patients with systemic lymphoma who have visual symptoms and of comprehensive staging studies in patients with documented vitreoretinal lymphoma.

**T. Milman, MD**

## Multicolor Flowcytometric Immunophenotyping Is a Valuable Tool for Detection of Intraocular Lymphoma

Missotten T, Tielemans D, Bromberg JE, et al (The Rotterdam Eye Hosp, The Netherlands; Univ Med Ctr, Rotterdam, The Netherlands)
*Ophthalmology* 120:991-996, 2013

*Objective.*—Intraocular lymphoma (IOL) is a rare condition and frequently difficult to distinguish from uveitis or other uveitis-masquerading syndromes. The diagnosis is confirmed by cytologic examination of ocular fluid specimens and more recently by molecular-immunoglobulin heavy chain

(IGH) translocation or cytokine analysis. However, some of these more recent methods have not been validated by follow-up studies.

*Design.*—Evaluation of a diagnostic test.

*Participants.*—In a cohort of 51 consecutive patients with a clinical suspicion of IOL, vitreous analysis was performed via multicolor flowcytometric immunophenotyping.

*Methods.*—Multicolor flowcytometric immunophenotyping was performed with CD45, CD3, CD19, CD20, anti-SmIgκ, and anti-SmIgλ antibodies. The presence of a clear B-cell population showing a disequilibrium of Igκ versus Igλ expression was used to confirm the diagnosis of non-Hodgkin lymphoma (NHL). Patients were followed for a minimum of 2 years (mean, 5.9 ± 2.0 years) to validate the accuracy of the method.

*Main Outcome Measures.*—The presence or absence of IOL during follow-up.

*Results.*—In 14 of 51 patients, a clinical diagnosis of IOL was confirmed using flowcytometric analysis. Of these 14 patients, 11 had primary IOL and 3 had metastasized secondary lymphomas. In 3 of 51 patients who were diagnosed with (central nervous system) NHL during follow-up, the test failed to confirm the presence of a clonal B-cell population. In 18 of the 34 other patients, an infectious or well-defined immunologic disorder was established during follow-up. The remaining 16 patients, with a minimal follow-up of 2 years, were diagnosed with idiopathic uveitis.

*Conclusions.*—Multicolor flowcytometric analysis had 82.4% sensitivity and 100% specificity in patients with suspected IOL. This is comparable to the reported vitreous interleukin (IL)-6/IL-10 testing sensitivity of 0.8 and sensitivity of 0.65 to 0.95 by immunoglobulin heavy chain (IGH) gene arrangement testing in clinical cohorts. Because flowcytometric tests are readily performed in hematologic laboratories, this can be regarded as a useful method for confirming the clinical diagnosis of IOL (Figs 1 and 2).

▶ In this retrospective case series, Missotten and colleagues evaluated 51 consecutive patients with (pseudo) uveitis, who underwent diagnostic vitrectomy. The investigators utilized multicolor flow cytometric analysis using 4 to 6 antibodies (CD45, CD3, CD19, CD20, anti-SmIgκ, and anti-SmIgλ). Polymerase chain reaction (PCR) for rearrangements within immunoglobulin heavy chain and TCR genes was performed on selected vitreous samples to determine B-cell and T-cell clonality, respectively. The patients were followed up for at least 2 years.

In the study population, 10 patients had prior diagnosis of non-Hodgkin lymphoma (NHL) (1 primary central nervous system lymphoma [PCNS] lymphoma and 9 systemic [visceral] lymphomas). Flow cytometric analysis confirmed presence of lymphoma in 2 of 10 patients (Fig 1). Infectious etiology was found in 4 patients. The other 4 patients had idiopathic uveitis.

In the remaining 41 patients with suspected intraocular lymphoma and no prior history of lymphoma, flow cytometric analysis confirmed the presence of lymphoma in 12 patients. Oncologic workup identified 11 primary intraocular

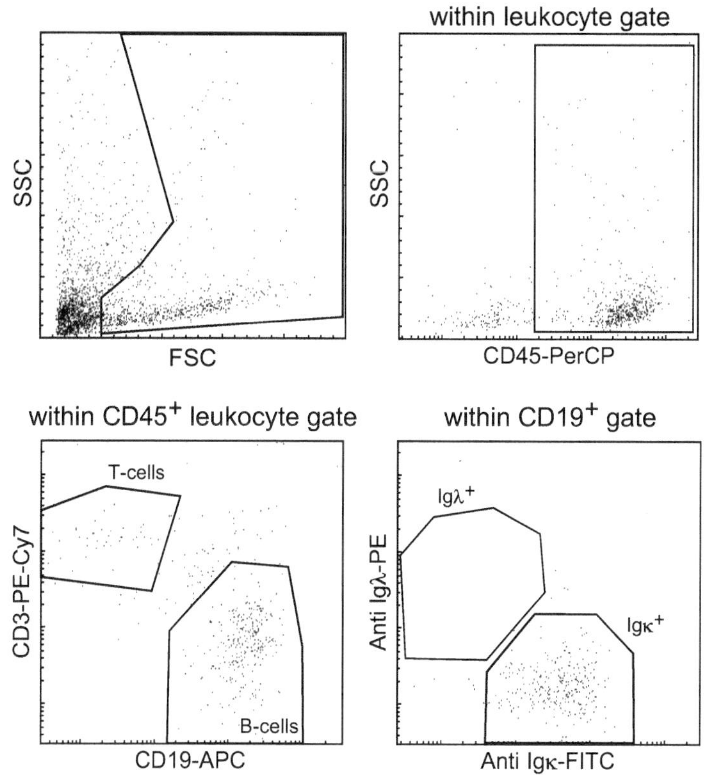


**FIGURE 1.**—Representative example of 6-color flowcytometric immunophenotyping analysis of a vitreous sample from a patient with clinically proven primary intraocular lymphoma (PIOL). After identification of CD19+ B lymphocytes and CD3+ T lymphocytes within the CD45+ leukocyte cell population, further analysis revealed a clonal SmIgκ+ CD19+ B-lymphocyte population, in keeping with the PIOL diagnosis. APC = allophycocyanin; FITC = fluorescein isothiocyanate; FSC = forward scatter; Ig = immunoglobulin; PE = phycoerythrin; SSC = side scatter. (Reprinted from Missotten T, Tielemans D, Bromberg JE, et al. Multicolor flowcytometric immunophenotyping is a valuable tool for detection of intraocular lymphoma. *Ophthalmology.* 2013;120:991-996, Copyright 2013, with permission from the American Academy of Ophthalmology.)

lymphomas (PIOLs) and 1 metastatic systemic lymphoma (secondary IOL). In 5 of these 12 patients, repeated flow cytometric analyses were performed on vitreous samples acquired during therapeutic vitrectomies. In 2 patients, the primary sample did not contain enough cells for a definitive diagnosis, whereas the secondary sample was positive. In 3 patients, no positive NHL diagnosis could be made using flow cytometric analysis of the vitreous sample, although subsequent magnetic resonance imaging confirmed the presence of PCNS lymphoma.

In the remaining 26 of the 41 patients who did not show clonal population suggestive of lymphoma (Fig 2), no IOL was found at the end of follow-up. In 14 of these 26 patients, a specific uveitis or masquerade diagnosis could be reached during follow-up of 6.1 +/− 2.1 years (range, 3.8–11.4 years). In the remaining 12 of the 26 patients, no specific etiology was found on a follow-up

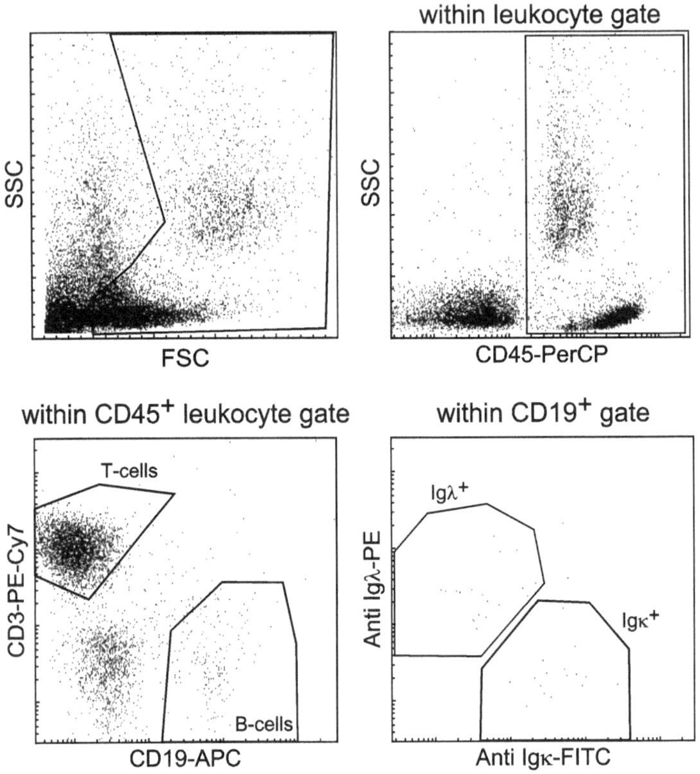


FIGURE 2.—Representative example of 6-color flowcytometric immunophenotyping analysis of a vitreous sample from a patient without clinical intraocular lymphoma. Within the CD45+ leukocyte population, CD19+ B lymphocytes and CD3+ T lymphocytes are observed. Further analysis of the CD19+ B-lymphocyte population shows a normal distribution of SmIgκ+ and SmIgλ+ cells. APC = allophycocyanin; FITC = fluorescein isothiocyanate; FSC = forward scatter; Ig = immunoglobulin; PE = phycoerythrin; SSC = side scatter. (Reprinted from Missotten T, Tielemans D, Bromberg JE, et al. Multicolor flowcytometric immunophenotyping is a valuable tool for detection of intraocular lymphoma. *Ophthalmology.* 2013;120:991-996, Copyright 2013, with permission from the American Academy of Ophthalmology.)

of 6.3 +/− 2.1 years (range 3–11.9 years), and the diagnosis of idiopathic uveitis was rendered.

Missotten and colleagues estimate that the sensitivity and specificity of multicolor flow cytometry using 4 to 6 antibodies are 82.4% and 100%, respectively. These are exciting results showing the continued refinement of flow cytometric analysis, which, thus far, has been fraught with challenges because of the low cellularity of intraocular fluid samples. Despite these encouraging results, they have to be interpreted with caution given several study limitations. The authors do not provide the data on cellularity of the vitreous biopsy and cell viability, which is crucial. The authors also do not provide the data on whether confirmatory PCR for B-cell clonality was performed on all vitreous fluid samples found to be polyclonal on flow cytometry. Additionally, the cytology data are not available, and interleukin studies were not performed. Lastly, it should be noted that diffuse large B-cell lymphomas are notorious for absence of light chain restriction by both immunohistochemical and flow cytometric analysis methods. The frequency of this phenomenon is even higher in studies performed on body fluids as opposed to tissues. Although most patients with vitreoretinal lymphoma develop CNS lymphoma and rapidly succumb to the disease, a subset of patients can have prolonged survival. Thus, it is possible that the patients with idiopathic uveitis may progress in time to a full-blown lymphoma.

**T. Milman, MD**

## Conjunctival melanoma: a review of conceptual and treatment advances

Lim LA, Madigan MC, Conway RM (The Univ of Sydney, New South Wales, Australia)

*Clin Ophthalmol* 7:521-531, 2013

The aim of this study was to review the available literature and identify recent advances in the classification and management of conjunctival melanoma (CM) for clinicians working in this field. English-based articles were

**TABLE 1.**—Pathologic Tumor (T) Staging (Extent of Disease Through Completion of Definitive Surgery) for Conjunctival Melanoma (CM)

| Pathologic Stage | Stage Category Definition |
|---|---|
| pTX | pT cannot be assessed |
| pT0 | No evidence of pT |
| pTis | Melanoma confined to the conjunctival epithelium |
| | Less than or equal to one quadrant[a] |
| | Melanoma confined to the conjunctival epithelium, melanoma in situ (includes the term primary acquired melanosis) |
| | • Atypia replacing >75% of normal epithelial thickness |
| | • Epithelioid cytology including: |
| | ♣ Abundant cytoplasm |
| | ♣ Vesicular nuclei or prominent nucleoli |
| | ♣ And/or the presence of intraepithelial nests of atypical cells. |
| | * ≤1 quadrant |
| T1 | CM of the bulbar conjunctiva |
| pT1a | Thickness ≤0.5 mm with invasion of the substantia propria |
| | More than one but less than or equal to two quadrants[a] |
| pT1b | Thickness >0.5 and ≤1.5 mm with invasion of the substantia propria |
| | More than two but less than or equal to three quadrants[a] |
| pT1c | Thickness >1.5 mm with invasion of the substantia propria |
| | More than three quadrants[a] |
| T2 | CM of the nonbulbar conjunctiva (palpebral, forniceal, caruncular) region |
| pT2a | Thickness ≤0.5 mm with invasion of the substantia propria |
| pT2b | Thickness >0.5 and ≤1.5 mm with invasion of the substantia propria |
| pT2c | Thickness >1.5 mm with invasion of the substantia propria |
| pT3 | Melanoma invades the eye, eyelid, nasolacrimal system, sinuses, or orbit |
| pT4 | Melanoma invades the central nervous system |

*Abbreviation:* pT, primary tumor.
*Editor's Note*: Please refer to original journal article for full references.
[a]Quadrants are defined by clock hour, starting at the limbus (eg, 3, 6, 9, 12) extending from central cornea to and beyond the eyelid margins – this will bisect the caruncle. Used with the permission of the American Joint Committee on Cancer (AJCC), Chicago, Illinois. The original source for this material is the AJCC Cancer Staging Manual, Seventh Edition (2010) published by Springer Science and Business Media LLC, http://www.springerlink.com. Edge SB, Byrd DR, Compton CC, editors. *AJCC Cancer Staging Manual*. 7th ed. New York, NY: Springer; 2010.[34]

TABLE 2.—Poor Prognostic Features of Conjunctival Melanoma

| Reference | Prognostic Features<br>Local Recurrence | Regional Metastases | Distant Metastases and Death |
|---|---|---|---|
| Missotten et al[18] (population-based study) | Tumor location[a] | Tumor thickness<br>Tumor diameter | Tumor location[a]<br>Tumor diameter |
| Tuomaala et al[5] (population-based study) | Tumor locationa | – | Tumor location[a]<br>Tumor thickness<br>Tumor diameter<br>Local recurrence |
| Tuomaala and Kivelä[16] (population-based study) | – | Tumor thickness | Tumor location[a]<br>Tumor thickness<br>Initial systemic metastases (without lymph node metastases) |
| Tuomaala et al[17] (population-based study) | Tumor location[a]<br>Absence of epithelioid cells<br>Increasing mitotic count | – | Tumor location[a]<br>Tumor thickness<br>Tumor diameter<br>Local recurrence |
| Shields et al[24] | Tumor location[d]<br>Technique of initial surgery (univariate analysis only) | – | Tumor location[a]<br>Initial symptom lump<br>Tumors arising de novo without PAM |
| Werschnik and Lommatzsch[14] | Unfavorable location[b]<br>Surgical excision alone | – | Unfavorable location[b]<br>Age at time of diagnosis >55 years |
| Damato and Coupland[22] | Medial tumors | – | – |
| Anastassiou et al[20] | Grade of pigmentation<br>Grade of invasion<br>Epithelioid and mixed cells<br>Incomplete surgical resection | – | Tumor location[a]<br>– |
| Anastassiou et al[29] | – | – | Neural crest adhesion molecule |
| De Potter et al[23] | Surgical excision alone | – | Local recurrence |
| Paridaens et al[10] | – | – | Tumor location[a]<br>Tumor thickness<br>Tumor diameter<br>Pure epithelioid and mixed cell tumors<br>Lymphocytic invasion and inflammation |
| Seregard and Kock[13] (population-based study) | – | – | Unfavorable location[c]<br>Tumor thickness<br>Tumor diameter<br>High mitotic index<br>Epithelioid cells |
| Bobić-Radovanović et al[21] | – | – | High mitotic index<br>Lymphocytic invasion and inflammation |
| Folberg et al[25] | – | – | Tumor thickness in tumors with associated PAM<br>Associated PAM and its features |
| Esmaeli et al[15] | – | – | Local recurrence |
| Crawford[28] | – | – | High mitotic index |

*Abbreviation:* PAM, primary acquired melanosis.
*Editor's Note*: Please refer to original journal article for full references.
[a]Nonepibulbar/nonlimbal.
[b]Unfavorable location: palpebral conjunctiva, fornix, caruncle, corneal stroma, eyelid.
[c]Unfavorable location: tarsal conjunctiva, fornix, caruncle.
[d]Palpebral.

TABLE 3.—Summary of Concepts in the Current Literature: Conjunctival Melanoma (CM) Classification, Therapy, and Management

| Summary of concepts |
| --- |
| • The seventh edition of the tumor node metastasis staging classification[34] more accurately reflects current knowledge of prognostic factors, and it will hopefully serve to provide consistent and comparable data collection for CM across centers |
| • Surgical excision alone (ie, without adjuvant therapy) has been shown to be less efficacious for CM, regardless of stage[14,23,55] |
| • MMC may be useful as an alternative primary treatment for PAM with atypia and, especially, superficial, diffuse, or multifocal disease[61] |
| Subepithelial nests and nodular tumors have been noted to be MMC-resistant[61,62] |
| • Adjuvant radiotherapy reduces the incidence of local recurrence and may allow for more conservative resections with a reasonable side effect profile |
| • There are promising anecdotal data for the use of recombinant interferon-alpha 2b as adjuvant therapy, compared with MMC |
| • Sentinel lymph node biopsy may improve the detection of micrometastatic disease in a select group of patients with tumor thickness >2 mm[9,11,16,18,21] and diameter >10 mm,[18] although overall survival benefit is yet to be determined[74] |

*Abbreviations:* MMC, mitomycin C; PAM, primary acquired melanosis.
*Editor's Note*: Please refer to original journal article for full references.

identified using the MEDLINE® database, and additional cited works not detected in the initial search were also obtained. Articles were assessed according to the Australian National Health and Medical Research Council levels of evidence criteria. Review of the literature indicated that the current classification and management of CM is predominantly based upon primarily nonrandomized, single-institution, retrospective case series. While these studies provide the basis for the recent seventh edition of the tumor node metastasis staging classification, this classification more accurately reflects the current knowledge of prognostic factors for CM. Application of this revised classification system together with prospective trials will provide the opportunity for future consistent and comparable data collection across centers, and it will improve the quality of evidence upon which current classification and management of CM is based. Furthermore, the high risk of local recurrence with current standard management suggests that adjuvant therapy, particularly mitomycin C and/or brachytherapy, may improve outcomes regardless of clinical staging. Finally, the use of sentinel lymph node biopsy may have significant benefit for a select group of CM patients (Tables 1-3).

► In this review article Lim, Madigan, and Conway bring the reader up to date on the recent developments in the field of conjunctival melanoma and summarize the body of literature regarding the classification, management, and prognostication of this rare malignancy (Table 3). The authors discuss the controversies regarding the terminology of intraepithelial melanocytic neoplasia. They explain how the current seventh edition of the *American Joint Committee on Cancer* (AJCC) attempts to reconcile this conflict and provide the available clinical and histopathologic prognostic data, which contributed to the current TNM classification, staging, and grading of conjunctival melanoma (Tables 1 and 2). The roles and benefits of the currently available surgical and adjuvant therapies for conjunctival melanoma, including radiotherapy, recombinant interferon-$\alpha$2b, and sentinel lymph node biopsy are also discussed. The authors update the readers on the recent advances in molecular genetics of conjunctival melanoma, such as *BRAF* mutations, and discuss the role for potential targeted therapies.

**T. Milman, MD**

---

**Vismodegib as Eye-Sparing Adjuvant Treatment for Orbital Basal Cell Carcinoma**

Kahana A, Worden FP, Elner VM (Univ of Michigan, Ann Arbor)

*JAMA Ophthalmol* 2013 [Epub ahead of print]

---

*Background.*—Disfigurement, blindness, or even death can occur when basal cell carcinoma (BCC) invades the orbit. The treatment is often limited to orbital exenteration, which is also disfiguring and blinding. A hedgehog pathway inhibitor, vismodegib, has recently been approved by the US Food and Drug Administration for the oral treatment of basal cell nevus syndrome and locally advanced or metastatic BCC. A patient with BCC invading the medial orbit was treated with oral vismodegib.

*Case Report.*—Man, 79, developed left lower eyelid retraction 10 years after having BCC excision. His vision was normal and there was no external skin lesion, but he had limited left ductions, increased left tear lake, and left medial canthal fullness. Biopsy identified aggressive-growth-pattern BCC, with magnetic resonance imaging (MRI) finding a 2.7 × 1.6 × 1.9-cm medial orbital mass. Medical treatment with vismodegib, 150 mg/day orally, was started a month later. Over the next 5 months the patient experienced occasional nausea and diarrhea along with progressively worsening muscle spasms. These were all recognized adverse effects associated with vismodegib. After 4 months of treatment, MRI revealed the tumor had shrunk to 0.7 × 0.7 × 0.5 cm. The painful muscle spasms led the patient to opt for surgical excision rather than continue vismodegib. The residual orbital mass was excised en bloc and medial rectus muscle release was done with frozen-section control. Histopathological assessment found all margins were clear. In addition, the residual squamous cells showed degenerative cytologic features and failed to demonstrate nuclear immunoreactivity for the proliferation marker Ki-67, indicating virtual loss of tumor cell proliferation potential after vismodegib treatment. The patient had complete resolution of treatment adverse effects within 2 months of discontinuing vismodegib therapy.

*Conclusions.*—Oral vismodegib may be considered for patients who have eye-threatening orbital BCC. Although further experience is needed to better assess the risks of treatment and to develop optimal treatment criteria, it appears that this agent damages tumor cells sufficiently to inhibit further proliferation. En bloc excision with margin control may be needed when the adverse effects of vismodegib therapy become unbearable to the patient (Figs 1 and 2).

▶ Vismodegib, an oral small molecule inhibitor of the hedgehog signaling pathway that is activated in basal cell carcinoma (BCC), has been approved recently for treatment of locally aggressive, inoperable, or refractory to radiation BCC and for treatment of metastatic BCC. This medication has been shown to have response rates of 30% to 60% in 2 clinical trials. Initial response, followed by subsequent tumor recurrence and progression, has been noted in some patients, consistent with development of drug resistance. The side effect profile can be debilitating for some patients and includes nausea, diarrhea, taste disturbance, alopecia, muscle spasms, and weight loss. Lastly, the costs can be prohibitive: $75 000 for 10 months of treatment.

Kahana et al describe their experience with one patient treated with vismodegib eye-sparing adjuvant therapy for unresectable BCC. The side effects of therapy (nausea, diarrhea, and muscle spasms) ultimately led to en block excision of residual orbital mass. The authors noted presence of residual tumor in the biopsied tissue, but instead of cellular, infiltrative BCC with areas of squamoid differentiation in prevismodegib biopsy, there were single or small clusters of squamous-appearing cells, which lacked evidence of proliferative activity by

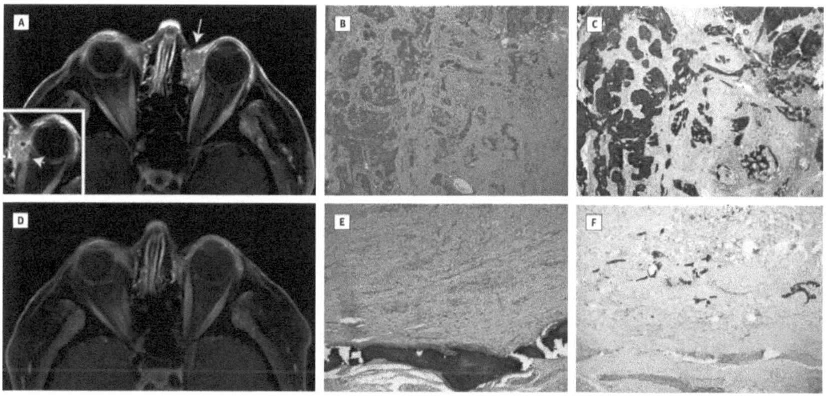


**FIGURE 1.**—Treatment with vismodegib results in reduction in the size of a left medial orbital basal cell carcinoma. Before vismodegib treatment, magnetic resonance imaging shows a left medial orbital basal cell carcinoma (arrows) (A and inset of A), and hematoxylin-eosin staining (original magnification ×40) (B) and immunohistochemistry with K903 antibody staining (original magnification ×40) (C) for high-molecular-weight keratin show tumor cell content. Following vismodegib treatment, magnetic resonance imaging reveals a reduction in size (D), while hematoxylin-eosin staining (original magnification ×40) (E) and immunohistochemistry with K903 antibody staining (original magnification ×40) (F) reveal reduction in tumor cell content. (Reprinted from Kahana A, Worden FP, Elner VM. Vismodegib as eye-sparing adjuvant treatment for orbital basal cell carcinoma. *JAMA Ophthalmol.* 2013 [Epub ahead of print].)

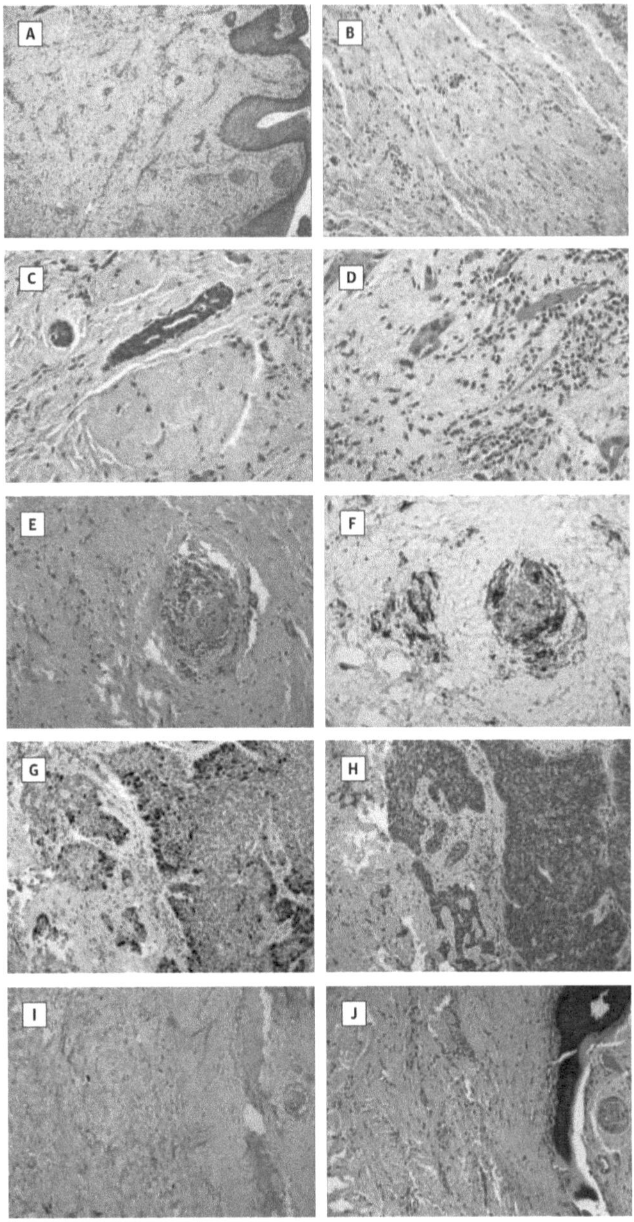


FIGURE 2.—Histologic and immunohistochemical analysis of the excised residual tumor. Histologic analysis of the excised residual tumor with hematoxylin-eosin staining reveals predominant pattern fibrosis (original magnification ×40 [A] and ×100 [B]) and degenerative nests (original magnification ×200) (C) with a lymphocytic infiltrate (original magnification ×200) (D). Leukocyte phagocytosis of degenerated cells is noted on hematoxylin-eosin staining (original magnification ×100) (E) and CD68 immunohistochemistry (original magnification ×100) (F). In contrast to a high pretreatment proliferative index as indicated by extensive nuclear immunostaining for Ki67 (original magnification ×100) (G), posttreatment tumor shows virtual absence of immunoreactivity (original magnification ×100) (I, representing the only area of the excised tumor with any hint of Ki67 staining). Histologic analysis of corresponding adjacent sections was performed with hematoxylin-eosin staining (original magnification ×100) (H and J). (Reprinted from Kahana A, Worden FP, Elner VM. Vismodegib as eye-sparing adjuvant treatment for orbital basal cell carcinoma. *JAMA Ophthalmol.* 2013 [Epub ahead of print].)

ki-67 immunostain and ghost cells devoid of nuclei (Figs 1 and 2). There was no evidence of recurrence of tumor at 2 months' follow-up. Despite the apparent low proliferative capacity in residual neoplastic cells, the authors recommend en block excision with margin control.

Kahana et al's observations parallel those of Iarrobino et al,[1] who noted emergence of predominantly squamous cell carcinoma with minor BCC differentiation in the region of biopsy-confirmed metastatic BCC. Although the authors did not perform ki-67 immunostaining for proliferative index, they noted enlargement of the mass despite the initial shrinkage with vismodegib therapy, consistent with tumor recurrence and suggestive of drug resistance. The authors proposed 3 possible mechanisms for their observations: (1) selection for an already present subpopulation of squamous cell carcinoma cells, (2) alterations in signaling of the BCC to favor squamous differentiation, and (3) progression of original BCC population to a less differentiated, drug resistant phenotype.

These reports show residual and, possibly, recurrent tumor after vismodegib therapy. Presence of scattered neoplastic cells and nests, separated by large areas of fibrosis, may pose a potential challenge for confirmation of pathologic clearance of margins. Thus, although the results with vismodegib therapy are encouraging, careful patient selection and caution is necessary when deciding to embark on this therapeutic path.[2,3]

**T. Milman, MD**

*References*


1. Iarrobino A, Messina JL, Kudchadkar R, Sondak VK. Emergence of a squamous cell carcinoma phenotype following treatment of metastatic basal cell carcinoma with vismodegib. *J Am Acad Dermatol.* 2013;69:e33-e34.
2. Cowey CL. Targeted therapy for advanced Basal-cell carcinoma: vismodegib and beyond. *Dermatol Ther (Heidelb).* 2013;3:17-31.
3. Poggi L, Kolesar JM. Vismodegib for the treatment of basal cell skin cancer. *Am J Health Syst Pharm.* 2013;70:1033-1038.


---

**Perilipin and adipophilin expression in sebaceous carcinoma and mimics**

Boussahmain C, Mochel MC, Hoang MP (Massachusetts General Hosp and Harvard Med School, Boston)

*Hum Pathol* 2013 [Epub ahead of print]

---

Although adipophilin has been reported to be a sensitive marker for sebaceous carcinoma, others have noted its expression in squamous cell carcinoma and a variety of noncutaneous tumors, suggesting that lipid droplet accumulation is a frequent feature of neoplastic cells. We investigated the expression of adipophilin and perilipin in 101 cutaneous carcinomas. They included 30 cases of sebaceous carcinoma, 28 squamous cell carcinoma with clear cell change (18 invasive and 10 in situ tumors), 8 hidradenocarcinomas, 1 spiradenocarcinoma, 10 porocarcinomas, 4 malignant chondroid syringomas, 1 malignant cylindroma, 7 apocrine carcinomas, 6 eccrine carcinomas, 5 aggressive digital papillary adenocarcinomas, and 1 pilomatrical carcinoma. Adipophilin stained the rim of cytoplasmic lipid droplets in various tumor types, including sebaceous carcinomas (30/30, 100%), squamous cell carcinoma with clear cell change (21/28, 75%), and eccrine-apocrine carcinomas (25/43, 58%). On the other hand, perilipin

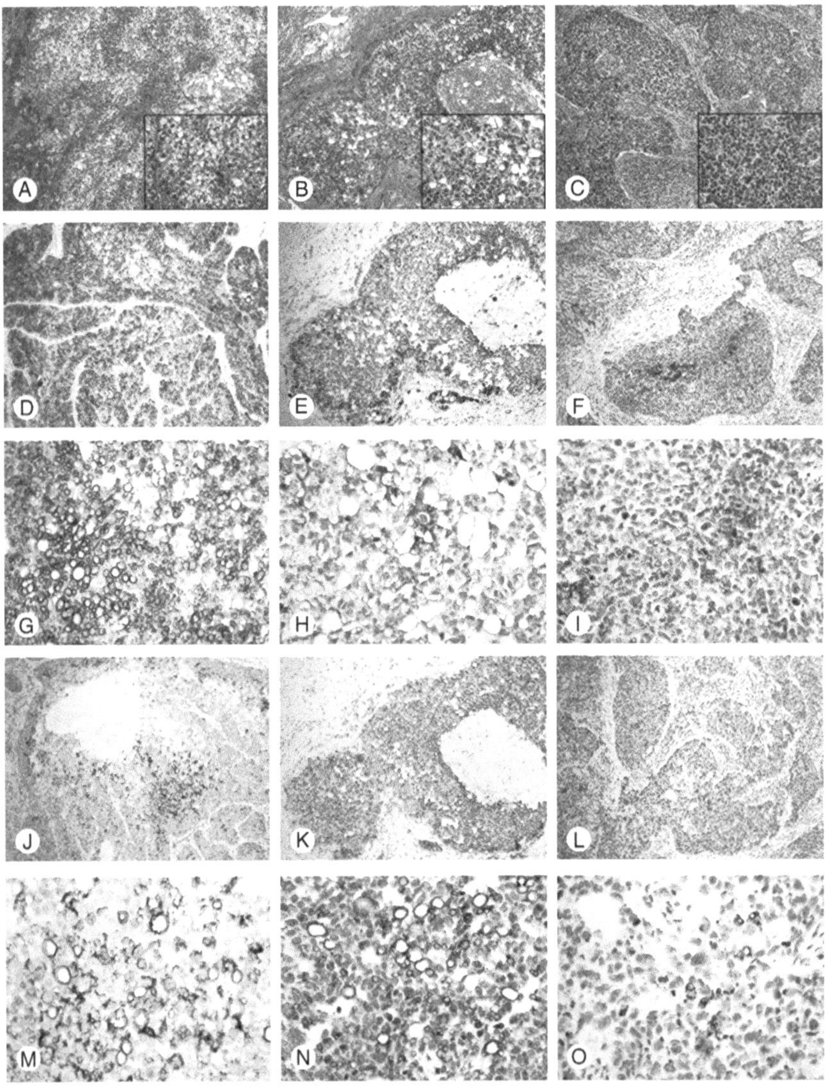


FIGURE 1.—In well (A), moderately (B), and poorly (C) differentiated sebaceous carcinomas, 3+ (D and G), 2+ (E and H), and 1+ (F and I) adipophilin expression as well as 3+ (J and M), 2+ (K and N), and 1+ (L and O) perilipin expression were noted, respectively (original magnification ×100 for A-F and J-L; ×400 for inset of A, inset of B, inset of C, G-I, and M-O). (Reprinted from Human Pathology. Boussahmain C, Mochel MC, Hoang MP. Perilipin and adipophilin expression in sebaceous carcinoma and mimics. *Hum Pathol.* 2013 [Epub ahead of print], Copyright 2013, with permission from Elsevier.)

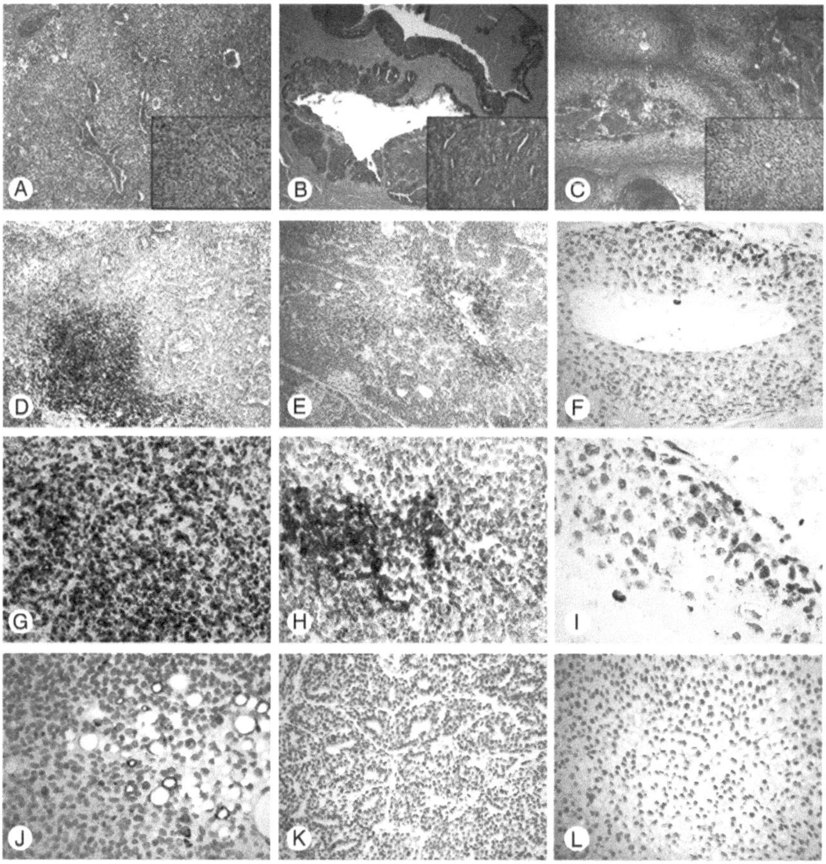


FIGURE 2.—In hidradenocarcinoma (A), aggressive digital papillary adenocarcinoma (B), and SCC with clear cell change (C), 2+ (D and G), 2+ (E and H), and 2+ (F and I) adipophilin expression was seen, respectively. However, 1+ perilipin expression was seen in only the hidradenocarcinoma (J), whereas perilipin expression was absent in the remaining 2 tumors (K and L) (original magnification ×100 for A-F; ×200 for G-L; and ×400 for inset of A, inset of B, and inset of C). (Reprinted from Human Pathology. Boussahmain C, Mochel MC, Hoang MP. Perilipin and adipophilin expression in sebaceous carcinoma and mimics. *Hum Pathol.* 2013 [Epub ahead of print], Copyright 2013, with permission from Elsevier.)

expression was seen in 13 (43%) of 30 sebaceous carcinoma and only 1 hidradenocarcinoma. The remaining 28 squamous cell carcinomas with clear cell change and 42 eccrine-apocrine carcinomas were negative. Although specific for invasive sebaceous carcinoma, perilipin expression was not helpful in distinguishing sebaceous carcinoma in situ from squamous cell carcinoma in situ with clear cell change. The expression of adipophilin seen in variety of cutaneous tumors suggests that the biosynthesis of lipid is altered in these neoplasms (Figs 1 and 2, Table 1).

▶ In this retrospective case series, Boussahmain et al investigated the expression of lipid droplet-associated proteins, adipophilin and perilipin, in 30

**TABLE.—Summary of Adipophilin and Perilipin Immunostaining**

| Tumor Types | n | Adipophilin Negative (%) | Positive (%) | 1+ | 2+ | 3+ | Perilipin Negative (%) | Positive (%) | 1+ | 2+ | 3+ |
|---|---|---|---|---|---|---|---|---|---|---|---|
| Sebaceous carcinoma | 30 | 0 (0) | 30 (100) | | | | 17 (57) | 13 (43) | | | |
| Invasive | 26 | 0 | 26 (100) | 10 | 9 | 7 | 13 (50) | 13 (50) | 7 | 4 | 2 |
| in situ | 7[a] | 1 (14) | 6 (86) | 5 | 1 | 0 | 7 (100) | 0 | 0 | 0 | 0 |
| SCC with clear cell change | 28 | 7 (25) | 21 (75) | | | | 28 (100) | 0 (0) | | | |
| Invasive | 18 | 3 (17) | 15 (83) | 9 | 5 | 1 | 18 (100) | 0 | 0 | 0 | 0 |
| in situ | 10 | 4 (40) | 6 (60) | 3 | 2 | 1 | 10 (100) | 0 | 0 | 0 | 0 |
| Eccrine-apocrine carcinoma | 43 | 18 (42) | 25 (58) | | | | 42 (98) | 1 (2) | | | |
| Hidradenocarcinoma | 8 | 2 (25) | 6 (75) | 3 | 3 | 0 | 7 (88) | 1 (12) | 1 | 0 | 0 |
| Spiradenocarcinoma | 1 | 0 | 1 (100) | 1 | 0 | 0 | 1 | 0 | 0 | 0 | 0 |
| Porocarcinoma | 10 | 6 (60) | 4 (40) | 3 | 1 | 0 | 10 | 0 | 0 | 0 | 0 |
| Malignant chondroid syringoma | 4 | 1 (25) | 3 (75) | 2 | 0 | 1 | 4 | 0 | 0 | 0 | 0 |
| Malignant cylindroma | 1 | 0 | 1 (100) | 1 | 0 | 0 | 1 | 0 | 0 | 0 | 0 |
| Apocrine carcinoma | 7 | 6 (86) | 1 (14) | 1 | 0 | 0 | 7 | 0 | 0 | 0 | 0 |
| Eccrine carcinoma | 6 | 2 (33) | 4 (67) | 4 | 0 | 0 | 6 | 0 | 0 | 0 | 0 |
| Aggressive digital papillary adenocarcinoma | 5 | 0 | 5 (100) | 2 | 3 | 0 | 5 | 0 | 0 | 0 | 0 |
| Pilomatrical carcinoma | 1 | 1 (100) | 0 | 0 | 0 | 0 | 1 | 0 | 0 | 0 | 0 |
| Total | 101 | | | | | | | | | | |

[a]Four were in situ carcinomas, and the remaining 3 were in situ components of invasive tumor.

sebaceous carcinomas and 71 cutaneous carcinomas with potential to mimic sebaceous carcinoma. The authors noted 100% sensitivity of adipophilin for detection of sebaceous carcinoma, but they lamented the low specificity of 35%. Conversely, perilipin had the specificity of 98% in distinguishing invasive sebaceous carcinoma from other tumors but much lower sensitivity of 43%. In addition, perilipin was not helpful in distinguishing intraepidermal spread of sebaceous carcinoma from squamous carcinoma in situ (Figs 1 and 2, Table).

These findings are contrary to the previous experience with adipophilin immunostain in sebaceous carcinoma reported by Ostler et al,[1] Ansai et al,[2] and Muthusamy et al.[3] According to Ostler et al,[1] adipophilin immunostain has sensitivity of 90% and specificity of 100% when "non-specific granular staining" is disregarded in nonsebaceous carcinomas. Ostler et al[1] proposed that this granular staining represents cross-reactivity of adipophilin with keratohyalin granules and lysosome-bound polarized lipid-rich structures, called *lamellar* (*Odland*) *bodies*. Boussahmain et al, conversely, suggested that granular staining, in fact, represents minute lipid droplets and reflects presence of steatogenesis in neoplastic cells. Boussahmain's theory is corroborated by the recent studies by Straub et al[4] and other investigators, which show upregulation of steatogenesis in metabolically and neoplastically altered cells and confirm presence of lipid droplet-associated proteins coating the minute intracytoplasmic lipid vacuoles in these cells.

Our experience is concordant with Boussahmain's observations on upregulated steatogenesis in nonsebaceous periocular carcinomas. We note frequent presence of small, rare vacuoles and abundant granules in squamous cell carcinoma of skin and conjunctiva, in basal cell carcinoma, and in many other tumors. However, we agree with Ostler's observations that presence of numerous large vacuoles and overall intense pattern of immunostaining is helpful in predicting true sebaceous differentiation.

Unfortunately, no immunostain at this point can serve as a gold standard for diagnosis of sebaceous carcinoma, and careful histologic observations still remain the cornerstone of diagnosis.

**T. Milman, MD**

*References*


1. Ostler DA, Prieto VG, Reed JA, Deavers MT, Lazar AJ, Ivan D. Adipophilin expression in sebaceous tumors and other cutaneous lesions with clear cell histology: an immunohistochemical study of 117 cases. *Mod Pathol.* 2010;23:567-573.
2. Ansai S, Takeichi H, Arase S, Kawana S, Kimura T. Sebaceous carcinoma: an immunohistochemical reappraisal. *Am J Dermatopathol.* 2011;33:579-587.
3. Muthusamy K, Halbert G, Roberts F. Immunohistochemical staining for adipophilin, perilipin and TIP47. *J Clin Pathol.* 2006;59:1166-1170.
4. Straub BK, Herpel E, Singer S, et al. Lipid droplet-associated PAT-proteins show frequent and differential expression in neoplastic steatogenesis. *Mod Pathol.* 2010;23:480-492.


## Sturge–Weber Syndrome and Port-Wine Stains Caused by Somatic Mutation in *GNAQ*


Shirley MD, Tang H, Gallione CJ, et al (Johns Hopkins School of Medicine, Baltimore, MD; Duke Univ Med Ctr, Durham, NC; et al)



*N Engl J Med* 368:1971-1979, 2013


*Background.*—The Sturge-Weber syndrome is a sporadic congenital neurocutaneous disorder characterized by a port-wine stain affecting the skin in the distribution of the ophthalmic branch of the trigeminal nerve, abnormal capillary venous vessels in the leptomeninges of the brain and choroid, glaucoma, seizures, stroke, and intellectual disability. It has been hypothesized that somatic mosaic mutations disrupting vascular development cause both the Sturge–Weber syndrome and port-wine stains, and the severity and extent of presentation are determined by the developmental time point at which the mutations occurred. To date, no such mutation has been identified.

*Methods.*—We performed whole-genome sequencing of DNA from paired samples of visibly affected and normal tissue from 3 persons with the Sturge–Weber syndrome. We tested for the presence of a somatic mosaic mutation in 97 samples from 50 persons with the Sturge–Weber syndrome, a port-wine stain, or neither (controls), using amplicon sequencing and SNaPshot assays, and investigated the effects of the mutation on downstream signaling, using phosphorylation-specific antibodies for relevant effectors and a luciferase reporter assay.

*Results.*—We identified a nonsynonymous single-nucleotide variant (c.548G→A, p.Arg183Gln) in *GNAQ* in samples of affected tissue from 88% of the participants (23 of 26) with the Sturge–Weber syndrome and from 92% of the participants (12 of 13) with apparently nonsyndromic port-wine stains, but not in any of the samples of affected tissue from 4 participants with an unrelated cerebrovascular malformation or in any of the samples from the 6 controls. The prevalence of the mutant allele in affected tissues ranged from 1.0 to 18.1%. Extracellular signal-regulated kinase activity was modestly increased during transgenic expression of mutant $G\alpha_q$.

*Conclusions.*—The Sturge–Weber syndrome and port-wine stains are caused by a somatic activating mutation in *GNAQ*. This finding confirms a long-standing hypothesis. (Funded by the National Institutes of Health and Hunter's Dream for a Cure Foundation.) (Tables 1 and 2)

▶ The Sturge–Weber syndrome, also known as "encephalofacial angiomatosis," is a neurocutaneous disorder that occurs as a sporadic congenital condition. It is characterized by a port-wine mark (cutaneous capillary malformation) that affects the skin in the distribution of the ophthalmic branch of the trigeminal nerve (Fig 1A and B in the original article) and is associated with venous-capillary abnormalities of the leptomeninges (Fig 1D-F in the original article) and the eye. A long-standing, but until this study unproven, hypothesis was that the Sturge–Weber syndrome and port-wine stains are caused by the same underlying somatic mosaic mutation with the precise clinical manifestations dependent on where and when in the developing fetus the mutation occurs. Mutations in early embryogenesis are lethal, mutations in early fetal development result in severe cerebral and cutaneous malformations, and mutations in later fetal development may manifest as isolated cutaneous vascular malformations.

Shirley et al tested this hypothesis through whole-genome sequencing of affected and unaffected tissues of 3 patients with Sturge–Weber syndrome to identify the causative somatic mutation. This resulted in the identification of a c.548G→a nucleotide transition in *GNAQ* on chromosome 9q21, encoding guanine nucleotide-binding protein (G protein), q polypeptide ($G\alpha_q$). The variant is predicted to result in the amino acid substitution, p.Arg-183Gln. The researchers then analyzed the skin and brain samples of other patients with Sturge–Weber syndrome and normal controls and identified the same mutation in 100% (9 of 9) of Sturge–Weber–related port-wine stains and 92% (12 of 13) of apparently nonsyndromic port-wine stains, whereas 86% of participants (6 of 7) with the syndrome were negative for the mutation in visibly normal skin (Table 1). The mutation was present in the brain samples from 83% of participants (15 of 18) with the Sturge–Weber syndrome, whereas 100% of brain samples (6 of 6 samples) from normal controls and 100% of brain samples from people with unrelated cerebrovascular malformation were negative (Table 2).

The researchers then performed cell culture studies and found that *GNAQ* mutation identified in Sturge–Weber patients activates mitogen-activated

**TABLE 1.**—Somatic Mutation of GNAQ in Skin Samples*

| Patient No. | Mutation Present† | PWS | SWS | Mutant Allele Frequency‡ *percent* | Total No. of Samples Assayed |
|---|---|---|---|---|---|
| 1 | Yes | Yes | Yes | 3.60 | 1 |
| 1 | No | No | Yes | 0.11 | 1 |
| 2 | Yes | Yes | Yes | 3.17 | 1 |
| 2 | No | No | Yes | 0.13 | 1 |
| 3 | Yes | Yes | Yes | 6.06–6.46 | 2 |
| 3 | No | No | Yes | 0.62–0.93 | 2 |
| 4 | Yes | Yes | Yes | 3.50–4.51 | 2 |
| 4 | No | No | Yes | 0.13–0.90 | 2 |
| 5 | Yes | Yes | Yes | 3.38 | 1 |
| 5 | No | No | Yes | 0.11 | 1 |
| 6 | Yes | Yes | Yes | 3.99 | 1 |
| 7 | Yes | Yes | Yes | 2.05–2.16 | 2 |
| 7 | Yes | No | Yes | 0.09–2.00 | 2 |
| 8 | Yes | Yes | Yes | 4.08 | 1 |
| 8 | No | No | Yes | 0.06 | 1 |
| 9 | Yes | Yes | No | 5.58 | 1 |
| 10 | Yes | Yes | No | 2.76 | 1 |
| 10 | Yes | No | No | 1.14 | 1 |
| 11 | Yes | Yes | No | 6.70 | 1 |
| 12 | No | Yes | No | 0.00 | 1 |
| 13 | Yes | Yes | No | 5.90 | 1 |
| 14 | Yes | Yes | No | 6.20 | 1 |
| 15 | Yes | Yes | No | 14.20 | 1 |
| 16 | Yes | Yes | No | 1.70 | 1 |
| 17 | Yes | Yes | No | 4.50 | 1 |
| 18 | Yes | Yes | No | 5.30 | 1 |
| 19 | Yes | Yes | No | 4.70 | 1 |
| 20 | Yes | Yes | No | 4.30 | 1 |
| 21 | Yes | Yes | No | 18.10 | 1 |
| 22 | Yes | Yes | Yes | 5.00 | 1 |

*Data are shown for c.548G→A, which results in the p.Arg183Gln amino acid substitution. This position corresponds to position 80,412,493 on chromosome 9 (Genome Reference Consortium Human Build 37). PWS denotes port-wine stains, and SWS Sturge–Weber syndrome.

†The p.Arg183Gln substitution was considered to be present if the mutant allele frequency was more than 1%.

‡The mutant allele frequency was calculated as the percentage of mutant alleles divided by total alleles (with ranges shown in the case of multiple samples).

protein kinase pathway, similar to somatic substitutions in *GNAQ* encoding p.Gln209Leu, which are found in patients with uveal melanoma. They noted, however, that the effect of p.Arg183Gln appeared to be both weaker and less promiscuous with respect to the activation of downstream effectors than the effect of the substitution of p.Gln209Leu (Fig 2 in the original article).

How does one put this all together? It is believed that neural crest contributes in part to the blood vessel development of leptomeninges and can potentially contribute to the blood vessels in perineural location (eg, in the distribution of V1). Furthermore, vasculogenesis, just like neural crest-derived melanocyte development, is dependent on the G protein-coupled receptor endothelin signaling. Thus, dysregulation of this G protein-coupled receptor as a result of the $G\alpha_q$ p.Arg183Gln mutation in persons with the Sturge-Weber syndrome and those with nonsyndromic port-wine stains may also bring about vascular

TABLE 2.—Somatic Mutation of GNAQ in Brain-Tissue Samples*

| Patient No. | Mutation Present | SWS | Mutant Allele Frequency *percent* | Total No. of Samples Assayed |
|---|---|---|---|---|
| 7 | Yes | Yes | 5.57–5.63 | 2 |
| 23 | Yes | Yes | 5.56–5.78 | 2 |
| 24 | Yes | Yes | 2.67–3.51 | 2 |
| 25 | No | Yes | 0.02–0.10 | 2 |
| 26 | Yes | Yes | 0.13–3.06 | 4 |
| 27 | Yes | Yes | 2.19–5.12 | 2 |
| 28 | Yes | Yes | 6.95–8.13 | 4 |
| 29 | Yes | Yes | 6.04–11.15 | 5 |
| 30 | Yes | Yes | 4.14 | 1 |
| 31 | Yes | Yes | 4.78 | 1 |
| 32 | Yes | Yes | 0.22–1.48 | 4 |
| 33 | Yes | Yes | 4.04–5.74 | 2 |
| 34 | No | Yes | 0.05–0.12 | 2 |
| 35 | Yes | Yes | 0.05–1.51 | 7 |
| 36 | Yes | Yes | 0.35–6.03 | 5 |
| 37 | Yes | Yes | 5.74–6.49 | 2 |
| 38 | No | Yes | 0.03–0.05 | 2 |
| 39 | Yes | Yes | 1.83 | 1 |
| 40 | No | No | 0.11 | 1 |
| 41 | No | No | 0.05 | 1 |
| 42 | No | No | 0.08 | 1 |
| 43 | No | No | 0.09 | 1 |
| 44 | No | No | 0.04 | 1 |
| 45 | No | No | 0.04 | 1 |
| 46 | No | No, CCM | 0.00 | 1 |
| 47 | No | No, CCM | 0.00 | 1 |
| 48 | No | No, CCM | 0.00 | 1 |
| 49 | No | No, CCM | 0.00 | 1 |

*Data are shown for c.548G→A, which results in the p.Arg183Gln amino acid substitution. Samples were obtained from persons with SWS, normal controls, and patients with a cerebral cavernous malformation (CCM).

malformation. It would be interesting to evaluate the diffuse and circumscribed choroidal hemangiomas for presence of *GNAQ* mutation.

**T. Milman, MD**

## Adenoid Cystic Carcinoma of the Lacrimal Gland: *MYB* Gene Activation, Genomic Imbalances, and Clinical Characteristics

von Holstein SL, Fehr A, Persson M, et al (Univ of Copenhagen, Denmark; Univ of Gothenburg, Sweden; et al)
*Ophthalmology* 120:2130-2138, 2013

*Purpose.*—To investigate genetic alterations in lacrimal gland adenoid cystic carcinomas (ACCs) with emphasis on the *MYB-NFIB* fusion oncogene and its downstream targets, *MYB* rearrangements, and copy number alterations in relation to clinical data and survival.

*Design.*—Experimental study.

*Participants and Controls.*—Fourteen patients with primary lacrimal gland ACC were included. As a control, we also studied the expression of *MYB-NFIB* in 19 non-ACC lacrimal gland tumors.

*Methods.*—The expression and identity of *MYB-NFIB* fusion transcripts were studied using reverse transcriptase polymerase chain reaction (RT-PCR) and nucleotide sequence analyses. Quantitative polymerase chain reaction (PCR) and immunohistochemistry were used to evaluate the expression of *MYB/MYB-NFIB* target genes. High-resolution array-based comparative genomic hybridization (arrayCGH) and fluorescence in situ hybridization were used to study copy number alterations and *MYB* rearrangements.

*Main Outcome Measures.*—mRNA or protein expression of MYB-NFIB, MYB, and its down stream targets; copy number alterations; and genomic rearrangements.

*Results.*—The median age of the patients was 43 years (equal gender distribution), and the median time of survival was 8.6 years. The MYB-NFIB fusion was expressed in 7 of 14 ACCs. In contrast, all non-ACC tumors were fusion-negative. All 13 ACCs tested stained positive for the MYB protein, and for the *MYB* targets KIT and BCL2, 12 were positive for MYC and CCNE1, and 9 were positive for CCNB1. Rearrangements of *MYB* were detected in 8 of 13 cases, including 2 cases with gain of an apparently intact MYB gene. The arrayCGH analysis revealed recurrent copy number alterations with losses involving 6q23-q27, 12q12-q14.1, and 17p13.3-p12, and gains involving 19q12, 19q13.31-qter,

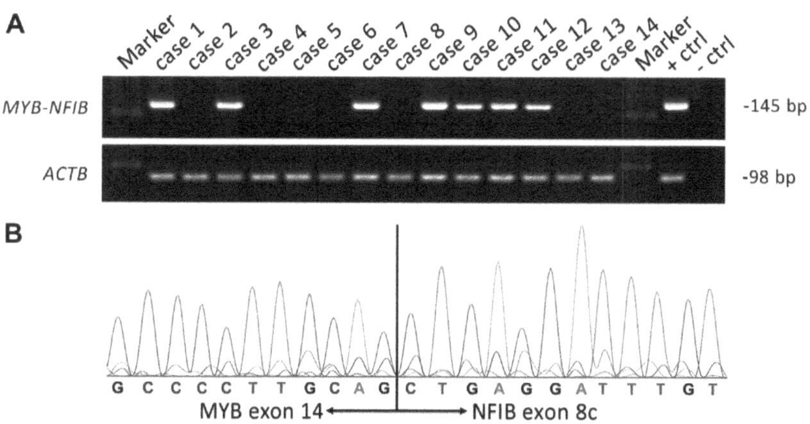


FIGURE 2.—Reverse transcription polymerase chain reaction (PCR) analysis of *MYB-NFIB* fusion transcripts in 14 lacrimal gland adenoid cystic carcinomas (ACCs). **A**, Detection of *MYB-NFIB* fusion transcripts in Formalin-fixed paraffin-embedded (FFPE) tumor tissues from 7 of 14 ACCs. *ACTB* was used as an internal control to test for intact RNA and cDNA. The sizes of the amplified fragments are indicated. **B**, Nucleotide sequence analysis of the PCR product generated from case 3 confirmed that it corresponded to a chimeric transcript consisting of *MYB* exon 14 fused to *NFIB* exon 8c. (Reprinted from von Holstein SL, Fehr A, Persson M, et al. Adenoid cystic carcinoma of the lacrimal gland: *MYB* gene activation, genomic imbalances, and clinical characteristics. *Ophthalmology.* 2013;120:2130-2138, Copyright 2013, with permission from the American Academy of Ophthalmology.)

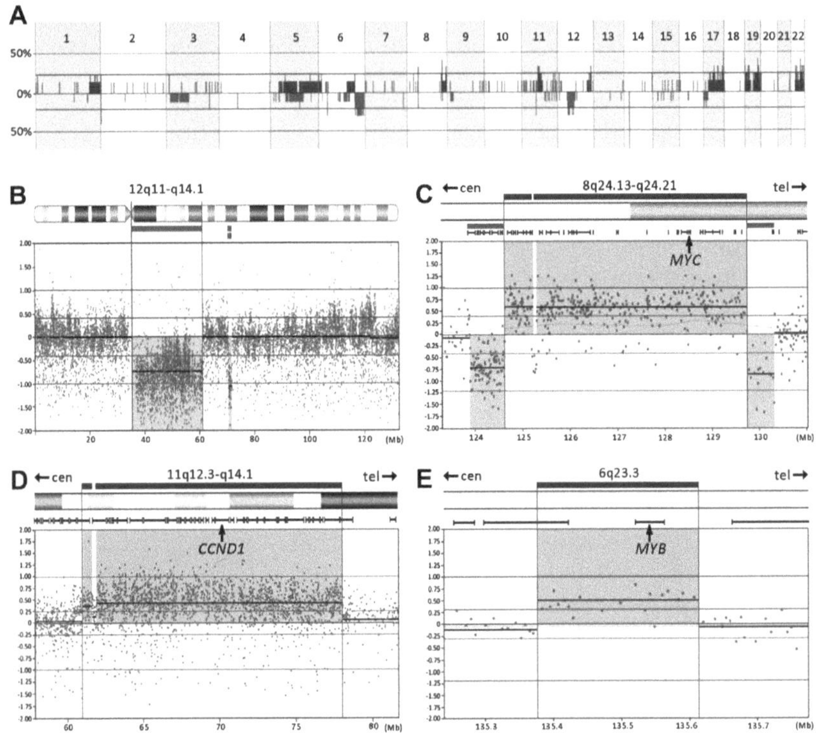


FIGURE 3.—The arrayCGH analysis of 10 lacrimal gland adenoid cystic carcinomas (ACCs). **A**, Genome-wide frequency plot of all copy number alterations detected in the 10 tumors. A total of 27 gains (blue) and 26 losses (red) were identified across the whole genome (sex chromosomes excluded). **B–E**, The arrayCGH profiles of lacrimal gland ACCs demonstrating (**B**) loss of 12q11-q14.1 (case 12), (**C**) gain of 8q24.13-q24.1 including the MYC locus (case 3), (**D**) gain of 11q12.3-q14.1 including the *CCND1* gene (case 9), and (**E**) gain of 6q23.3 including an apparently intact MYB gene (case 7). For Interpretation of the references to color in this figure legend, the reader is referred to web version of this article. (Reprinted from von Holstein SL, Fehr A, Persson M, et al. Adenoid cystic carcinoma of the lacrimal gland: *MYB* gene activation, genomic imbalances, and clinical characteristics. *Ophthalmology.* 2013;120:2130-2138, Copyright 2013, with permission from the American Academy of Ophthalmology.)

8q24.13-q24.21, 11q12.3-q14.1, and 6q23.3. Neither *MYB-NFIB* fusion nor any copy number alteration correlated with survival.

*Conclusions.*—Lacrimal gland ACCs are frequently positive for the *MYB-NFIB* fusion, overexpress *MYB* and its downstream targets, and have genomic profiles characterized by losses involving 6q, 12q, and 17p, and gains involving 19q, 8q, and 11q. Our findings show that lacrimal gland ACCs are genetically and clinically similar to their salivary gland counterparts and that MYB-NFIB is a clinically useful diagnostic biomarker for ACC. Our data also suggest that MYB and its downstream targets are potential therapeutic targets for these tumors (Figs 2 and 3, Table 1 and 3).

▶ Adenoid cystic carcinoma (ACC) of the lacrimal gland is a rare epithelial malignancy with approximately 80% 15-year mortality rate. Unfortunately, the

**TABLE 1.**—Clinical Data, *MYB-NFIB* Fusion Status, MYB Gene Rearrangement/Gain, MYB Protein Expression, and Genomic Imbalances in 14 Lacrimal Gland Adenoid Cystic Carcinomas

| Case No. | Age (yrs)/Sex | Grade | TNM* | Follow-up (yrs) | *MYB-NFIB* Fusion Status | MYB R/G | MYB Protein Expression | Genomic Imbalances *Gains* | Genomic Imbalances *Losses* |
|---|---|---|---|---|---|---|---|---|---|
| 1 | 41/M | I | T4b† | DM (4), TRD (5) | + | – | + | 3q13.13 | |
| 2 | 67/M | II | T4c‡ | DOC (3) | – | + | + | NDA | |
| 3 | 56/F | I | T4§ | LR (2), TRD (12) | + | + | + | 6pter-p24.1, 6q21-q23.3, 8q24.13-q24.1 | 1q32.1, 6q23.3-qter, 8q24.13, 8q24.21 |
| 4 | 45/M | II | T4c‡ | DM (1), TRD (1) | – | + | + | 1q32.1-qter | 6q23.3-qter |
| 5 | 26/M | I | T4b‡ | DM (4), TRD (4) | – | NDA | NDA | NDA | |
| 6 | 66/M | III | T2‡ | DM (5), TRD (9) | – | + | + | 7pter-p22.2, 11, 19 | 6q23.2, 6q23.3, 9p23-p21.3 |
| 7 | 32/F | II | T2‡ | NED (14) | + | + | + | 5p13.2-q21.1, 5q21.3-qter, 6q23.3, 8q24.13-qter, 17p11.2-q25.3, 19 | 5p13.3-p13.2, 6q13, 6q14.1, 6q16.1-q21, 6q21-q22.2, 6q24.2-q25.1, 6q25.1-q26, 6q27, 17p13.2-p11.2 |
| 8 | 57/F | II | T2‡ | LR+DM (5), TRD (6) | – | – | + | 17, 19, 22 | 3p25.1-p12.1, 5q11.2-q23.2 |
| 9 | 23/F | II | T4a‡ | LR (4), DM (5), TRD (5) | + | + | + | 8, 11q12.3-q14.1, 12p, 12q14. 1-qter, 17q | 11q14.2-qter, 12q12-q14.1, 17p13.3-p12 |
| 10 | 41/M | I | T3‡ | LR (2), NED (7) | + | + | + | 9p23-p22.3, 19q12, 19q13.31-qter | 12q12-q15 |
| 11 | 41/M | II | T2† | LR (3), NED (8) | + | + | + | 22 | |
| 12 | 24/F | III | T4a‡ | DM (2), TRD (15) | + | – | + | 22 | 12q11-q14.1, 15q23-q24.1, 15q25.1 |
| 13 | 64/F | II | T4a† | NED (27) | – | – | + | NDA | |
| 14 | 67/F | I | T2‡ | NED (7) | – | – | + | NDA | |

DM = distant metastases; DOC = dead of other causes; LR = local recurrence; NED = no evidence of disease; NDA = no data available; R/G = rearrangement/gain; TNM = tumor, node, and metastasis; TRD = tumor-related death.

*None of the patients had lymph node or distant metastases at the time of diagnosis.

†Tumor size <2.5 cm.

‡Tumor size >2.5 cm.

§Tumor size not known.

TABLE 3.—Recurrent Copy Number Changes (Minimal Common Regions of Gains and Losses) in 10 Lacrimal Gland Adenoid Cystic Carcinomas

| Cytoband Location | Chromosome Region (bp) | Region Length (bp) | Copy Number Change | No. of Tumors | No. of Genes | Potential Target Genes |
|---|---|---|---|---|---|---|
| 6q23.3 | Chr6: 135,377,625-135,614,043 | 236,418 | Gain | 2 | 2 | MYB |
| 6q23.3 | Chr6: 137,085,474-137,872,891 | 787,417 | Loss | 3 | 12 | |
| 6q24.2-25.1 | Chr6: 143,638,308-150,305,814 | 6,667,506 | Loss | 3 | 65 | *LATS1, PLAGL1* |
| 6q25.1-q26 | Chr6: 151,436,540-161,876,246 | 10,436,706 | Loss | 3 | 96 | *PARK2, WTAP* |
| 6q27 | Chr6: 164,714,653-167,867,112 | 3,152,459 | Loss | 3 | 31 | *RPS6KA2, RNASET2* |
| 8q24.13-q24.21 | Chr8: 124,624,995-129,751,417 | 5,126,421 | Gain | 3 | 50 | *MYC, PTV1* |
| 11q12.3-q14.1 | Chr11: 62,989,903-77,828,132 | 14,838,229 | Gain | 2 | 419 | *CCND1, ESRRA, FOSL1, RELA, RIN1* |
| 12q12-q14.1 | Chr12: 37,941,004-60,662,390 | 22,721,386 | Loss | 3 | 452 | *LIMA1, NR4A1* |
| 17p13.3-p12 | Chr17: 3,039,487-11,800,908 | 8,761,421 | Loss | 2 | 290 | *TP53, MYBBP1A* |
| 19q12 | Chr19: 34,305,176-35,950,763 | 1,645,587 | Gain | 4 | 14 | *CCNE1* |
| 19q13.31-qter | Chr19: 48,617,748-63,811,651 | 15,193,903 | Gain | 4 | 867 | *FOSB, RELB, RRAS, BCL3* |

bp = base pair.

data on its molecular genetic alterations, which can potentially lead to targeted therapies, are limited. An important breakthrough in the understanding of the molecular pathogenesis of ACC of the breast and neck was recently made when it was shown that the ACC-specific t(6;9)(q22-23;p23-24) chromosomal translocation results in an *MYB-NFIB* fusion oncogene. Subsequent studies have found that *MYB-NFIB* or *MYB* is overexpressed in more than 85% of ACCs, leading to activation of the *MYB* oncogene and of *MYB* target genes associated with cell growth, apoptosis, transcriptional regulation, and cell cycle control. In addition to activation of *MYB*, salivary ACCs also are characterized by recurrent genomic imbalances, including losses involving 1p, 5q, 6q, 11q, 12q, and 14q, and gains involving 1q and 22q.

This prompted von Holstein et al to conduct a retrospective study on 14 lacrimal gland ACCs and 19 non-ACC epithelial tumors of the lacrimal gland (12 pleomorphic adenomas, 2 adenocarcinomas, 2 carcinoma-ex-pleomorphic adenomas, 1 mucoepidermoid carcinoma, 1 ductal carcinoma, and 1 squamous cell carcinoma) to investigate the expression of *MYB-NFIB*, *MYB*, and their downstream target genes; to study genomic imbalances and *MYB* rearrangements; and to correlate the findings with clinical data and survival. The investigators found *MYB-NFIB* fusion transcript in half of lacrimal gland ACCs and in none of non-ACC tumors. They also noted increased expression of *MYB* and its downstream targets BCL2 and KIT in all 13 ACCs tested. In addition, there were recurrent chromosomal copy number alterations, including losses of 6q and 12q and gains of 19q, 8q, and 11q. The authors found that ACC stage, histologic grade, and therapy did not correlate with survival. Additionally, *MYB-NFIB* fusion status and genomic alterations did not correlate with tumor size or patient survival (Tables 1 and 3, Figs 2 and 3).

Demonstration of frequent *MYB-NFIB* fusion and increased *MYB* expression in ACCs irrespective of anatomic location suggests that it might be a driver mutation in this tumor. This opens the possibility for MYB and its downstream targets to become novel candidates for therapeutic intervention in selected ACCs.

**T. Milman, MD**

---

**Functional lacrimal gland regeneration by transplantation of a bioengineered organ germ**

Hirayama M, Ogawa M, Oshima M, et al (Keio Univ, Shinjuku-ku, Tokyo, Japan; Tokyo Univ of Science, Noda, Chiba, Japan; et al)

*Nat Commun* 4:2497, 2013

---

The lacrimal gland has a multifaceted role in maintaining a homeostatic microenvironment for a healthy ocular surface via tear secretion. Dry-eye disease, which is caused by lacrimal gland dysfunction, is one of the most prevalent eye diseases that cause corneal epithelial damage and results in significant loss of vision and a reduction in the quality of life. Here we demonstrate orthotopic transplantation of bioengineered lacrimal gland germs into adult mice with an extra-orbital lacrimal gland defect, a mouse model that mimics the corneal epithelial damage caused by lacrimal gland dysfunction. The bioengineered lacrimal gland germs and harderian gland germs both develop *in vivo* and achieve sufficient physiological functionality, including tear production in response to nervous stimulation and ocular

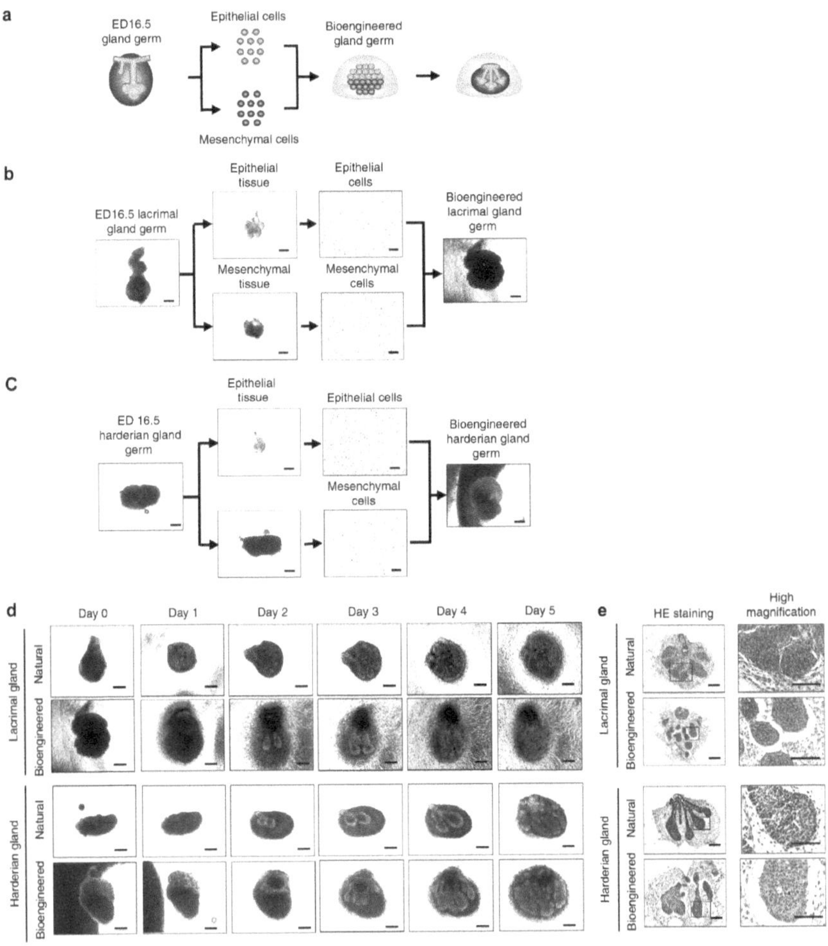


FIGURE 1.—Development and engraftment of the bioengineered gland. (a) Schematic representation of the methods used to generate a bioengineered lacrimal or harderian gland germ. (b) Phase-contrast images of the regeneration of the bioengineered lacrimal gland germ by the organ germ method. Scale bar, 100 μm. (c) Phase-contrast images of the development of harderian gland germ in organ culture. Scale bar, 100 μm. (d) Phase-contrast images of the development of natural and bioengineered lacrimal gland germ (upper) and harderian gland germ (lower) in organ culture. Scale bar, 100 μm. (e) Light microscopic images of HE-stained organ cultures of a natural and a bioengineered lacrimal gland germ (upper) and a harderian gland germ (lower) on day 3 and corresponding higher magnification images (right). Scale bar, 100 μm. (Reprinted from Hirayama M, Ogawa M, Oshima M, et al. Functional lacrimal gland regeneration by transplantation of a bioengineered organ germ. *Nat Commun.* 2013;4:2497, with permission from Macmillan Publishers Limited.)

surface protection. This study demonstrates the potential for bioengineered organ replacement to functionally restore the lacrimal gland.

▶ Several therapeutic approaches have been developed to restore lacrimal gland function, including heterotopic salivary gland transplantation and regenerative therapy methods with lacrimal gland-derived progenitor stem cells. In addition, a novel concept for organ replacement regenerative therapy has been

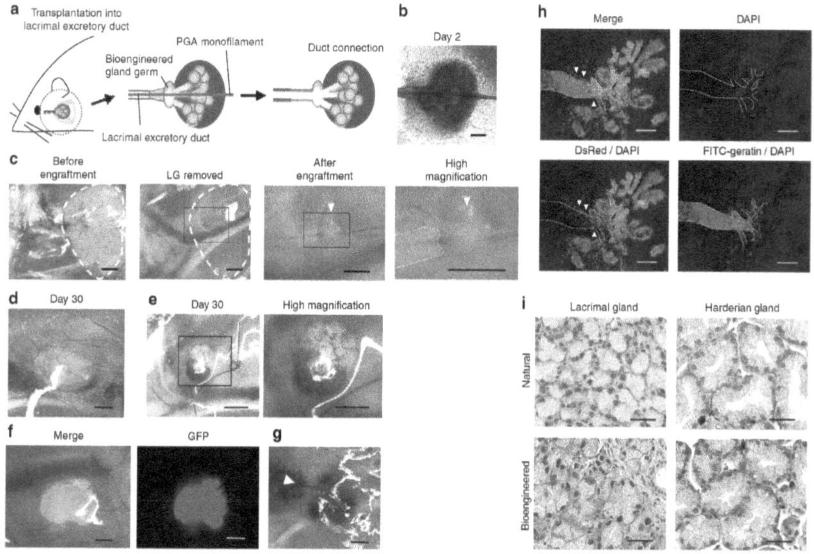


FIGURE 2.—Engraftment of the bioengineered gland germ. (**a**) Schematic representation of the methods used to engraft a bioengineered germ into an adult lacrimal gland-defect mouse. (**b**) Phase-contrast images of bioengineered lacrimal gland germs with a PGA monofilament inserted after 2 days of culture. Scale bar, 100 μmm. (**c**) Photographs of procedures for bioengineered gland germ engraftment. The extra-orbital lacrimal gland was completely removed (left, centre-left, white dotted line). The boxed area in the centre-left panel is the engraftment site shown at a higher magnification in the centreright panel. The boxed area in the centre-right panel is shown at a higher magnification in the right panel. The PGA monofilament was inserted into the host lacrimal excretory duct (centre-right, right). The white dotted line in the right panel indicates the host lacrimal duct. The arrowhead in the centre-right and right panels indicates the engrafted bioengineered lacrimal gland with a PGA monofilament. Scale bar, 1 mm. (**d**) Photographs of bioengineered lacrimal glands at 30 days after engraftment (left). Scale bar, 500 μm. (**e**) Photographs of a bioengineered harderian gland at 30 days after engraftment (left). The boxed area in the left panel is shown at a higher magnification in the right panel. Scale bar, 500 μm. (**f**) Photographs of a bioengineered lacrimal gland reconstituted using epithelial cells and mesenchymal cells from GFP-transgenic mice. A merged image (left) and a fluorescent image (right) are shown. Scale bar, 500 μm. (**g**) Analysis of the duct connection using Evans blue dye injection. The arrowhead indicates the injection site. Scale bar, 500 mm. (**h**) Histological analysis of the duct connection. 3D images of the bioengineered lacrimal gland reconstituted between DsRed transgenic mice-derived epithelial cells (red) and normal mice-derived mesenchymal cells. Bioengineered lacrimal glands developed in vivo with the correct connection (arrowhead) to the recipient lacrimal excretory duct. FITC-gelatin conjugate (green), DAPI (blue) and excretory duct (dotted line) are shown. Scale bar, 100 μm. (**i**) HE-stained lacrimal gland (left) and harderian gland (right). A natural (upper) and bioengineered (lower) gland after 30 days of engraftment are shown. Scale bar, 50 μm. For Interpretation of the references to color in this figure legend, the reader is referred to web version of this article. (Reprinted from Hirayama M, Ogawa M, Oshima M, et al. Functional lacrimal gland regeneration by transplantation of a bioengineered organ germ. *Nat Commun.* 2013;4:2497, with permission from Macmillan Publishers Limited.)

recently proposed to replace organs lost or damaged by disease, injury, or aging. In this article, Hirayama et al report functional bioengineered lacrimal gland replacement via an orthotopic engraftment of a bioengineered lacrimal gland germ into an extra-orbital lacrimal gland defect mouse model, a model that mimics ocular surface damage by lacrimal gland dysfunction. The bioengineered lacrimal and harderian gland germs, both developed in vivo, achieved sufficient physiologic functions, including tear production in response to pilocarpine and menthol stimulation and ocular surface protection.

The researchers first reconstituted in vivo lacrimal and harderian glands by using dissociated single cells from the epithelial and mesenchymal tissues of embryonic murine-lacrimal gland and harderian gland germs (Fig 1). This was followed by engraftment of the bioengineered germ into the extra-orbital

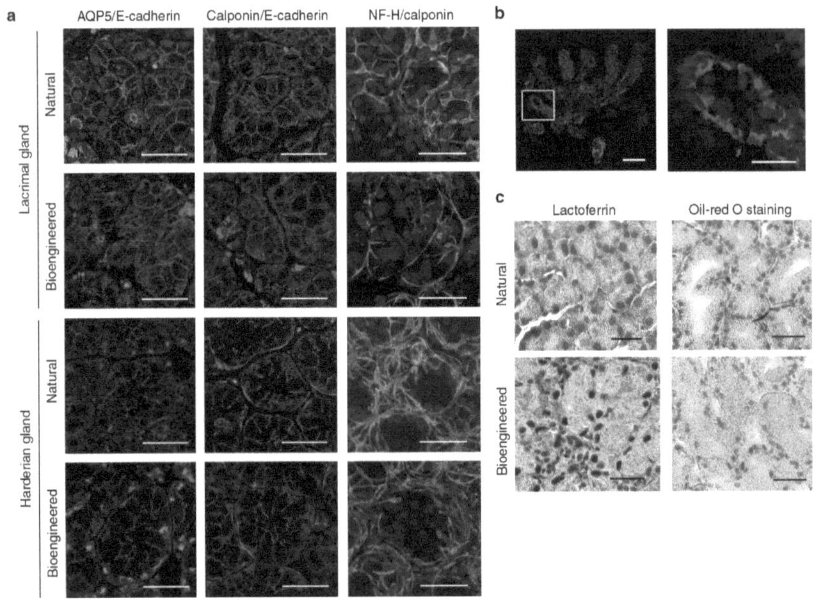


FIGURE 3.—Histological analysis of a bioengineered gland. (a) Immunohistochemical analysis of the acinar and duct cells in natural or bioengineered lacrimal and harderian glands. Their respective acini were analysed by immunostaining with specific antibodies for AQP5(red, in left panels), calponin (red, in centre and left panels), neurofilament-H (NF-H, green, in right panels) and E-cadherin (green, in left and centre panels). Nuclei were stained using Hoechst 33342 dye (blue). Scale bar, 50 µm. (b) Immunohistochemical analysis of a bioengineered lacrimal gland reconstituted between H2B-GFP-transgenic mice-derived epithelial cells and normal mice-derived mesenchymal cells. Green fluorescence indicates the nuclei of epithelial cells isolated from H2B-GFP-transgenic mice. The myoepithelial cells were analysed by immunostaining with specific antibodies for calponin (red). The boxed area in the left panel is shown at a higher magnification in the right panel. Scale bar, 50 µm in the upper panel, 20 µm in the lower panel. (c) Photomicrographs showing lactoferrin (left) in the acini of a natural lacrimal gland (upper) and a bioengineered lacrimal gland (lower). Lipids (right) in the natural harderian gland (upper) and bioengineered harderian gland (lower) acini were revealed by oil-red O staining. Scale bar, 50 µm. For Interpretation of the references to color in this figure legend, the reader is referred to web version of this article. (Reprinted from Hirayama M, Ogawa M, Oshima M, et al. Functional lacrimal gland regeneration by transplantation of a bioengineered organ germ. *Nat Commun*. 2013;4:2497, with permission from Macmillan Publishers Limited.)

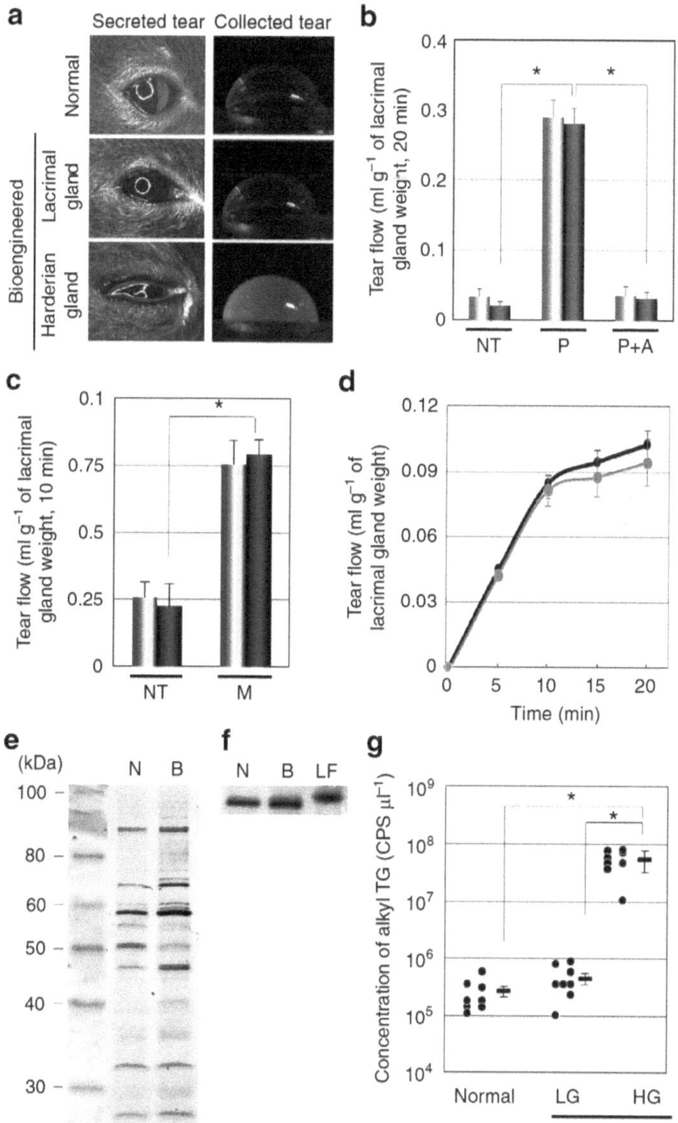


FIGURE 4.—Functional analysis of the bioengineered gland. (a) Photographs of eyes after pilocarpine stimulation (left) and the collection of tear fluid (right), including a normal lacrimal gland (upper), a bioengineered lacrimal gland that was engrafted into a mouse (centre) and a bioengineered harderian gland that was engrafted into a mouse (lower). (b) Assessment of the tear flow in normal (light bars) and bioengineered (dark bars) lacrimal glands that were engrafted into mice at 30 days after surgery. Tear flow without pilocarpine stimulation (NT), with pilocarpine stimulation (P) and with pilocarpine and atropine stimulation (P+A) are shown. Error bars represent the s.e.m. ($n = 5$). $*P = 0.0001$ was regarded as statistically significant (Student's t-test). NT, no-treatment; P, pilocarpine; and A, atropine. (c) Assessment of the tear flow and the response of normal (light bars) and bioengineered (dark bars) lacrimal glands that were engrafted into mice at 30 days after surgery. Tear flow without ocular surface stimulation (NT) and with ocular surface stimulation by menthol (M). Error bars represent the s.e.m. ($n = 6$). $*P = 0.0005$ was

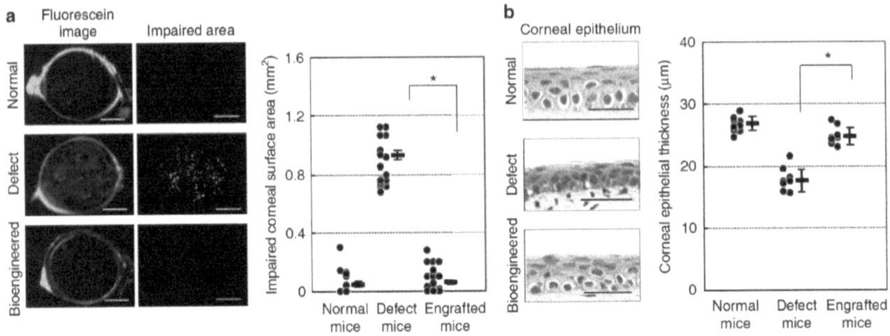


**FIGURE 5.**—Ocular-surface protection function of the bioengineered lacrimal gland. (**a**) Representative images (left) of the corneal surface of a normal lacrimal gland (upper), a lacrimal gland-defect mouse (centre) and a bioengineered lacrimal gland-engrafted mouse (lower). The punctate staining area in the 2.5-mm central corneal zone was measured using the Imaris software (right). Assessment of the impaired corneal surface area of a normal control (left), a lacrimal gland-defect mouse (centre) and a bioengineered lacrimal gland-engrafted mouse (right). The data are presented as the median and the mean ± s.e.m. ($n = 20$ for normal and the lacrimal gland-defect mice, 35 for the bioengineered lacrimal gland-engrafted mice). $^*P < 0.0001$ was regarded as statistically significant (Student's t-test). Scale bar, 1 mm. (**b**) Representative microscopic images of the corneal epithelium at 60 days after surgery, including a same week-old control (upper), a lacrimal gland-defect mouse (centre) and a bioengineered lacrimal gland-engrafted mouse (lower). Scale bar, 25 µm. Assessment of the corneal epithelial thickness of the central cornea of the control (left), the lacrimal gland-defect mouse (centre) and the bioengineered lacrimal gland-engrafted mouse (right). The data are shown as the median and the mean ± s.e.m. ($n = 11$ for normal, 8 for the lacrimal gland-defect mice and the bioengineered lacrimal gland-engrafted mice). $^*P < 0.0001$ was regarded as statistically significant (Student's t-test). (Reprinted from Hirayama M, Ogawa M, Oshima M, et al. Functional lacrimal gland regeneration by transplantation of a bioengineered organ germ. *Nat Commun*. 2013;4:2497, with permission from Macmillan Publishers Limited.)

lacrimal gland defect adult mouse model (Fig 2A–F). The success rates for the development of engrafted bioengineered lacrimal and harderian glands were 77.8% and 73.7%, respectively. The investigators were able to document the presence of connection between the engrafted bioengineered lacrimal gland and the excretory lacrimal duct of the recipient mouse (Fig 2G,H). Histologic studies on the transplanted bioengineered glands showed acinar and duct cells in correct 3-dimensional orientation with expected immunohistochemical profile and with evidence of innervation (Fig 3). In addition, Hirayama and colleagues documented functionality of the transplanted bioengineered lacrimal glands by noticing increase in lacrimation in mice in response to pilocarpine

regarded as statistically significant (Student's *t*-test). NT, no-treatment; M, ocular-surface stimulation by menthol. (**d**), The time course of tear flow in response to ocular-surface stimulation using menthol. The time course of tear flow for normal (black line) and bioengineered lacrimal glands (red line) after ocular-surface stimulation using menthol. Error bars represent the s.e.m. ($n = 6$). (**e**) Tear proteins in secreted tear fluid were analysed using SDS-PAGE. N, normal; B, bioengineered. (**f**) Lactoferrin in tear fluid secreted from bioengineered lacrimal glands was detected using western blot analysis. N, normal; B, bioengineered; LF, recombinant lactoferrin. (**g**) The concentration of alkyl triglycerides in tear fluid secreted from normal mice, bioengineered lacrimal gland-engrafted mice and the bioengineered harderian gland-engrafted mice are shown. The data are presented as the median and the mean ± s.e.m. ($n = 8$). $^*P$-values = 0.0001 were regarded as statistically significant (Student's *t*-test). CPS, count per second; LG, lacrimal gland; HG, harderian gland. For Interpretation of the references to color in this figure legend, the reader is referred to web version of this article. (Reprinted from Hirayama M, Ogawa M, Oshima M, et al. Functional lacrimal gland regeneration by transplantation of a bioengineered organ germ. *Nat Commun*. 2013;4:2497, with permission from Macmillan Publishers Limited.)

stimulation, inhibition of lacrimation in response to atropine, and increase in lacrimation in response to ocular surface cooling stimulation with menthol. They also noted the presence of expected tear proteins, including lactoferrin, in the secreted tear fluid (Fig 4). Lastly, the investigators showed that the bioengineered lacrimal gland tear secretion was able to restore and maintain normal, healthy corneal surface in the lacrimal gland defect mouse (Fig 5).

This meticulous study provides the exciting potential for bioengineered lacrimal gland replacement to restore lacrimal gland function. For additional information regarding organ replacement regenerative therapy, please read the article by Hirayama et al.[1]

**T. Milman, MD**

*Reference*

1. Hirayama M, Oshima M, Tsuji T. Development and prospects of organ replacement regenerative therapy. *Cornea*. 2013;32:S13-S21.

---

**Reactive Retinal Astrocytic Tumors (So-called Vasoproliferative Tumors): Histopathologic, Immunohistochemical, and Genetic Studies of Four Cases**

Poole Perry LJ, Jakobiec FA, Zakka FR, et al (Harvard Med School, Boston, MA; et al)

*Am J Ophthalmol* 155:593-608.e1, 2013

---

*Purpose.*—To evaluate the cellular nature of and diagnostic terminology used in connection with acquired retinal "vasoproliferative tumors."

*Design.*—Retrospective clinicopathologic study.

*Methods.*—Clinical records and microscopic slides of 4 enucleated globes were reviewed. Special stains and immunohistochemical probes for CD31, CD34, p53, glial fibrillary acidic protein (GFAP), CD163, and Ki67 (cell replication) were employed; ultrastructural and fluorescence in situ hybridization (FISH) analyses were performed.

*Results.*—Tumors were located inferotemporally in middle-aged patients. They were uniformly composed of compacted elongated, GFAP-positive spindle cells (due to intermediate filaments identified ultrastructurally) with a Ki67 index of less than 1%. Rosenthal fibers and eosinophilic granular bodies were observed. Hyalinized periodic acid-Schiff-positive vessels were widely separated. CD31 and CD34 revealed a sparse microvasculature. Tumor-associated exudate spread predominantly subretinally. The retinal pigment epithelium had undergone extensive placoid fibrous metaplasia with focal ossification. P53 upregulation, *BRAF-KIAA* gene rearrangement, and *IDH1 R132H* mutation typically associated with low-grade astrocytic neoplasms were absent.

*Conclusions.*—Retinal "vasoproliferative" tumors have been mischaracterized, because they actually display a paucity of microvessels. Proliferating fibrous astrocytes with a very low proliferation index predominate, without immunohistochemical or genetic evidence favoring a neoplasm.

Subretinal exudate appeared capable of provoking widespread fibrous metaplasia of the pigment epithelium that was mainly responsible for secondary retinal damage. The term "reactive retinal astrocytic tumor" is proposed as more appropriate for this entity. In carefully selected progressive

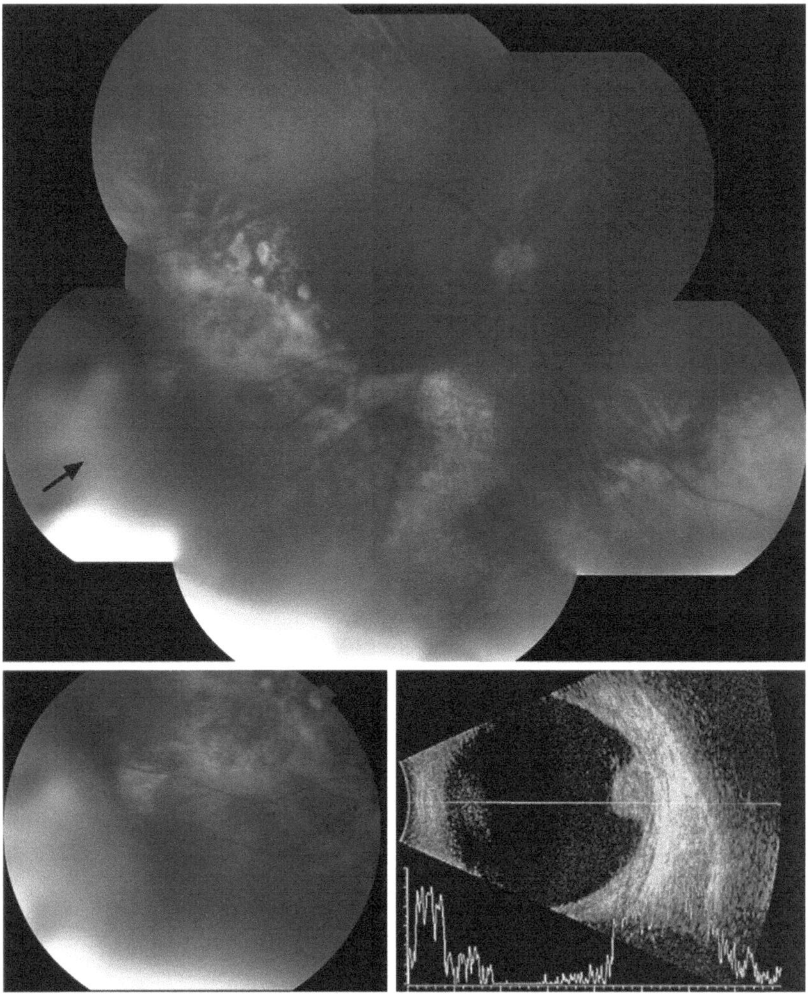

FIGURE 1.—Clinical features of reactive retinal astrocytic tumor. (Top) Photomontage of right fundus: appearance of an elevated lesion in the far retinal periphery (arrow) with extensive surrounding exudate including in the inferonasal quadrant. Note that there are no large feeding and draining vessels, in contrast to a von Hippel lesion (hemangioblastoma). (Bottom left) Somewhat blurred view (due to difficulty in focusing on peripheral lesion) of pink-yellow to orange retinal lesion toward the left. (Bottom right) B-scan ultrasonogram displays a well-circumscribed retinal mass that measured 5 mm in elevation without choroidal or scleral acoustic excavation. The superimposed A-mode ultrasonogram shows moderate and uniform intralesional internal acoustic reflectivity without spikes that might suggest calcification. (Reprinted from American Journal of Ophthalmology. Poole Perry LJ, Jakobiec FA, Zakka FR, et al. Reactive retinal astrocytic tumors (so-called vasoproliferative tumors): histopathologic, immunohistochemical, and genetic studies of four cases. *Am J Ophthalmol*. 2013;155:593-608.e1, Copyright 2013, with permission from Elsevier.)

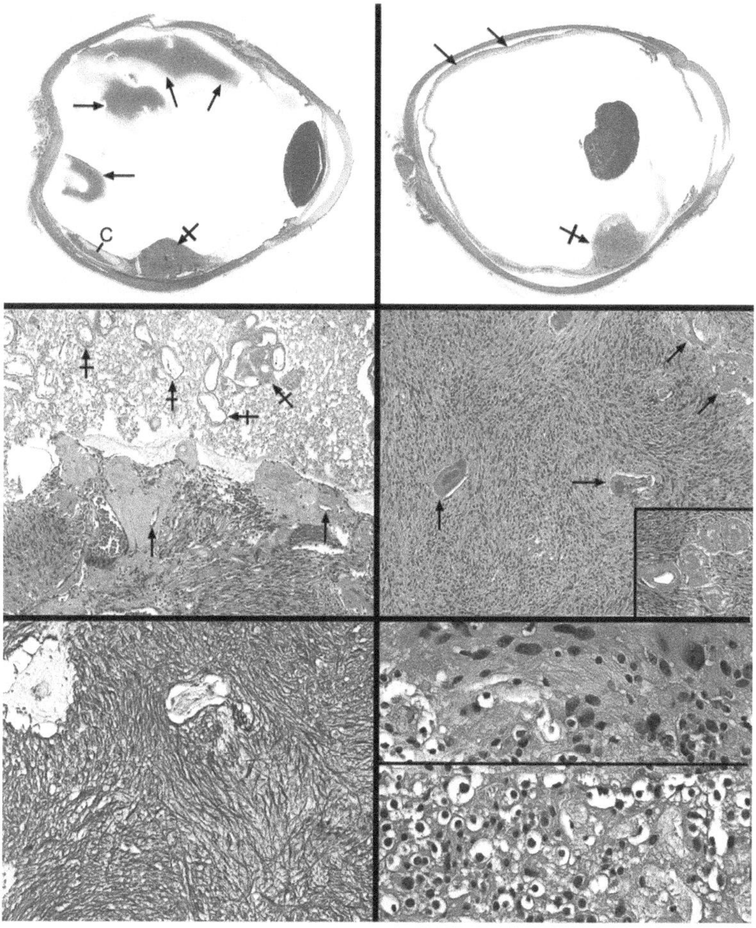


FIGURE 2.—Histopathologic features of reactive retinal astrocytic tumors. (Top left) Enucleated globe containing inferotemporal moderately elevated tumor (crossed arrow) with eosinophilic exudate present in the vitreous cavity (arrows). A large intraretinal cyst (C) is present immediately posterior to the mass. (Top right) Another example of a reactive astrocytic tumor (crossed arrow) with an area of apical necrosis. Contralateral to the tumor is an area of diffuse placoid fibrous thickening in the subretinal space (arrows) corresponding to areas of metaplasia of the retinal pigment epithelium. (Middle left) There is no inflammation within the necrotic area of the tumor present in the top right panel. Ghost-like vascular outlines (crossed arrows) are clearly identifiable. At the bottom is the interface with viable tumor showing massively sclerotic vessels with barely discernible lumens (arrows). (Middle right) All of the tumors were composed of interweaving bundles of bipolar spindle cells with regularly spaced sclerotic vessels (arrows), shown in a small cluster in the inset. (Bottom left) Glial fibrillary acidic protein (GFAP) intensely and diffusely immunostains the highly elongated (pilocytic) fibrous astrocytes composing the lesions. (Bottom right) Top panel: Two of the lesions displayed cells with mildly atypical nuclei consisting of hypochromasia, more rounded than elongated nuclear forms, and occasional nucleoli. Bottom panel: In 1 tumor there was an area at the periphery abutting the adjacent retina with honeycombed cells having clear cytoplasm and resembling oligodendroglial cells. Some of these cells were synaptophysin- and neurofilament-positive, indicating that they were probably persistent entrapped elements of the preexisting retina being replaced by the tumor. (Top left and Top right, hematoxylin-eosin [H&E], ×7; Middle left, H&E, ×7; Middle right, H&E, ×100, inset ×100; Bottom left, immunoperoxidase reaction, diaminobenzidine chromogen, ×200; Bottom right, H&E, top panel ×500, bottom panel ×400.). (Reprinted from American Journal of Ophthalmology. Poole Perry LJ, Jakobiec FA, Zakka FR, et al. Reactive retinal astrocytic tumors (so-called vasoproliferative tumors): histopathologic, immunohistochemical, and genetic studies of four cases. *Am J Ophthalmol.* 2013;155:593-608.e1, Copyright 2013, with permission from Elsevier.)

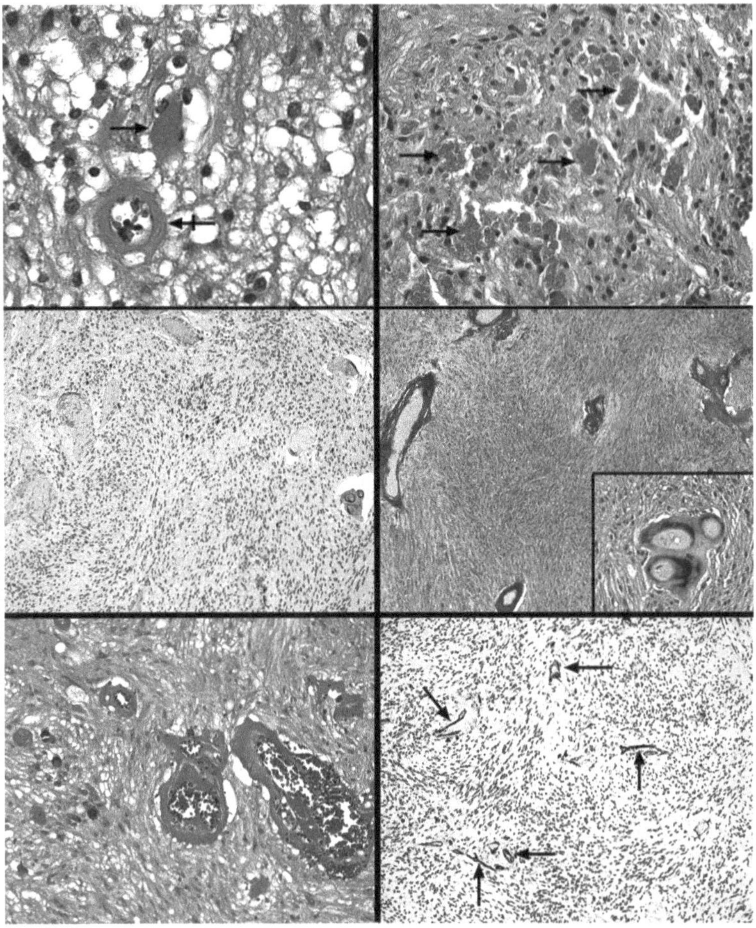

FIGURE 3.—Histopathologic figures of reactive retinal astrocytic tumors. (Top left) A homogeneous eosinophilic intracytoplasmic inclusion (arrow), called a Rosenthal fiber, is present in this more loosely textured field. The crossed arrow indicates a mildly sclerotic blood vessel. (Top right) Numerous collections of eosinophilic granular bodies (arrows) are distributed among the astrocytic cells. (Middle left) Ki67 stains a minimal number of cells (fewer than 1%) within the tumors. (Middle right) The tumors feature widely spaced sclerotic vessels, which are endowed with periodic acid–Schiff (PAS)-positive, thickened walls. The inset depicts the trichrome positivity signifying collagen in the vascular walls. (Bottom left) Rare cluster of proliferating blood vessels within the tumors. Note the eosinophilic granular bodies on the left. (Bottom right) CD31 immunostains a sparsity of microvessels within the tumor (arrows). (Top left, hematoxylin-eosin [H&E], ×500; Top right, H&E, ×400; Middle left, immunoperoxidase reaction, diaminobenzidine chromogen, ×100; Middle right, PAS, ×100, inset, Masson trichrome, ×200; Bottom left, H&E, ×400; Bottom right, immunoperoxidase reaction, ×100.). (Reprinted from American Journal of Ophthalmology. Poole Perry LJ, Jakobiec FA, Zakka FR, et al. Reactive retinal astrocytic tumors (so-called vasoproliferative tumors): histopathologic, immunohistochemical, and genetic studies of four cases. *Am J Ophthalmol.* 2013;155:593-608.e1, Copyright 2013, with permission from Elsevier.)

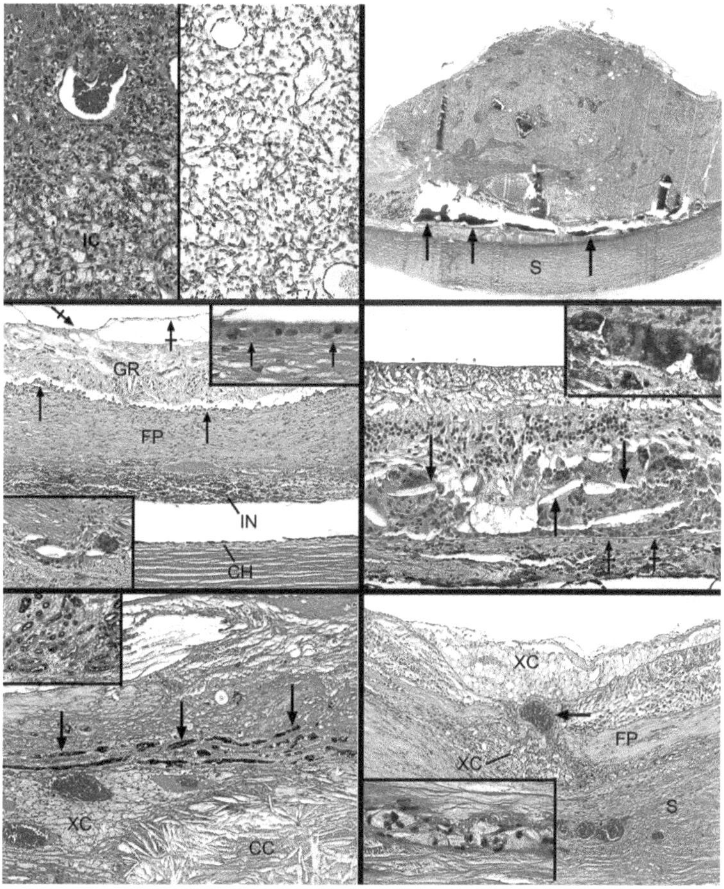


FIGURE 4.—Histopathologic features of reactive retinal astrocytic tumors. (Top left) The left panel illustrates a hemangioblastoma (von Hippel lesion) with lipidized interstitial cells (IC). The right panel shows CD31 immunostaining of a rich background microvasculature, in contrast to the minimal microvasculature of reactive retinal glial astrocytic tumors (see Fig 3, Bottom right). (Top right) Osseous metaplasia of the retinal pigment epithelium (arrows) underlies a reactive astrocytic tumor (S, sclera). (Middle left) Diffuse placoid fibrous metaplasia of the retinal pigment epithelium in a zone contralateral to where the astrocytic tumor was located. On the surface of the fibrous plaque (FP) is a layer of loosely adherent histiocytic cells (arrows). The overlying retina shows a preretinal gliotic membrane (closed arrows), disorganization, loss of ganglionic and photoreceptor cells, and mild intraretinal gliosis. The underlying choroid exhibits a moderately intense lymphocytic infiltrate (IN). The inset in the upper right demonstrates a monolayer of epithelioid histiocytes (arrows) on the surface of the fibrous plaque. The inset on the bottom left demonstrates entrapped multinucleated and mononucleated epithelioid histiocytes within the plaque. (Middle right) There are myriad mononucleated and multinucleated granulomatous cells in the subretinal space above the pigment epithelium (crossed arrows) engulfing cholesterol clefts (arrows). The inset displays intense periodic acid–Schiff (PAS) positivity in the cytoplasm of the histiocytes, mimicking the appearance of Whipple cells. (Bottom left) Pseudoadenomatous proliferation where the pigment epithelium (arrows and inset) begins to undergo metaplasia into a fibrous plague. In the choroid there are masses of cholesterol clefts (C) and a collection of fully lipidized xanthoma cells (XC). (Bottom right) A blood vessel is present in the deep retina (arrow), having originated from the choroid and migrated through a break in the metaplastic fibrous plaque (FP). The vessel is surrounded by xanthoma cells (XC), which are also present in the retina above. (S, sclera.) The inset displays intralamellar histiocytes within the sclera. (Top left, left panel, hematoxylin-eosin [H&E], ×200, right panel, immunoperoxidase reaction, diaminobenzidine chromogen, ×200; Top right, H&E, ×20; Middle left, H&E, ×100, insets ×200 and ×400; Middle right, H&E, ×200, inset, PAS, ×400; Bottom left, H&E, ×100, inset ×100; Bottom right, H&E, ×100, inset ×400.) (Reprinted from American Journal of Ophthalmology. Poole Perry LJ, Jakobiec FA, Zakka FR, et al. Reactive retinal astrocytic tumors (so-called vasoproliferative tumors): histopathologic, immunohistochemical, and genetic studies of four cases. *Am J Ophthalmol.* 2013;155:593-608.e1, Copyright 2013, with permission from Elsevier.)

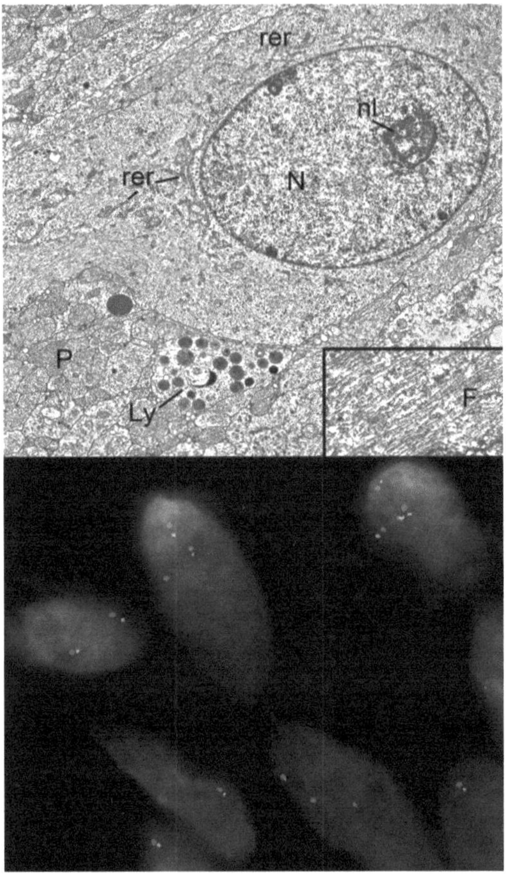


FIGURE 5.—Ultrastructural and genetic features of reactive retinal astrocytic tumors. (Top) Transmission electron micrograph of a tumor cell reveals short profiles of rough-surfaced endoplasmic reticulum (rer) in the perikaryon region. The cell has straight borders without basement membranes. Adjacent small cellular processes (P), some of which contain lysosomes (Ly), are clustered toward the bottom left and upper left. The inset highlights intermediate cytoplasmic filaments that correspond to the glial fibrillary acid protein positivity of the tumor cells. There are no villous processes suggestive of Müller cells. (Bottom) Fluorescence in situ hybridization analysis failed to reveal a BRAF-KIAA fusion because probes BRAF (red) and KIAA (green) were nonoverlapping. (Top, ×11 000, inset ×15 000; Bottom, ×1000.) For Interpretation of the references to color in this figure legend, the reader is referred to web version of this article. (Reprinted from American Journal of Ophthalmology. Poole Perry LJ, Jakobiec FA, Zakka FR, et al. Reactive retinal astrocytic tumors (so-called vasoproliferative tumors): histopathologic, immunohistochemical, and genetic studies of four cases. *Am J Ophthalmol.* 2013;155:593-608.e1, Copyright 2013, with permission from Elsevier.)

lesions, consideration should be given to earlier surgical intervention before extensive subretinal exudate accumulates and pigment epithelial proliferation with fibrous metaplasia ensues (Figs 1-5).

► Acquired tumors containing vascular and glial components were first described by Shields et al in 1983 in a series of 12 cases and termed "presumed acquired nonfamilial retinal hemangiomas." In 1995, a larger cohort of 113 eyes was evaluated by Shields et al, and classification of this tumor was proposed with specific delineation of the clinical features and related underlying ocular conditions. It was recognized that this vascular mass involved not only the retina but occasionally the retinal pigment epithelium and choroid, so this tumor was renamed "vasoproliferative tumor (VPT) of the retina." In the most recent series from Shields' oncology practice, the authors describe their clinical experience with 295 eyes with retinal VPTs.[1] Eighty percent of patients had primary tumors without identifiable predisposing conditions, whereas 20% of patients had underlying ocular disease, including retinitis pigmentosa, pars planitis, Coats disease, previous retinal detachment surgery, idiopathic peripheral retinal vasculitis, and familial exudative vitreoretinopathy. When compared with secondary VPTs, primary tumors generally presented in older patients; were more frequently solitary, unilateral, and pre-equatorial in location; caused less severe visual impairment; and were less frequently associated with intraocular inflammation. A notable finding in the study by Shields et al was the prevalence of a visually damaging effect of peripheral VPT on macular function. Visual acuity at presentation was 20/60 or worse in 39% of patients and 20/200 or worse in 18% of patients from macular exudation, macular edema, epiretinal membrane, or retinal traction.

Despite the wealth of clinical information on these lesions, the histopathologic data are sadly lacking. Several small, clinical-pathologic case series describe proliferation of vascular, glial, and retinal pigment epithelial elements in retinal VPTs consistent with reactive process[2,3]; thus, several other terms have been proposed to reflect these observations, including the "reactionary retinal glioangiosis." In their painstakingly detailed retrospective clinicopathologic case series of 4 patients with retinal VPTs, Poole Perry et al focus primarily on histopathologic, immunohistochemical, and molecular biologic findings of these lesions. They note that the masses were dominated by glial cell proliferations histopathologically reminiscent of pilocytic astrocytoma, although the immunohistochemical and molecular diagnostic investigations have convincingly excluded the diagnosis of astrocytoma in these tumors. Poole Perry et al noted relative paucity of vascular elements in these lesions and suggest that vascular proliferation in the tumors is a secondary phenomenon driven by the primary glial proliferative process. The ultrastructural studies on these tumors led authors to conclude that astrocytes, rather than Müller cells, are responsible for the glial proliferation (Figs 1-5). Thus, the authors propose yet another term for this lesion: "retinal reactive astrocytic tumor or RRAT."

The strength of the study by Poole Perry et al lies in the detailed histopathologic observations and ancillary pathologic studies on these rare lesions. Despite this additional information, there is still considerable ambiguity regarding these tumors. The clinical data on the eyes in Poole Perry's study are not provided in detail; therefore, it is difficult to correlate histopathologic observations with the clinical findings. What were the inciting clinical factors predisposing to development of these lesions? What were the primary pathologic events?

**T. Milman, MD**

*References*

1. Shields CL, Kaliki S, Al-Dahmash S, et al. Retinal vasoproliferative tumors: comparative clinical features of primary vs secondary tumors in 334 cases. *JAMA Ophthalmol.* 2013;131:328-334.
2. Saito W, Kase S, Fujiya A, Dong Z, Noda K, Ishida S. Expression of vascular endothelial growth factor and intravitreal anti-vegf therapy with bevacizumab in vasoproliferative retinal tumors. *Retina.* 2013 [Epub ahead of print].
3. Irvine F, O'Donnell N, Kemp E, Lee WR. Retinal vasoproliferative tumors: surgical management and histological findings. *Arch Ophthalmol.* 2000;118:563-569.

---

**Ciliary Body Medulloepithelioma: Analysis of 41 Cases**

Kaliki S, Shields CL, Eagle RC Jr, et al (Thomas Jefferson Univ, Philadelphia, PA; et al)

*Ophthalmology* 1-8, 2013

---

*Purpose.*—To describe the clinical features, histopathology, treatment, and outcomes of ciliary body medulloepithelioma.

*Design.*—Retrospective study.

*Participants.*—Forty-one patients with medulloepithelioma.

*Intervention.*—Cryotherapy, plaque radiotherapy, external beam radiotherapy, tumor removal by partial lamellar sclerouvectomy (PLSU), or enucleation.

*Main Outcome Measures.*—Metastasis and death.

*Results.*—Of 41 patients with ciliary body medulloepithelioma, the median age at diagnosis was 5 years. The mean tumor basal diameter was 11 mm, and the mean tumor thickness was 7 mm. Related features included secondary glaucoma (n = 18, 44%), iris neovascularization (n = 21, 51%), cataract (n = 19, 46%), lens subluxation (n = 11, 27%), lens coloboma (n = 8, 20%), retrolental neoplastic cyclitic membrane (n = 21, 51%), intratumoral cysts (n = 25, 61%), and extraocular extension (n = 4, 10%). There was systemic association with pleuropulmonary blastoma in 2 cases (5%). Primary tumor treatment included enucleation (n = 21, 60%), tumor removal by PLSU (n = 8, 23%), plaque radiotherapy (n = 3, 9%), external beam radiotherapy (n = 1, 3%), cryotherapy (n = 1, 3%), or palliative chemotherapy (n = 1, 3%). In 1 case, medulloepithelioma was diagnosed histopathologically after inadvertent evisceration for blind painful eye. Subsequent treatment for residual or recurrent tumor in cases treated conservatively/inappropriately (n = 15) was necessary in 7 cases (47%). Histopathology disclosed benign features in 6 cases (20%), malignant features in 24 cases (80%), teratoid features in 11 cases (37%), and nonteratoid features in 19 cases (63%). In the 26 enucleated eyes, other features included retrolental neoplastic cyclitic membrane (n = 18, 69%), neoplastic epiretinal membrane (n = 6, 23%), and persistent hyaloid artery (n = 6, 23%). Systemic metastasis occurred in 3 cases (8%) over a mean follow-up of 49 months, all of whom presented with extrascleral extension of tumor due to mean delay in diagnosis by 39 months.

*Conclusions.*—Medulloepithelioma most commonly occurs in children. Systemic association with pleuropulmonary blastoma rarely is found. Patients with extrascleral medulloepithelioma are at risk for metastasis.

▶ In their retrospective case series of 41 patients with medulloepithelioma diagnosed at the Wills Eye Hospital and L.V. Prasad Eye Institute, Kaliki et al confirmed prior observations from several smaller case series. The investigators noted that the median age at the time of diagnosis was 5 years and that approximately half of the tumors were associated with iris neovascularization and secondary glaucoma, cataract, retrolental neoplastic cyclitic membrane, and intratumoral cysts (Fig 1 in the original article). From the standpoint of histopathology, four-fifths of the tumors were classified as malignant and approximately one-third had teratoid features (Figs 2-4 in the original article). Systemic metastases occurred in 3 patients (8%), all of whom had delay in diagnosis and extrascleral tumor extension. Interestingly, there was a systemic association with an earlier diagnosed pleuropulmonary blastoma in 2 patients (5%).

Pleuropulmonary blastoma is a rare embryonic tumor of early childhood that occurs in the lungs and pleura. It is believed to arise from primitive pleuropulmonary mesenchyme and is the pulmonary analogue of retinoblastoma, neuroblastoma, medulloepithelioma, and Wilms' tumor. One-third of the patients with pleuropulmonary blastoma have a familial cancer syndrome caused by dicer-1 mutation on chromosome 14q31. Dicer-1 directs production of small RNA molecules controlling gene expression, and mutations in this gene have been associated with a geographic atrophy variant of macular degeneration. In addition, germline loss of dicer-1 function can result in multiple familial pleuropulmonary blastomas, lung cysts, neuroblastoma, cystic nephroma, Wilms' tumor, and rhabdomyosarcoma. Medulloepithelioma is another association. A 2011 review of 299 patients in the International Pleuropulmonary Blastoma Registry found 3 patients who also had ciliary body medulloepithelioma and one patient whose parent had medulloepithelioma. All patients had lung tumor diagnosed before the age of 3. Thus, knowledge of this association may allow for earlier diagnosis and treatment of medulloepithelioma, for oncologic screening for other malignancies, and for genetic counseling.

**T. Milman, MD**

---

**American Joint Committee on Cancer Classification of Posterior Uveal Melanoma (Tumor Size Category) Predicts Prognosis in 7731 Patients**

Shields CL, Kaliki S, Furuta M, et al (Thomas Jefferson Univ, Philadelphia, PA)
*Ophthalmology* 120:2066-2071, 2013

---

*Purpose.*—To evaluate the clinical features and prognosis of posterior uveal (ciliary body and choroid) melanoma based on the American Joint Committee on Cancer (AJCC) classification (7th edition) of primary tumor (T).

*Design.*—Retrospective, interventional case series.
*Participants.*—Seven thousand seven hundred thirty-one patients.
*Intervention.*—Ocular management including plaque radiotherapy, enucleation, local resection, or laser therapy.
*Main Outcome Measures.*—Melanoma-related metastasis and death.
*Results.*—Of 7731 patients with posterior uveal melanoma, the AJCC classification based on T was category T1 in 3557 (46%), T2 in 2082 (27%), T3 in 1599 (21%), and T4 in 493 (6%). Based on tumor categories T1, T2, T3, and T4, respectively, features that showed significant increase with tumor category included patient age at presentation (57, 58, 58, and 61 years; $P < 0.001$), tumor base (8, 12, 15, and 20 mm; $P < 0.001$), tumor thickness (3.5, 5.2, 8.9, and 11.4 mm; $P < 0.001$), mushroom configuration (8%, 20%, 38%, and 39%; $P < 0.001$), associated subretinal fluid (64%, 80%, 82%, and 83%; $P < 0.001$), intraocular hemorrhage (5%, 12%, 17%, and 18%; $P < 0.001$), rupture of Bruch's membrane (9%, 24%, 40%, and 40%; $P < 0.001$), and extraocular extension (1%, <1%, 4%, and 12%; $P < 0.001$). After therapy, Kaplan-Meier estimates of metastasis at 5, 10, and 20 years were 8%, 15%, and 25% for category T1, 14%, 25%, and 40% for category T2, 31%, 49%, and 62% for category T3, and 51%, 63%, and 69% for category T4, respectively ($P < 0.001$). Kaplan-Meier estimates of death at 5, 10, and 20 years were 4%, 8%, and 11% for category T1, 8%, 13%, and 24% for category T2, 19%, 27%, and 36% for category T3, and 30%, 43%, and 51% for category T4, respectively ($P < 0.001$). Compared with category T1, the hazard ratio for metastasis and death for T2 was 1.8 and 1.9, respectively, that for T3 was 4.5 and 4.7, respectively, and that for T4 was 8.2 and 8.8, respectively.
*Conclusions.*—Based on the AJCC classification, increasing tumor category was associated with older age, larger tumor, and greater incidence of subretinal fluid, hemorrhage, and extraocular extension. Compared with uveal melanoma classified as T1, the rate of metastasis and death was 2 times greater for T2, 4 times greater for T3, and 8 times greater for T4. The risk for metastasis and death increased 2-fold with each increasing melanoma category (Figs 1-3).

▶ The current seventh edition of the American Joint Committee on Cancer (AJCC) staging manual provides a detailed classification for uveal melanoma with the intent of improving understanding and prognostication of this malignancy. The tumor is classified incrementally according to size, based on a combination of basal diameter and thickness as T1, T2, T3, and T4 categories (Fig 1). Subclassification within each category is determined by the absence or presence of ciliary body involvement and extraocular extension and by the extent of extraocular extension. In addition, the tumors are histologically graded as G1, G2, and G3 depending on the percentage of spindle and epithelioid melanoma cells.

In this retrospective, nonrandomized, noncomparative, interventional case series of 7731 patients with posterior uveal melanoma, Shields at al explored the correlation of melanoma clinical features and melanoma-related metastasis and death with the AJCC classification. The investigators found good correlation

| Melanoma thickness (mm) | Category | | | | | | |
|---|---|---|---|---|---|---|---|
| >15 | | | | | 4 | 4 | 4 |
| 12.1-15 | | | | 3 | 3 | 4 | 4 |
| 9.1-12 | | 3 | 3 | 3 | 3 | 3 | 4 |
| 6.1-9 | 2 | 2 | 2 | 2 | 3 | 3 | 4 |
| 3.1-6 | 1 | 1 | 1 | 2 | 2 | 3 | 4 |
| ≤3 | 1 | 1 | 1 | 1 | 2 | 2 | 4 |
| | ≤3 | 3.1-6 | 6.1-9 | 9.1-12 | 12.1-15 | 15.1-18 | >18 |
| | Melanoma basal diameter (mm) | | | | | | |

FIGURE 1.—American Joint Commission on Cancer, 7th edition, classification of uveal melanoma (ciliary body and choroidal melanoma) into 4 tumor categories defined by tumor thickness and basal diameter. (Reprinted from Shields CL, Kaliki S, Furuta M, et al. American Joint Committee on Cancer classification of posterior uveal melanoma (tumor size category) predicts prognosis in 7731 patients. *Ophthalmology.* 2013;120:2066-2071, Copyright 2013, with permission from the American Academy of Ophthalmology.)

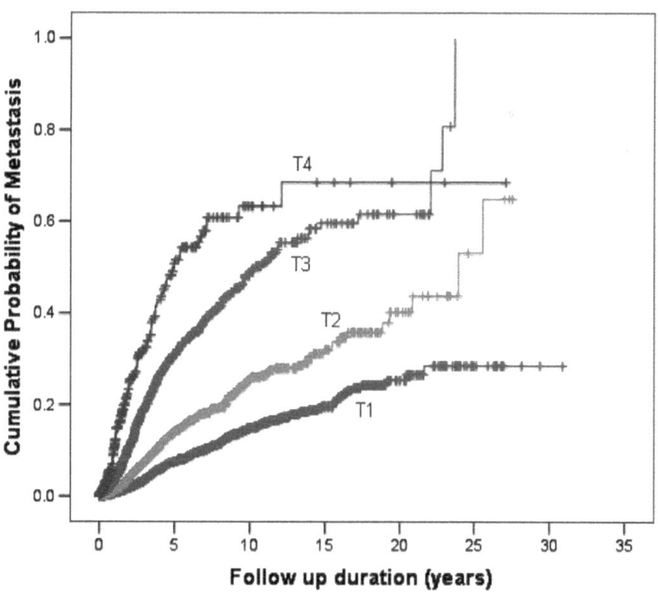


FIGURE 2.—Kaplan-Meier estimate of metastasis in posterior uveal melanoma based on the American Joint Committee on Cancer classification. T = tumor. (Reprinted from Shields CL, Kaliki S, Furuta M, et al. American Joint Committee on Cancer classification of posterior uveal melanoma (tumor size category) predicts prognosis in 7731 patients. *Ophthalmology.* 2013;120:2066-2071, Copyright 2013, with permission from the American Academy of Ophthalmology.)

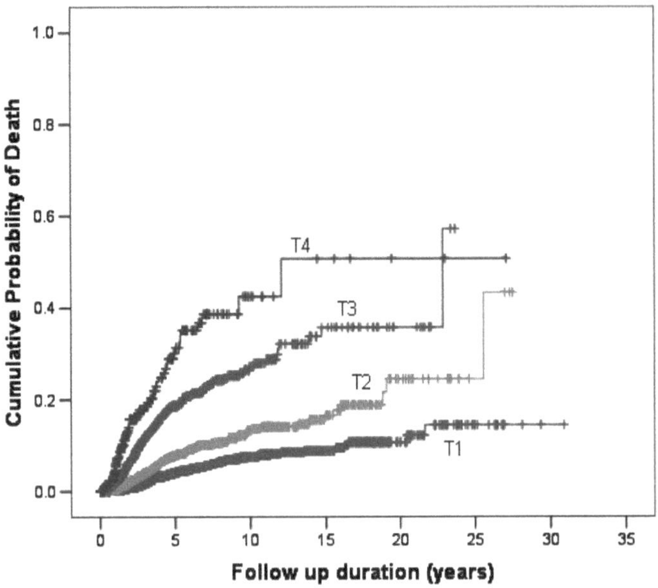


FIGURE 3.—Kaplan-Meier estimate of melanoma-related death in posterior uveal melanoma based on the American Joint Committee on Cancer classification. T = tumor. (Reprinted from Shields CL, Kaliki S, Furuta M, et al. American Joint Committee on Cancer classification of posterior uveal melanoma (tumor size category) predicts prognosis in 7731 patients. *Ophthalmology.* 2013;120:2066-2071, Copyright 2013, with permission from the American Academy of Ophthalmology.)

between T categories and subcategories and patient survival: the 10-year rate of metastasis was 15% for T1, 25% for T2, 49% for T3, and 63% for T4 (Figs 2 and 3). In multivariate analysis, the factors predictive of metastasis per T category were older age, ciliary body involvement, and increasing tumor base for T1; older age, multiquadrant location, dome or plateau configuration, and nonpigmented melanoma for T2; older age, inferior location, close proximity to foveola, increasing tumor base, nonpigmented melanoma, and intraocular hemorrhage for T3; and increasing tumor thickness, plateau configuration, and mixed pigmentation for T4. These high-risk features could be useful in prognostication and may be incorporated into future modifications of AJCC classification.

The authors recognize that the presumption that each therapeutic method imparted equivalent control for melanoma and did not affect systemic metastasis is a potential limitation of the study. Future directions may include validation of the current AJCC uveal melanoma grading system and incorporation of molecular genetic analysis into prognostication.

**T. Milman, MD**

## Molecular Histopathology Using Gold Nanorods and Optical Coherence Tomography

Prabhulkar S, Matthews J, Rawal S, et al (Univ of Miami-Bascom Palmer Eye Inst, FL; Univ of Miami-Miller School of Medicine, FL)
*Invest Ophthalmol Vis Sci* 54:1192-1200, 2013

*Purpose.*—To examine the novel application of a commercially available optical coherence tomography (OCT) system toward molecular histopathology using gold nanorod (GNR) linked antibodies as a functionalized contrast agent to evaluate ocular surface squamous neoplasia (OSSN).

*Methods.*—GNRs were synthesized and covalently attached to anti–glucose transporter-1 (GLUT-1) antibodies via carbodiimide chemistry. Three specimens from each of three distinct categories of human conjunctival tissue were selected for analysis, including conjunctiva without epithelial atypia (controls); conjunctival intraepithelial neoplasia, carcinoma in situ (CIS); and conjunctival squamous cell carcinoma (SCC). Tissue sections were incubated initially with GNR tagged anti–GLUT-1 antibodies and then with a fluorescent-tagged secondary antibody. Immunofluorescence and OCT imaging of the tissue was performed and the results were correlated to the light microscopic findings on traditional hemotoxyin and eosin stained sections.

*Results.*—No binding of the functionalized GNRs was observed within the epithelium of three normal conjunctiva controls. While immunofluorescence disclosed variable binding of the functionalized GNRs to atypical epithelial cells in all six cases of OSSN, the enhancement of the OCT signal in three cases of CIS was insufficient to distinguish these specimens from normal controls. In two of three cases of SCC, binding of functionalized GNRs was sufficient to produce an increased scattering effect on OCT in areas correlating to atypical epithelial cells which stained intensely on immunofluorescence imaging. Binding of functionalized GNRs was sufficient to produce an increased scattering effect on OCT in areas correlating to regions of erythrocytes and hemorrhage which stained intensely on immunofluorescence imaging within all nine tested samples.

*Conclusions.*—We have demonstrated the use of OCT for molecular histopathology using functionalized gold nanorods in the setting of OSSN. Our results suggest a threshold concentration of functionalized GNRs within tissue is required to achieve a detectable enhancement in scattering of the OCT signal.

▶ The image quality and axial resolution of the optical coherence tomography (OCT) technique has undergone a remarkable evolution. Much recent work has focused on metallic nanoparticles, particularly gold nanorods (GNRs), as potential molecular imaging adjuncts to OCT.[1] GNRs have demonstrated the remarkable capacity to absorb and scatter light at visible and near-infrared regions. The principle of using OCT for GNR detection relies on the local collective in phase electron oscillation, known as the surface plasmon resonance effect, caused by the incident OCT light. GNRs are preferred over other shapes of nanoparticles because their plasmon-resonant wavelength can be precisely tuned to the central wavelength of the OCT beam. They have excellent biocompatibility, are nontoxic, and are not susceptible to photo bleaching. The surfaces of GNRs can be modified to allow for antibody conjugation, which enables the use of GNRs as functionalized OCT contrast agents with molecular specificity (Fig 1 in the original article).

In this retrospective case series, Prabhulkar and colleagues have applied the properties of GNRs conjugated to anti–glucose transporter-1 (Glut-1), which has been shown to be overexpressed in ocular surface squamous neoplasia (OSSN), to image normal conjunctiva, pterygia, and varying degrees of conjunctival dysplasia and squamous cell carcinoma. The researchers observed that although there was variable binding of the functionalized GNRs to atypical epithelial cells in all 6 cases of OSSN, the enhancement of the OCT signal in 3 cases of conjunctival intraepithelial neoplasia was insufficient to distinguish these specimens from normal controls. The study was more promising in squamous cell carcinomas, for which in 2 of 3 cases, binding of functionalized GNRs was sufficient to produce an increased scattering effect on OCT in areas correlating to atypical epithelial cells. In addition, Glut-1 strongly highlighted the inflammatory cells and erythrocytes (Figs 2-4 in the original article). The authors conclude that a threshold concentration of functionalized GNRs within tissue is required to achieve a detectable enhancement in scattering of the OCT signal.

This study has several important limitations. The methodology was applied to formalin-fixed, deparaffinized, rehydrated tissue samples, and therefore the results cannot be generalized to in vivo studies. Second, the choice of Glut-1 as a molecular marker is problematic because of the lack of sensitivity and specificity. The Ki-67, a proliferation marker, although nonspecific, may potentially be assessed for conjugation with GNRs because dysplastic lesions will generally have different ki-67 immunoreactivity profiles from reactive processes. Another possibility is conjugation of 2 markers to GNRs: an epithelial marker (cytokeratin) and ki-67. Lastly, applying GNR methodology to the ultra-high-resolution OCT technique, pioneered at the authors' institution, may additionally increase the sensitivity and specificity of this imaging modality.

Despite its limitations, this model has potential advantages. GNR-OCT methodology can be used to monitor specific disease load by conjugating an appropriate targeting molecule to the GNR. In addition to allowing the diagnosis and monitoring of disease on a molecular level, this methodology could potentially be used for targeted therapies.

**T. Milman, MD**

*Reference*

1. Kieval JZ, Karp CL, Abou Shousha M, et al. Ultra-high resolution optical coherence tomography for differentiation of ocular surface squamous neoplasia and pterygia. *Ophthalmology.* 2012;119:481-486.

# Article Index

## Chapter 1: Cataract Surgery



## Chapter 2: Refractive Surgery

## Chapter 3: Glaucoma

## Chapter 4: Cornea



## Chapter 5: Retina

## Chapter 6: Oculoplastic Surgery

## Chapter 7: Pediatric Ophthalmology



## Chapter 8: Neuro-ophthalmology

## Chapter 9: Imaging



## Chapter 10: Ocular Oncology



## Chapter 11: Pathology

# Author Index

## A



## B



## C



## D



## E



## F



## G



## H

## R



## S



## T



## U



## V



## W



## Y



## Z